# PORTRAIT THERAPY

*of related interest*

**Art Therapy with Physical Conditions**
*Edited by Marian Liebmann and Sally Weston*
ISBN 978 1 84905 349 5
eISBN 978 0 85700 911 1

**The Creative Arts in Palliative Care**
*Edited by Nigel Hartley and Malcolm Payne*
ISBN 978 1 84310 591 6
eISBN 978 1 84642 802 9

**Art Therapy and Substance Abuse**
Enabling Recovery from Alcohol and Other Drug Addiction
*Libby Schmanke*
ISBN 978 1 84905 734 9
eISBN 978 1 78450 118 1

**Complicated Grief, Attachment, and Art Therapy**
Theory, Treatment, and 14 Ready-to-Use Protocols
*Edited by Briana MacWilliam*
ISBN 978 1 78592 738 6
eISBN 978 1 78450 458 8

**Digital Art Therapy**
Material, Methods, and Applications
*Edited by Rick L. Garner*
ISBN 978 1 84905 740 0
eISBN 978 1 78450 160 0

# Portrait Therapy

*Resolving Self-Identity Disruption in Clients with Life-Threatening and Chronic Illnesses*

SUSAN M. D. CARR

Jessica Kingsley *Publishers*
London and Philadelphia

On page 18, *Out of this World* by John D. Edwards, copyright © John D. Edwards 1999, is used with kind permission of John D. Edwards; further details on this image can be found at john.d.edwards.co.uk. On page 39 and Colour Plate vii, *Last Portrait of Mother* by Daphne Todd, copyright © Daphne Todd 2009, is used with kind permission of Daphne Todd. On page 40, *Lucy's Kingdom* by Juliet Chenery-Robson, copyright © Juliet Chenery-Robson 2010, is used with the kind permission of Juliet Chenery-Robson. On page 41, *Portrait of Phillip* by Juliet Chenery-Robson, copyright © Juliet Chenery-Robson 2016, is used with the kind permission of Juliet Chenery-Robson. On page 42, *Jo Spence, Narratives of Disease (Included)* by Jo Spence and Tim Sheard, copyright © the Estate of Jo Spence 1990, is used with the kind permission of the Estate of Jo Spence; image is provided courtesy of the Richard Salton Gallery, London. On page 63 and Coloured Plate viii, *Robin and Mardi* by Mark Gilbert, copyright © Mark Gilbert 2007, is used with kind permission of Mark Gilbert. On page 65, *Barry C* by Mark Gilbert, copyright © Mark Gilbert 1999, is used with kind permission of Mark Gilbert. On page 67 and Coloured Plate ix, *Evelyn* by Heath Roselli, copyright © Heath Roselli 1997, is used with kind permission of Heath Roselli. On page 68 and Colour Plate x, *Steve* by Antonia Rolls, copyright © Antonia Rolls 2007, is used with kind permission of Antonia Rolls. On page 68, *Julia* by Antonia Rolls, copyright © Antonia Rolls 2013, is used with kind permission of Antonia Rolls. On page 69 and Coloured Plate xi, *Dead Man Posing, Portrait of Philip Ledbury* by David Fisher, copyright © David Fisher 2009, is used with kind permission of Brenda Fisher.

First published in 2018
by Jessica Kingsley Publishers
73 Collier Street
London N1 9BE, UK
and
400 Market Street, Suite 400
Philadelphia, PA 19106, USA

*www.jkp.com*

Copyright © Susan M. D. Carr 2018

Front cover image source: *Bohemian Rhapsody*
by Susan M.D. Carr (co-designed by Rose), 2011.

All rights reserved. No part of this publication may be reproduced in any material form (including photocopying, storing in any medium by electronic means or transmitting) without the written permission of the copyright owner except in accordance with the provisions of the law or under terms of a licence issued in the UK by the Copyright Licensing Agency Ltd. www.cla.co.uk or in overseas territories by the relevant reproduction rights organisation, for details see www.ifrro.org. Applications for the copyright owner's written permission to reproduce any part of this publication should be addressed to the publisher.

Warning: The doing of an unauthorised act in relation to a copyright work may result in both a civil claim for damages and criminal prosecution.

**Library of Congress Cataloging in Publication Data**
A CIP catalog record for this book is available from the Library of Congress

**British Library Cataloguing in Publication Data**
A CIP catalogue record for this book is available from the British Library

ISBN 978 1 78592 293 0
eISBN 978 1 78450 605 6

Printed and bound in the United States

*This book is dedicated to Eileen and Hugh for being the inspiration for portrait therapy, and to Rose, Hilary, Peter and Mark, Bill, Susan, Norma and Paul, who were my patient-collaborators throughout. The delightful combination of humour, wisdom, courage and inspiration they brought to this project is reflected through their portraits, collages and prose poems and will be with me always, and hopefully, through sharing these portraits and stories of self-identity, with many others.*

# ACKNOWLEDGEMENTS

Particular acknowledgements and thanks go to my three PhD supervisors. During the first two years of this project Professor Alan Radley's clear vision on 'worlds' and 'works' of illness provided a foundation for portrait therapy. I also thank Alastair Adams, whose encouragement and guidance made it possible for me to overcome my anxieties about painting portraits, and his knowledge of, talent for and experience of portraiture in general was invaluable to the process. My third supervisor, Professor Sarah Pink, is thanked for her innovative suggestions and experience in ethnography and visual and sensory research methods, taking me into unthought-of areas of development and expertise. I also thank my drama therapist/supervisor Rachel, for her ongoing belief in this project and in me, and all the staff and volunteers who I worked with in the day-hospice, for sharing their wisdom and care with me and others in such a special way.

I thank my partner Terry, my parents Mary and David, and my sons James and Matthew, for all their love, support and encouragement during this time, and for understanding my preoccupation with 'yet another project'. I couldn't have done it without you!

# CONTENTS

## PART I: FOCUSING THE GAZE

1. Setting the Scene: Introducing Portraiture as a 'Third Hand' Intervention . . . . . . . . . . . . . . . . . . 15
2. Priming the Canvas: A Phenomenological Approach to Depicting Subjectivity . . . . . . . . . . . . . . . . . 34
3. Selecting the Medium: Portraiture as a Therapeutic Tool . . . . 55

## PART II: COLLABORATIVE CASE-STUDIES

4. Portrait Therapy as a Collaborative Intervention: Paint Me This Way!. . . . . . . . . . . . . . . . . . . 77
5. Increasing the Patients' Creative Capacity to Adapt to Illness. . 91
6. Mirroring and Attunement Through Portraiture: Intersubjective and Symbolic Ways of Knowing, Being and Relating . . . . 127
7. Making Special, Making Meaning: Homelike-being-in-the-world and Ontological Security. . . . . . . . . . . . . . 167

## PART III: PORTRAIT THERAPY PROTOCOL AND EVALUATION METHODS

8. A Therapist's Manual: The Three Phases of Portrait Therapy . . 209
9. Making Connections: Evaluating Portrait Therapy . . . . . . . 223
10. Afterword: Drawing Conclusions. . . . . . . . . . . . . . 236

*Appendix 1: Portrait Reference Album* . . . . . . . . . . . 252
*Appendix 2: Semi-structured End of Project Interview Questions.* . . . . . . . . . . . . . . . . . . . 255
*References* . . . . . . . . . . . . . . . . . . . . . . . 257
*Author biography.* . . . . . . . . . . . . . . . . . . . . 275
*Subject Index.* . . . . . . . . . . . . . . . . . . . . . 276
*Author Index* . . . . . . . . . . . . . . . . . . . . . . 291

# FIGURES

| | | |
|---|---|---|
| Figure 1.1 | *Out of This World* by John D. Edwards © 1999 (see also Coloured Plate vi) | 18 |
| Figure 1.2 | *Eileen Aged 10 Years*, 2007 | 28 |
| Figure 1.3 | *Eileen* by Susan Carr, 2007 | 29 |
| Figure 1.4 | *Hugh* | 31 |
| Figure 2.1 | *Last Portrait of Mother* by Daphne Todd © 2009 (see also Coloured Plate vii) | 39 |
| Figure 2.2 | *Lucy's Kingdom* by Juliet Chenery-Robson © 2010 | 40 |
| Figure 2.3 | *Portrait of Philip* by Juliet Chenery-Robson © 2016 | 41 |
| Figure 2.4 | *Jo Spence, from Narratives of Disease (Included)* by Jo Spence and Tim Sheard © 1990 | 42 |
| Figure 3.1 | *Robin and Mardi* by Mark Gilbert © 2007 (*Portraits of Care* Project) (see also Coloured Plate viii) | 63 |
| Figure 3.2 | *Barry C* by Mark Gilbert © 1999 (*Saving Faces* Project) | 65 |
| Figure 3.3 | *Evelyn* by Heath Rosselli © 1997 (see also Coloured Plate ix) | 67 |
| Figure 3.4 | *Steve* by Antonia Rolls © 2007 (see also Coloured Plate x) | 68 |
| Figure 3.5 | *Julia* by Antonia Rolls © 2013 | 68 |
| Figure 3.6 | *Dead Man Posing, Portrait of Philip Ledbury* by David Fisher © 2009 (see also Coloured Plate xi) | 69 |
| Figure 5.1 | *The Window* by Susan Carr (co-designed by Hilary), 2011 | 93 |
| Figure 5.2 | *The Heart of the Home* by Susan Carr (co-designed by Hilary), 2011 | 93 |
| Figure 5.3 | *A Proper Grandma* by Susan Carr, 2010 | 95 |
| Figure 5.4 | *Held by an Angel* by Susan Carr (co-designed by Hilary), 2011 (see also Coloured Plate i) | 97 |
| Figure 5.5 | *Broken Lungs* by Susan Carr (co-designed by Paul), 2013 (see also Coloured Plate ii) | 100 |
| Figure 5.6 | *Pin Hole Camera* by Susan Carr (co-designed by Susan), 2012 | 103 |
| Figure 5.7 | *Can't Breathe* collage by Susan Carr, 2011 | 107 |
| Figure 5.8 | *Mark, Charlie & Rusty* by Susan Carr (co-designed by Peter), 2011 | 107 |

| | | |
|---|---|---|
| Figure 5.9 | *RIP Mark & Rusty* collage by Susan Carr, 2011 (co-designed by Peter), 2011. | 108 |
| Figure 5.10 | *There's Something About Mark, RIP* by Susan Carr (co-designed by Peter), 2011. | 109 |
| Figure 5.11 | *Peter & Mark in Kenya* by Susan Carr (co-designed by Peter), 2011. | 110 |
| Figure 5.12 | *At the Races* by Susan Carr (co-designed by Peter), 2011. | 111 |
| Figure 5.13 | *My Mother Walked Out and Left Me* collage by Susan Carr, 2012. | 113 |
| Figure 5.14 | *Seven Holes in My Heart* collage by Susan Carr, 2012. | 113 |
| Figure 5.15 | *Unwelcome Contradictions of Death in Birth* by Susan Carr, 1999. | 114 |
| Figure 5.16 | *My Baby/My Self* by Susan Carr and Norma, 2012. | 116 |
| Figure 5.17 | Susan's post-diagnosis button task, 2012. | 117 |
| Figure 5.18 | *Back in That Box* collage by Susan Carr, 2012. | 118 |
| Figure 5.19 | *The Swan Island Book* by Susan Carr (co-designed by patient Susan), 2012. | 121 |
| Figure 5.20 | *Paint Me Like a Picasso* by Susan Carr (co-designed by Rose), 2011. | 122 |
| Figure 5.21 | *I'll Give It A Damn Good Try*, collage by Susan Carr, 2010. | 124 |
| Figure 6.1 | *Hard to Leave the House,* collage by Susan Carr, 2013. | 132 |
| Figure 6.2 | *At Home* by Susan Carr, 2013. | 134 |
| Figure 6.3 | *The Two Normas* by Susan Carr (co-designed by Norma/North Bear) 2012 (after *The Two Fridas* by Frida Kahlo, 1939). | 138 |
| Figure 6.4 | Montage of Rose's three portraits: *The Poppy Field, Paint Me Like a Picasso* and *Bohemian Rhapsody* by Susan Carr (co-designed by Rose), 2011. | 141 |
| Figure 6.5 | *All I Might Be Able To Do*, collage by Susan Carr, 2010. | 142 |
| Figure 6.6 | *I Climbed Mount Kilimanjaro* by Susan Carr, 2011. | 143 |
| Figure 6.7 | *Climbing Mt Kilimanjaro* by Susan Carr (co-designed by Peter), 2011. | 143 |
| Figure 6.8 | *Flying Ace* by Susan Carr, 2011 (co-designed by Bill), 2011 (see also Coloured Plate iii). | 145 |
| Figure 6.9 | *All My Plates Came Crashing Down*, collage by Susan Carr, 2010. | 147 |
| Figure 6.10 | Detail of the canary in the cage, from *Paint Me Like a Picasso* by Susan Carr (co-designed by Rose), 2011. | 148 |
| Figure 6.11 | *Idealised*, collage by Susan Carr, 2012. | 149 |
| Figure 6.12 | *I Lived in Fear of Him*, collage by Susan Carr, 2012. | 150 |
| Figure 6.13 | *Over Protected*, collage by Susan Carr, 2012. | 150 |
| Figure 6.14 | *Catch 22* by Susan Carr (co-designed by Susan), 2012. | 151 |
| Figure 6.15 | *The Cupboard of Imagination and Dreams* by Susan Carr (co-designed by Susan), 2012. | 153 |

| | | |
|---|---|---|
| Figure 6.16 | *Being Pandora* (after Rossetti, 1828–1882) by Susan Carr (co-designed by patient Susan), 2012.. . . . . . . . . . . | 155 |
| Figure 6.17 | *Saying Goodbye to the Sea* by Susan Carr (co-designed by Susan), 2012. . . . . . . . . . . . . . . | 161 |
| Figure 6.18 | *Lost* by Susan Carr (co-designed by Norma), 2012. . . . . | 163 |
| Figure 6.19 | *Fish Out of Water* by Susan Carr (co-designed by Norma), 2012 (see also Coloured Plate iv).. . . . . . . . . . . . . | 164 |
| Figure 7.1 | *I Don't Want to Just Disappear*, collage by Susan Carr, 2010. | 170 |
| Figure 7.2 | Montage of Hilary's three portraits: *The Window*, *The Heart of the Home*, and *Held by an Angel* by Susan Carr (co-designed by Hilary), 2011. . . . . . . . . . . . . . . . . | 171 |
| Figure 7.3 | 'Baby' detail from *My Baby/My Self* by Susan Carr and Norma, 2012.. . . . . . . . . . . . . . . . . . . . . . . | 172 |
| Figure 7.4 | *North Bear* by Susan Carr (co-designed by Norma), 2012. | 175 |
| Figure 7.5 | *Bill's Gunga Din* by Susan Carr, 2012. . . . . . . . . . . . | 179 |
| Figure 7.6 | *Sacrifice* by Susan Carr, 2012. . . . . . . . . . . . . . . . | 180 |
| Figure 7.7 | Montage of Bill's first three portraits: *The Flying Ace*, *Pegasus Bridge* and *The Veteran* by Susan Carr (co-designed by Bill), 2011. . . . . . . . . . . . . . . . . . . . . . . | 181 |
| Figure 7.8 | *Mentioned in Despatches*, collage by Susan Carr, 2012. . . . | 182 |
| Figure 7.9 | *Mentioned in Despatches* by Susan Carr (co-designed by Bill), 2011. . . . . . . . . . . . . . . . . . . . . . . . | 182 |
| Figure 7.10 | *Bohemian Rhapsody* by Susan Carr (co-designed by Rose), 2011.. . . . . . . . . . . . . . . . . . . . . . . . . . . | 184 |
| Figure 7.11 | *English Gothic* by Susan Carr (co-designed by Paul), 2013. | 186 |
| Figure 7.12 | *The Paper Dress* by Susan Carr (co-designed by Susan), 2012.. . . . . . . . . . . . . . . . . . . . . . . . . . . | 188 |
| Figure 7.13 | Montage of Susan's four portraits: *Little Susan*, *Saying Goodbye to the Sea*, *Being Pandora* and *The Library* by Susan Carr (co-designed by PR Susan), 2012.. . . . . . . . . . . | 190 |
| Figure 7.14 | *The Rainbow Snake* by Susan Carr, 2012.. . . . . . . . . . | 192 |
| Figure 7.15 | *The Poppy Field* by Susan Carr (co-designed by Rose), 2011 (see also Coloured Plate v) . . . . . . . . . . . . . . . | 195 |
| Figure 7.16 | *Trapped*, collage by Susan Carr, 2012.. . . . . . . . . . . . | 200 |
| Figure 7.17 | *Virtual Paul* by Susan Carr (co-designed by Paul), 2013. . | 201 |
| Figure 10.1 | *RIP Peter*. . . . . . . . . . . . . . . . . . . . . . . . . . | 251 |

# COLOURED PLATES

Coloured Plate i  *Held by an Angel* by Susan Carr (co-designed by Hilary), 2011.
Coloured Plate ii  *Broken Lungs* by Susan Carr (co-designed by Paul), 2013.
Coloured Plate iii  *Flying Ace* by Susan Carr (co-designed by Bill), 2011.
Coloured Plate iv  *Fish Out of Water* by Susan Carr (co-designed by Norma), 2012.
Coloured Plate v  *The Poppy Field* by Susan Carr (co-designed by Rose), 2011.
Coloured Plate vi  *Out of This World* by John D. Edwards © 1999.
Coloured Plate vii  *Last Portrait of Mother* by Daphne Todd © 2009.
Coloured Plate viii  *Robin and Mardi* by Mark Gilbert © 2007 (*Portraits of Care* Project).
Coloured Plate ix  *Evelyn* by Heath Rosselli © 1997.
Coloured Plate x  *Steve* by Antonia Rolls © 2007.
Coloured Plate xi  *Dead Man Posing, Portrait of Philip Ledbury* by David Fisher © 2009.

# TABLES

Table 9.1 Six steps for the Arts-based Life/World
 Phenomenological Analysis (ALPHA). . . . . . . . . . . 227
Table 9.2 Example of how to 'extract the essences'
 from the portraits . . . . . . . . . . . . . . . . . . . . . 229
Table 9.3 Example of identifying themes found in the
 analysis in the EPI data . . . . . . . . . . . . . . . . . . 233

— PART I —

# FOCUSING THE GAZE

— Chapter 1 —

# SETTING THE SCENE

## *Introducing Portraiture as a 'Third Hand' Intervention*

I wanted to begin this book with a story that succinctly described how portrait therapy grew out of the issues presented by the patients I worked with over many years in palliative care, something thoughtful and profound, or at least something that showed my insight and sensitivity to these issues. Yet as I sit here at the computer my mind refuses to give forth its profound thoughts, and instead reminds me of my awkward and embarrassing moments. My first experience of working in palliative care was as an art therapy student over 12 years ago, it was during the second week of my placement and I was sat around a table with five patients, their faces all looking at me expectantly. 'What are we going to do today then?' asked one lady. 'I can't draw a straight line!' joked another. 'Well,' I said nervously, 'today I think we shall begin by painting a picture of how our week has been…' As I spoke I was filling some pallets with some very liquid poster paint, newly bought for the group, but the yellow paint was proving particularly stubborn and refused to flow from the narrow plastic spout in the lid.

In hindsight just squeezing harder on the belly of the bottle was obviously a mistake, because at that moment the whole lid decided to fly off and the contents of this lurid yellow paint flew in all directions, splattering these severely ill patients from head to foot in yellow spots. After a second or two of stunned silence hilarious laughter broke forth, as the patients turned around and looked at each other, tears of laughter running down their cheeks mingling with the yellow paint. Needless to say, this story went around the hospice causing much hilarity; however, later that day I overheard one elderly lady say that the art therapy group was 'the best medicine' she'd had all week and that she 'couldn't wait to get home and tell her husband all about the yellow paint!' This was, I guess, my first experience of 'painting' my patients…

Despite my inauspicious start, at the end of my training I was offered a position as an art therapist at this same hospice, and my journey towards the development of portrait therapy began. My art therapy practice is based on the 'studio art therapy' model outlined by Catherine Moon (2002), and other art therapists concerned with keeping the focus on 'art' within art therapy (Allen 1992, 2001a, 2001b; Brown 2008b; Cahn 2000; Malchiodi 1999a; McNiff 1986; Robbins 2000; Wix 2000). This model aims to avoid the 'clinification' of art therapy (Allen 1992, p.23), something that art therapist and writer Pat Allen says 'neglects to employ the very specialized knowledge that derives from our background in art making itself'. Allen's (1992) open studio model works on the premise that it is part of the art therapist's role to pursue his or her own art making as a way to create 'a bridge to and from her core self to her role as therapist' (ibid., p.26). And as Reason (2006, p.188) says:

> If we start from the idea that creating knowledge is a practical affair, we will start not, as in traditional academic research, from an interesting theoretical question, but from what concerns us in practice, from the presenting issues in our lives.

Within portrait therapy, I acknowledge that my *therapist* and *artist* identities merge, and as an art(ist)-therapist I believe in the power of art to heal, challenge, and transform meaning (Adamson 1984; Stuckley and Nobel 2010), and to build bridges between our *discursive* and *non-discursive* selves (O'Brien 2004). The creation of art has played an important role in all known cultures around the world (Dissanayake 1988) and there is extensive anecdotal and growing empirical evidence that art therapy and the arts have a contribution to make in the health and well-being of those living with life-threatening and chronic illnesses (Connell 1992, 1998; Hill 1945, 1951; Kramer 1971, 2004; Luzzatto 1998; Malchiodi 1999b, 2007; McNiff 1992, 2004; Pratt and Wood 1998; Waller and Sibbett 2005).

Portrait therapy is grounded within the 'holistic' paradigm, with its focus on the *physical, emotional, psychosocial* and *spiritual* aspects of a person's experience of illness (Saunders 1976, 1990). Central to the ethos of palliative care is the improvement of patients'/clients' 'quality of life' (Bell 2008, p.354), and this, along with the empowerment of individuals, is the overarching aim of portrait therapy. As Judith Herman says (1992, p.133), 'The first principle of recovery is the empowerment of the survivor. She must be the author of her own recovery. Others may offer advice, support, assistance, affection and care, but not cure.'

Within portrait therapy an attempt is made to equalise the relationship between art therapist and patients through the development of a collaborative intersubjective relationship. Within this relationship the patients, in a series of negotiations, co-design their own portraits directing how they wish to be portrayed. The co-designing process and viewing of the portraits provide a unique way of looking at the phenomena of disrupted self-identity and embodiment, enabling patients to see themselves through the eyes of an empathic and attuning 'other'. This, therefore, is the foundation for the collaborative and intersubjective relationship: *'Paint me this way!'*

## What is self-identity disruption?

My interest in using portraiture as an intervention developed from a growing recognition and concern for the *disruption* to self-identity caused by life-threatening and chronic illnesses that many of my patients talked about on a daily basis. Self-identity *disruption* is characterised by statements such as 'I don't know who I am any more', or 'I'm not the person I used to be', and 'I look in the mirror and I say "who's that?"' Indeed, patients often describe the impact of their diagnosis, treatment and illness as having changed their sense of self-identity beyond all recognition (Charmaz 1983).

Very early in this research process I discovered this quote describing identity disruption, by counselling researcher Mitchell B. Young (1988, p.32). He said:

> To have one's identity disrupted is to travel without a compass...

This captures the essence of self-identity disruption, describing succinctly a sense of *displacement, disorientation* and *disempowerment*, of not knowing which way to turn, or who they are now they are ill (Corbin and Strauss 1987). This sense of disorientation clearly causes problems in all aspects of a person's life/world, impacting on decision-making, relationships with significant others and most importantly their relationship with themselves. As Bolen (1996, p.14) says:

Illness is both soul-shaking and soul-evoking for the patient and for all others for whom the patient matters. We lose an innocence, we know vulnerability, we are no longer who we were before this event, and we will never be the same.

The diagnosis of a life-threatening illness and the steady deterioration of a chronic illness also negatively impacts upon a person's 'creative capacity' to adapt to illness (Reeve *et al.* 2010), and their quality of life (Carel 2011; Crewe 1980; Mathieson and Stam 1995; Toombs 1988). It can cause: increased stress, loss and grief; loss of meaning and disruption to future goals (Falvo 1999), and commonly results in depression and social isolation (Rodin *et al.* 1991). Research has demonstrated that aside from all the other stresses faced by those living with life-threatening and chronic illnesses, social isolation on its own can reduce immune function, cause depression and shorten life expectancy (Jaremka *et al.* 2012), suggesting the importance of developing effective interventions such as portrait therapy, where the relational aspects of self-identity can be validated.

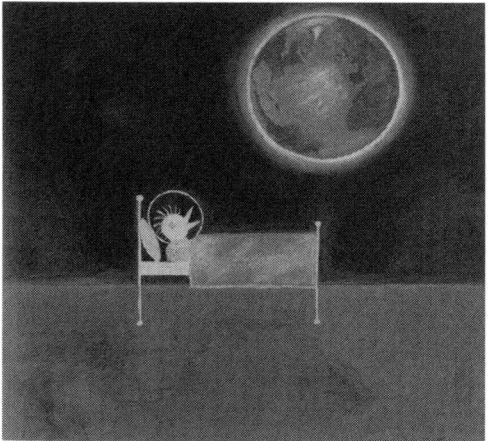

Figure 1.1 *Out of This World* by John D. Edwards © 1999
(see also Coloured Plate vi).

In this painting called *Out of This World* (Figure 1.1) artist John D. Edwards (2007) conveys his experience of social isolation and disruption to his life and self-identity caused by his experience of cancer. Edwards' experience is echoed by Claire Smith (2008), talking about her own experience of 'deep illness' (Frank 1997):

> I live in a bubble and I watch the world revolve around me from within it. No one sees my bubble, but it is there, a film deadening the noise and commotions of the world, as life goes on everywhere else. (Smith 2008, p.11)

Edwards' painting clearly depicts an experience of 'liminality' (Sibbett 2004, 2005a, 2005b, 2005c) often expressed by people living with life-threatening and chronic illnesses. Liminality is described as a place where feelings of 'limbo, ambiguity, embodied experience, chaos…expression and transition' are manifest, as well as being a place of creativity and adaption where rites of passage are played out (Sibbett 2005a, p.68). What is characterised by Young's (1988, p.22) quote is that people living with a diagnosis of life-threatening and chronic illness often find themselves suddenly, and earth shatteringly, transported into this liminal 'betwixt and between' threshold space (Sibbett 2004, 2005a, 2005b; Turner 1969), an unknown world or landscape without a 'compass' to guide them. It is a place where social stigma and 'the sick role' cause feelings of shame and distress, and people are described in passive terms as 'dependent' (Fraser and Gordon 1994) or 'disabled', thus further disrupting self-identity. My aim in developing portrait therapy is that the portraits created *for* patients will become *points of reference* within the journey into this unknown and liminal space (liminality will be discussed in more detail in Chapter 2).

## Illness as unhomelike being-in-the-world

When researching the impact of chronic illness on self-identity I discovered the writings of university professor and philosopher Havi Carel (2004, 2007, 2008, 2011, 2012, 2014; Carel *et al.* 2016), who writes about her own experience of living with a chronic illness. Carel writes about being 'unable to transcend the social barrier created by illness' (2008, p.50), about a 'bitterness' which is 'verboten', and the pressures of being manoeuvred into being courageous and uncomplaining (ibid. p.55):

> …first I am set up in a social context that forbids me from talking about my illness. Then, when I turn to other topics, I discover the social reward: I am seen as brave, graceful, a good sport… This is how you are seen once you conform to the demands and expectations

of society: once your 'sick role' (as Talcott Parsons called it) is validated by those around you.

Carel (2008, p.50) also talks about how illness brings with it a distinct change in self-perception, which is mirrored by changes in social perception; she says:

> ...the thought that was truly novel for me was this: I will never get better. All the usual rules that governed my life – that trying hard yields results, that looking after yourself pays off, that practice makes perfect – seemed inoperative here. It was the first instance, for me, of unconditional, uncontrollable failure. No matter what I did, I would only get worse. The inevitability of decline was the only principle governing my life. (Carel 2008, p.63)

The disruption caused by illness also impacts upon the way patients think *others* perceive them:

> ...I became aware that I had fallen from a position of respect, friendship and admiration, to one of pity, pitied by all, admired by none. An instant and unwelcome change. Who am I now? (Smith 2008, p.7)

These accounts describe a double betrayal by the body, first in becoming the container for 'disease' and second in 'revealing' that disease, through the dysfunction and dis-ability of the body.

Bodies which have been compromised by illness also change how life is experienced, which can result in a profound disruption to a person's sense of self (Carel 2011, p.36). The French phenomenological philosopher Merleau-Ponty (1908–1961) wrote extensively about how the body is central to the way we perceive experience and interpret the world, indeed, he believed that it is the whole reason we have a world to experience (Matthews 2006; Merleau-Ponty 2002). Portrait therapy therefore recognises the importance of the body in our experience of self-identity, and the embodied nature of all experience, especially within the experience of illness which can lead to feelings of 'unhomelikeness' (Svenaeus 2011, p.334).

Fredrik Svenaeus (professor of medical humanities and philosophy at Södertörn University, Sweden) has developed a phenomenological model of illness within which he defines the 'otherness' of the ill-body and the 'enforced inhabitation of an alien world' as 'unhomelikeness' (2011, p.334). He believes that diseases and the over-medicalisation and objectification of the body are therefore a direct threat to our 'homelike being-in-the-world', through their 'radical and dreadful otherness' (Svenaeus 2011, p.335).

> ...the unhomelike being-in-the-world of illness, in contrast to other forms of unhomelike being-in-the-world is characterized by a fatal change in the meaning-structures, not only of the world, but of the self... (Svenaeus 2011, p.337)

Within his seminal thesis on identity, philosopher Charles Taylor (1989) suggests that we all have a fundamental need for a sense of *meaning* in our lives. However, one of the key changes in thinking around self-identities, and that which has come to characterise a post-traditional or 'late modern' (Giddens 1991) society, is the problem of *meaninglessness*. Taylor says that this is caused by a Western move away from a belief in traditionalist frames of identity, such as religion and mythology, to an emphasis on materiality, science and technology. This general lack of meaning and connection in our late modern society has, I believe, compounded *self-identity disruption* for people living with life-threatening and chronic illnesses, with the core experiences of trauma – disconnection, disempowerment and disorientation (van der Kolk 1987, 1988, 2003) – being a key feature of 'unhomelike being-in-the-world' (Svenaus 2011).

Svenaeus suggests that healthcare professionals are duty bound to try to understand this 'unhomelike being-in-the-world' that patients experience, and to 'bring it back to homelikeness again, or at least, closer to home', where a 'reinterpretation of the self' can be achieved (ibid., pp.336–8). The problem is that a sense of meaning has also been lost within healthcare, and behavioural and clinical science have 'no category to describe suffering, no routine way of recording this most thickly human dimension of patients' and families' stories of experiencing illness' (Kleinman 1988, p.28). Through utilising compelling imagery, portrait therapy and art therapy can convey powerful messages that highlight the 'universality and timelessness' of an individual's suffering, as well as mediating between this and 'collective suffering', in order to bring about social action and change (Hocoy 2007, p.22).

The lack of consideration for a sense of meaning around illness is underlined by a general lack of attention paid by the medical profession to the underlying psychological needs of patients living with life-threatening and chronic illnesses (Waller and Sibbett 2005, p.xxix), and a tendency within palliative care and general medical practice to treat an emotional and physiological reaction to traumatic events as a medical issue. This has meant the widespread use of drugs such as antidepressants, given to patients as a way to 'blunt the impact' (Grau 2006). Within palliative care the rationale often used is that patients do not have 'time' for lengthy therapeutic encounters that an exploration of root causes might require. Antidepressants on their own may help some people, but they do not tackle the underlying problems of *self-identity disruption*, whereas therapeutic processes, such as those within portrait therapy, give patients the opportunity to *re-vision* facets of their past and present identities, enabling traumatic experiences to be *transformed* (Etherington 2008, p.53), and therefore deep healing and closure to occur. For patients, this may result in a reclaimed sense of meaning in their lives, a coherent sense of self and *a good death*, where patients die with a peaceful heart and mind (Cooper 2016).

## What are self-identities and disrupted self-identities?

Concepts of 'identity' and 'self' have been, and continue to be, a deeply contested and complex phenomena (Bauman 2004, p.77; Evans 2005b; Lawler 2008). Their meanings are elusive and ambivalent (Vecchi 2004, p.2) and yet remain topics of key interest across the social sciences (e.g. Elliott 2008, 2011; Gauntlett 2002, 2007; Gauntlett and Holzwarth 2006; Giddens 1991; Leary and Tangney 2012; Oyserman *et al.* 2012; Radley and Bell 2007; Taylor 1989, 1991). Defining self-identity is therefore 'problematic and cannot be the preserve of any single perspective, because it is not an objective entity and is subject to dynamic influences ultimately beyond the complete control of any individually identifiable agencies' (Evans 2005b, p.40). However, the patients' search for a cohesive sense of self-identity is something this intervention supports. Akhtar and Samuel (1996) describe a 'cohesive identity' as comprising 'a realistic body image, subjective self-sameness, consistent attitudes, temporality, gender, authenticity, and ethnicity'. My understanding of *self-identity* is closely aligned with writer Parker J. Palmer's description. He writes that identity is:

> ...an evolving nexus where all the forces that constitute my life converge in the mystery of self: my genetic makeup, the nature of the man and woman who gave me life, the culture in which I was raised, people who have sustained me and people who have done me harm,

the good and ill I have done to others and to myself, the experience of love and suffering...identity is a moving intersection of the inner and outer forces that make me who I am, converging in the irreducible mystery of being human. (Palmer 2007, p.14)

I therefore see self-identities as multifaceted and intrinsically relational, a 'reflexive project' (Giddens 1991, p.32), characterised by fluidity and change. Sociologists believe that self-identity is built through social interactions within a cultural construct, where each person is a 'child of their time and place' (Evans 2005b, p.40), and that 'definitions that value who and what we are, as persons, have been steadily diminishing over the last two centuries and now, at the start of the twenty-first century, have almost completely been eliminated' (Evans 2005a, p.7). Whilst such theories are contested I suggest that a lack of focus within the National Health Service (NHS) on *personalised care*, and the importance of recognising and working with unique individuals, highlights the need for new and innovative interventions to support people at end of life in ways that help them validate their sense of self-identity following the impact of illness and medicalisation.

I was reminded of this lack of 'personalised care' when I visited my local GP for an appointment recently. As I approached the receptionist's desk, instead of a welcoming human face I saw a large sign, on which was written, 'For all appointments, please sign yourself in on the interactive screen to the right, please do not disturb the receptionist.' I stood there dumbfounded, but obediently 'signed in' on the 'interactive screen'. As I sat waiting for my appointment I noticed the distress this notice caused to the elderly and the infirm, as they attempted and often failed to grapple with technology, and I felt the sadness and injustice of it all. Where can people go to get the recognition and self-identity validation they require to rebuild their self-identities, when every function is automated, and connection with humanity is lost?

## The formation of self-identity: Mirroring and attunement

When developing a theoretical basis for portrait therapy I discovered writer and psychoanalyst Kenneth Wright's (2009) theory of 'mirroring and attunement', which supports the idea of using portraiture as a way to *re-vision* self-identities. Wright's (2009) theory develops and connects Melanie Klein's (1952) *object relations theory*, Donald Winnicott's (1971) *mirroring*, with Daniel Stern's (1985) ideas about *attunement*, and applies them to the artist and the art object (Wright 2009). Building on the ideas of art critic Peter Fuller (1980), Wright argues that the surface of the canvas in a painting is 'derivative, or "analogue"' to the mother's expressive face in infancy, and functions in a similar way as 'a responsive and mirroring extension of the self' or 'surrogate adaptive mother' (Wright 2009, p.13). Within portrait therapy I have developed these ideas further to include the *portrait* painted *for* the patient as an embodied, mirroring device, which acts as the *attuning* (m)other, enabling the *revisioning*, *validation* and *integration* of aspects of a person's self-identity, as well as a process of *mourning* for perceived losses to self-identity (Carr 2014).

Stern's concept of *attunement* (1985) is an important theory for portrait therapy, as it describes the process whereby the (m)other reflects back her baby's affective states, in order to promote self-awareness, and therefore help the baby build a sense of self-identity. However, Stern observed that this is not a process only of mimesis or mirroring – but a process where the (m)other 'attunes' a response to the baby, which either validates the baby's experience or attempts to modify that experience. The (m)other does this by adding something of her *own* to the reflected experience – e.g. by downplaying distress or exaggerating surprise, therefore the *attunement* becomes 'a recasting, a restatement of a subjective state' (Stern 1985, p.61). Although writer and art therapist Sally Skaife (2001, p.40) suggests that object relations theory does not address the *adult* art-making process, Wright's (2009) ideas seem to offer such a process through the portrait becoming a *symbolic* (m)other's face, and although Stern was mainly concerned with the early mother–infant relationship, he believed that attunement is important *throughout a person's life* (ibid., p.23).

The theory of *containment* put forward by psychoanalyst Wilfred Bion (1962, 1967) is also important for portrait therapy as it describes the (m)other's/therapist's task of 'holding', 'containing' and 'transforming' the patient's unbearable anxiety, such as the fear of death. This allows the patient's lived experience to be temporarily held and contained by the therapist, and then transformed and transferred into the portraits, in a process that involves the 'empathic passage through the other – a passage during which each experience acquires a maternal form' (Wright 2005). The relationship between the 'container' and the 'contained' is an intersubjective one, and this combined experience becomes, in the portrait, a concrete, sensory and symbolic form (Langer 1953), offering a unique way to hold, contain and safeguard this attuned experience (Wright 2005). Within psychodynamic and psychoanalytic art therapy this attunement is indicated through the art therapist's verbal and facial responses and therefore, unlike portrait therapy, no concrete evidence remains of this mirroring and attunement for ongoing reflection by the patients.

It is important to note that within portrait therapy *object relations theory* is used, not as a way to identify something *lacking* in the patients' primary relationships (unless this is presented by the patients themselves), or in a Freudian sense to identify *unconscious fantasies* or *drives*, but as a way to *re-vision* and *re-integrate* aspects of the patients past, present and future self-identities, and therefore build a stronger, more coherent sense of self-identity (Carr 2014).

Interpretative language is also avoided within portrait therapy, something which is sometimes evident in psychodynamic and psychoanalytical analysis. Pathologising language, as implicated within the 'clinification' of art therapy (Allen 1992), is also avoided; instead the focus is on intersubjective, and therefore *co-created*, interpretation of meanings.

## What are portraits and how can they be used as a therapeutic intervention?

Defining what 'portraits' are, or can be, is almost as difficult as defining what 'art' is, so for the purposes of this book I will use Cynthia Freeland's definition. Freeland, Professor of Philosophy at the University of Houston and author of *Portraits and Persons*, describes portraits as:

> …visual artefacts that are made in order to draw attention to the depicted person as a subject with his or her own intentionality; the artefact itself thus manifests two distinct sorts of purposes (both intentional), that of the creator and that of the subject. (Freeland 2010, p.192)

Freeland (2010, p.99) uses a typology to further define a 'portrait', describing four key characteristics; these are: 'accuracy of likeness', 'testimony of presence', 'emotional characterization or evocations of personality, and revelation of a subject's uniqueness or their "air" (Barthes 1985)'. The first characteristic, 'accuracy of likeness', refers to a mimesis of the sitter's physical face/form. However, in portrait therapy, patients are given the opportunity to co-design portraits that deviate from this, through giving them the option to use photographic reference, perhaps choosing to be painted at a younger age, or by choosing imaginary images reflecting an inner reality or landscape (Carr 2011). This is in addition to the option of a portrait mirroring their current 'likeness'.

Within Freeland's second characteristic, 'testimonies of presence', she suggests that the portrait can be a powerful way of connecting with people even when they are not present, thereby providing a privileged contact with the dead or absent (Freeland 2007, p.101). Art critic and author Charlotte Mullins (2006, p.8) posits that portraits 'cheat death, and have the lure of immortalizing the sitter', and an 'ability to capture the essence of the sitter over the time it takes to paint it' giving these images 'much more authority than a single snapshot' (Mullins 2006, p.8).

The third characteristic is 'evocations of personality' which offers information about the sitter's personality, emotions or attitudes (Freeland 2007, p.101). As a fourth characteristic, Freeland uses Roland Barthes' (1985, p.102) term, 'the revelation of a subject's uniqueness or their "air"'. For Barthes, a person's 'air'…'is that exorbitant thing which induces from body to soul…a kind of intractable supplement of identity' (ibid., pp.109–110). I refer to this as a person's 'essence', which I understand to be the essential characteristics by which they are identified, combined with their 'presence' (West 2004, p.12).

Mullins (2006, p.8) argues that the portrait, with its inherent subjectivity, 'does not engage with universality'; however, if this were true, portraits in general would hold no interest to anyone except the person depicted and their family, which is belied by the huge numbers of people who visit the National Portrait Gallery every year. Rather it is the *universality* of human existence that draws people to examine the faces of others and lures them to the gallery as a place where one has permission to closely examine, and contemplate, the faces of others. As Freeland (2010, p.298) says, 'Among a world of meaningful objects, portraits are among the most engaging of all because they reveal to us subjects in which we are all inevitably interested: *persons*' (my emphasis). Portraits usually feature faces, and reading the face and facial expressions are key when attempting to understand another person's changing emotional state or inner world. The eyes are often described as windows to the soul and 'one of the most wonderful things in nature, where all is wonderful, is, the glance, or meeting of the eyes; …it transcends speech and action and…; it is the bodily symbol of identity…' (Ralph Waldo Emerson, quoted in Whicher *et al.* 1964, p.283). Also, the *face* is the most universally understood symbol for a person's identity (Bruce and Young 1986, p.305), and is used in all forms of identification, e.g. a passport without a photograph of the person it belongs to is of little use. Also, as human beings we are all highly attuned to recognise emotional and behavioural clues within facial expressions and body language, which indicates something important about the thoughts and feelings of the person (Freeland 2010, p.154).

Alastair Adams (2009), former president of the Royal Society of Portrait Painters, defines the painted portrait as something which, in the physicality of its creation, 'sifts through time', becoming a 'reflective space' achieved through 'sustained observation'. Freeland (2010, p.290) talks of the 'paradox of portraiture' and questions how 'something that is an artefact or object can ever succeed at capturing a person who is a living being, a subject?' This paradox encompasses *alchemy* or the *transformative* nature of art (Cauvel 1999), the way an artist uses inanimate objects, such as paint and canvas, to recreate the sense of a living person, with a 'distinctive soul, essence or air' (Freeland 2010, p.290). Marcia Pointon (2013, p.11), author of *Portrayal and the Search for Identity*, proposes that portraits are both '*effective*' and '*affective*', an 'instrumental art form, a kind of agency', meaning that they can be actively 'instrumental in changing lives', as well as moving and thought provoking for those who view them.

My interest in portraits and their power to heal began through my art therapy work with a patient called Eileen, several years before I even thought of developing portrait therapy. Eileen was an 82-year-old lady, diagnosed with terminal cancer and severe osteoarthritis; she lived with her husband and her only child, a daughter who still lived with them. One day Eileen brought an old photograph album into the day-hospice and through the photographs told me the story of her life, a life dedicated to looking after her husband and daughter. One particular photograph was of herself as a ten-year-old child (see Figure 1.2) and this tiny photograph resonated with me.

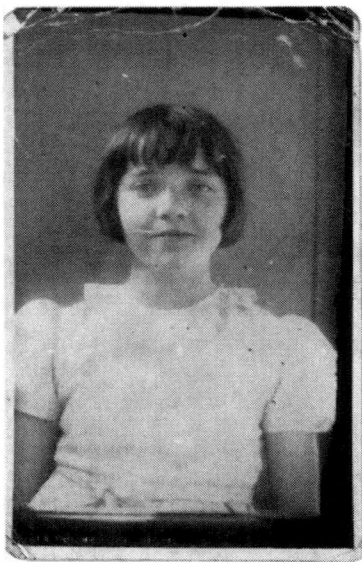

Figure 1.2 *Eileen Aged 10 Years*, 2007.

The photograph had clearly been taken in an early 'photo booth' and I was struck by the innocent beauty in this young face. Eileen said the dress she wore in the photograph was significant, as it had been her Christmas present that year. Due to financial constraints, Eileen had been asked by her parents to choose between a toy or a dress for her present and she chose the dress, made from pale green 'floaty' silk. The resonance I felt for the child in this photograph was, I believe, a recognition of the transitional moment of self-identity between childhood and young-adulthood captured within it, where Eileen had chosen the 'adult' *dress* over the 'childish' *toy*. I asked Eileen if I could copy the photograph to use as reference for a portrait, and she seemed genuinely pleased and excited at the idea, Eileen's only reservation being that it might be better if I painted her daughter instead of her; however, I assured her that her daughter would have a 'presence' of some sort within the portrait.

Over several weeks we co-designed the portrait together, and I took in photographs to show Eileen how the portrait was progressing, and to discuss its development. Eileen selected photographs of significant events in her life, including ones featuring her daughter, to be painted as if pinned to the wall behind her. This process of collaboration meant that our therapeutic relationship became very close, and Eileen trusted me with many of her fears and anxieties around her illness. As the weeks progressed, Eileen's health deteriorated and she was admitted to the hospice in-patient unit. Fearing she would die without seeing the finished painting, I took it in to show her (see Figure 1.3), and even in its unfinished state her delight was obvious. 'Oh,' she said, 'you have painted me beautiful! ... I love it!' 'You were a beautiful child,' I said. 'Well!' she said, 'I never knew that! I've lived for 82 years and I never knew that!'

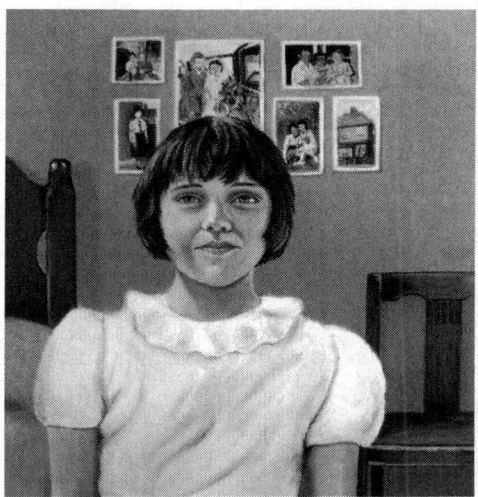

Figure 1.3 *Eileen* by Susan Carr, 2007.

Reflecting upon this conversation I realised that through the portrait, through mirroring and attuning the 'beauty' I had seen – a connection had formed for Eileen with something previously *unknown* about herself. Eileen's 'love' for this painting also reawakened a love for her 'self' as a vulnerable child, something she had become again through her illness, needing the constant care and support of others as her health deteriorated. Eventually Eileen slipped into a coma, and it struck me that even as I was painting her transitional moment from childhood to young adulthood, so Eileen had slipped into a transitional space between life and death.

The painting has been left unfinished since Eileen died, acknowledging the unfinished business that death brings, and in a way, it seemed that it had fulfilled its purpose. However, this experience of co-designing *with* and painting a portrait *for* a patient was the main genesis for this intervention and is therefore part of Eileen's ongoing legacy.

## Reversing the terms of engagement: Invoking Edith Kramer's concept of the art therapist's 'third hand'

Art therapy pioneer Edith Kramer (1971, 1986, 2000) described her 'third hand' model as 'an area of the art therapist's functioning wherein artistic competence and imagination are employed in the empathic service of others' (2000, p.48), and as 'a hand that helps the creative process along without being intrusive, without distorting meaning or imposing pictorial ideas or preferences alien to the client' (1986, p.71). Kramer's (1971, 1986) art therapy model also focused on 'sublimation', which she describes as the transformation of negative impulses or beliefs into something positive through art, with the view that changing 'chaos' into 'formed expressions' facilitated 'sublimation' and integration of uncontrolled affect (ibid.).

Kramer spent most of her career working with disturbed children and adolescents, and in 1971 she published *Art as Therapy with Children*. Within this Kramer describes using portraiture as a way to strengthen feelings of identity in her child clients, saying... 'they also loved it when, as a special treat, *I drew their portraits*. My actions seemed to reassure them and to *strengthen their feelings of identity*' (Kramer 1971, p.40 [my emphasis]). I query whether 'reassuring them' and 'strengthening their identity' should be termed 'a special treat', rather it seems to be a *fundamental* aspect of Kramer's therapeutic input (Carr 2014, p.57), and as such one of the key aims of portrait therapy.

I was also inspired to use a 'third hand' approach by a patient called Hugh, who attended the day-hospice not long after I began working there. Hugh was diagnosed with motor neuron disease (MND) and had become so severely disabled that he was virtually 'locked' within his own body, unable to speak or move, and it was difficult to see what benefit he gained from attending the day-hospice. I felt frustrated that I was unable to offer Hugh an accessible art therapy intervention. In an interview printed in a hospice brochure, Hugh reflected upon his fundamental need to reciprocate, and an understanding of how the physical embodiment of his illness could be used to help others, when all other function had been lost. Hugh said, 'If I can go to day-hospice and by my presence and by my own lack of function, make the other patients feel better about themselves, then I have achieved something.'

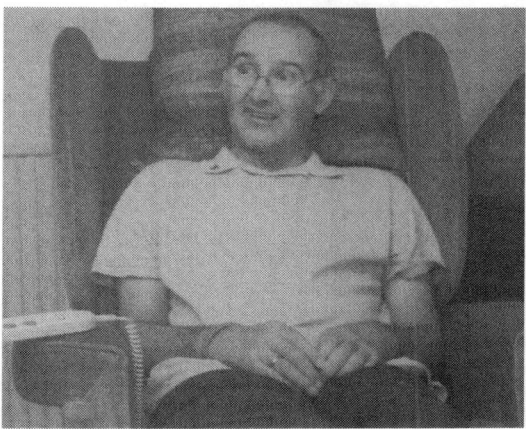

Figure 1.4 *Hugh*.

An expectation that patients will create artwork and talk about this within art therapy sessions does have some 'limitations' and 'problems' (Maclagan 2011, p.8), particularly in palliative care. As in Hugh's case patients are often too unwell, disabled or fatigued to make art themselves, and (as with clients in other fields of art therapy) for a variety of reasons some are unwilling or unable to make art, despite the expectation that they do so. These sessions then become reliant on 'talking therapy', which while beneficial in its own way is not the point of *art* therapy and does not harness the power of *art* to transform meanings and experience.

Engaging with art materials can be an exciting new challenge for some patients, but for others it can be an insurmountable obstacle and often no amount of reassurance, that they don't need to be 'an artist' or 'good at art', will suffice. I agree with art therapist and author Paola Luzzatto (1998) on this point when she says, 'In my mind I am on the side of the patients who feel empty, blocked and unimaginative, and I do not want to make them feel they "should" become visually creative.' Art therapist and author Michèle Wood (1998) observes that the act of self-representation through *creating their own artwork* can help patients to 'strengthen and validate their sense of identity' (ibid., p.2). I contend that through using the art therapist's 'third hand', and therefore at-once-removed from the creation of art, patients *are* still able to present themselves 'in their own terms' through the collaborative co-designing process and therefore 'strengthen and validate their sense of identity'.

Through using 'third hand' techniques to paint portraits *for* patients, this intervention provides the opportunity to reintroduce the creative, imaginative process of co-designing and viewing self-referential images, into what would otherwise be 'artistically barren' therapeutic encounters (Carr 2014, p.55). I realise that by painting portraits *for* patients, I am taking Kramer's 'third hand' model of art therapy to its extreme; however, this intervention is not intended in any way as a replacement for the many and varied art therapy theoretical models within which patients/clients create the art objects, rather it seeks to extend opportunities and knowledge by visiting the borderlands of art therapy practice and portraiture, as well as developing a specific intervention for a defined client group. However, I believe that portrait therapy has the potential to help people in many different ways and contexts that are as yet undiscovered or researched, leaving the way open for other art therapists to push the boundaries of this intervention.

That being said, early on in the development of portrait therapy I still had some anxieties and resistance around my own ability to paint portraits *for* patients, thinking that perhaps enabling patients to paint their own *self*-portraits would be a more therapeutic process. Taking these anxieties to my personal therapist/supervisor, she wisely instructed me to ask the patients what they thought, so I set up a focus group at the hospice inviting patients to talk about their experience of self-identity disruption and illness and my potential intervention ideas. I asked the patients if they would engage in an intervention where they were required to paint their own *self-portraits*. This question was met with immediate laughter and much shaking of heads. 'No,' they all said unanimously, 'we wouldn't take part!' 'It would be a joke,' said one lady, 'I can't even draw a tree, let alone myself.' Another held up her uncontrollably shaking hands saying, 'What could I do with these hands?' Then another lady said, 'Of course, if *you* painted the portrait then I would definitely take part!' This was followed up by general excitement and calls of 'Oh yes, so would I…' and 'Oh yes, paint me!'

Following this discussion with the patients I felt ready to embrace my own artistic identity and develop my 'third hand' abilities, remembering that I was doing this, not for my own benefit, but 'for the empathic service of others' (Kramer 2000, p.48), 'without being intrusive, without distorting meaning or imposing pictorial ideas or preferences alien to the client' (Kramer 1986, p.71). The collaboration between art(ist)-therapist and patient reminded me of Freeland's two distinct 'purposes of portraiture' (2010, p.192), i.e. the intentional act of the *creator* and the intentional act of the *subject*, and how these two intentional strands entwine together to create the portraits. I also found it empowering to recognise that through Wright's (2009) thesis the 'good enough (m)other' can also be translated into the 'good enough artist', and I felt liberated as a portrait artist through the recognition that I only needed to be 'good enough'.

## Calls for research in the fields of art therapy and life-threatening and chronic illnesses

Over the past decade there have been calls for the development of interventions that enhance, support and maintain patients' 'individual creative capacity' to adapt to illness, and those which explore the 'embodied' nature of self-identity and the illness experience (Reeve *et al.* 2010, p.190). Within art therapy literature there have been calls for more research studies to support the contribution art therapy plays in ameliorating suffering in those living with life-threatening and chronic illnesses (Waller and Sibbett 2005; Wood *et al.* 2011, p.144). More specifically Hubbard *et al.* (2010) explored the biographical work of people living with a diagnosis of cancer and concluded that there is a need for the development of interventions that 'support those people who experience cancer as an assault on their identity' (ibid., p.143). Portrait therapy therefore seeks to answer these calls through the development of a creative, flexible, inclusive and collaborative intervention.

A focus on *disrupted identities* is also a *non-pathologising* way of working with the many losses and changes to body, life and abilities, that people who suffer from life-threatening and chronic illnesses experience on a day-to-day basis. By collaborating with patients such as Eileen and becoming 'a brush for their (self)-portraits', the *art* in *art therapy* becomes accessible to those who choose not to make art or who are physically or psychologically unable to, offering an *inclusive* intervention at a time when *exclusion* has become a dominant theme in the lives of those most severely affected by life-threatening and chronic illnesses. It also becomes a way to develop and discover a sense of 'health within illness' (Carel 2008, p.17).

— Chapter 2 —

# PRIMING THE CANVAS

*A Phenomenological Approach to Depicting Subjectivity*

Over the years many patients have talked to me about their sense of shock and disbelief at diagnosis, even when they say they 'knew' something was wrong. The diagnosis story is usually the first thing a patient will tell me, and they are often still feeling traumatised by it, either because of the insensitive way they were told, or because of the time it took to get a diagnosis and treatment. However, this is understandable when one considers the nature of illness:

> Illness is the night side of life, a more onerous citizenship. Everyone who is born holds dual citizenship, in the kingdom of the well and in the kingdom of the sick. Although we all prefer to use the good passport, sooner or later each of us is obliged, at least for a spell, to identify ourselves as citizens of that other place. (Sontag 1991)

Finding ourselves citizens of 'that other place' is always a surprise...a shock...it is not somewhere we go willingly. Ultimately no one wants to be ill, and no one wants to inhabit or even visit for a time...'that other *liminal* place'. However, this liminal place is where art therapists and artists work, on the edges of society, helping people make sense of illness, and giving voice to their lived experience.

## The challenge of 'liminality' and the 'world of illness'

'Liminality' has been extensively researched by art therapist Caryl Sibbett (2004, 2005a, 2005b, 2005c), both through her own experiences of cancer and those of her art therapy clients. I suggest that within this 'liminal' space, portraits are 'made special' (Dissanayake 1988), and can be used by employing processes, materials and crafts, as ritualistic symbols. 'Making special' is a unique function of art, it speaks of the *alchemy* of art, and it is one of the reasons why we have dedicated 'cathedrals' of art, housed in the majestic and classical museums and national art galleries within this country and throughout the World. As Dissanayake says:

> One intends by making special to place the activity or artefact in a 'realm' different from the everyday… Both artist and perceiver often feel that in art they have an intimate connection with a world that is different from if not superior to ordinary experience. (1988, p.92)

This is similar to Sibbett's (2005a, p.68) descriptions of the *world of* liminality, a place where rites of passage are played out, where feelings of 'limbo, ambiguity, embodied experience, chaos…expression and transition' are manifest. O'Neill (2008, p.11) points out that when we merge the 'sensory/sensuous experience of storytelling with the sensory/sensuous immediacy of visual representations' we find ourselves in an 'in between space' which is 'dialogic, visual' and also a 'potential' (Winnicott 1971) or 'inter psychic space'.

Concepts of liminality originated within Van Gennep's seminal paper on *rites of passage* (1960), Turner's later work on *ritual* around rites of passage events (Turner 1969), and Little *et al.*'s (1998) linking of liminality to illness. Within Van Gennep's (1960) anthropological study he describes rites of passage as containing 'all the ceremonial patterns which accompany a passage from one situation to another or from one cosmic or social world to another' (ibid., p.10). Van Gennep studied major life events such as childbirth, marriage and death, suggesting that as these events provoke change and uncertainty they cause profound anxiety, and therefore rituals, such as baptisms, weddings and funerals, have grown up around these events to give people a framework within which to pass through and witness these transitions. Van Gennep's ideas are still used by contemporary researchers to understand and explain the experience of living with life-threatening and chronic illnesses (Blows *et al.* 2012; Meyer and Land 2003; Sibbett 2005a; Sibbett and Thompson 2008), and are therefore important to consider.

Art therapist, writer and academic Susan Hogan goes further, suggesting that people who inhabit the borderlands of 'life and death', or 'self and other', may be viewed as 'liminal entities' (2013, p.418), and interestingly Turner (1969, pp.128–9) also views *artists* as 'liminal and marginal people'. This may explain why artists often feel an affinity with, and seek to work alongside, those living with life-threatening and chronic illnesses, perhaps recognising fellow inhabitants of the *liminal* sphere. Little *et al.* (1998, p.1490) believe that liminality is a 'fundamental category of the experience of serious illness that needs separate recognition and examination in any account of serious illness...'

Turner (1969, p.109) suggests that 'liminars' or 'threshold people' are seen by unliminal people as 'others' and hence initiate feelings of *danger* or *distrust*, and hospices (even with the best of intentions) could be seen as liminal places that 'hide' or segregate people with 'unbounded bodies' (Evans 2005a, p.3; Lawton 1998, p.132), unconsciously adding to discourses that speak of 'dependence' (Fine and Glendinning 2005) and 'shame' (Street and Kissane 2001, p.169). Sibbett (2005c, p.69) warns that if healthcare professionals are unable to recognise the realities of their own 'unboundedness and death' then the 'vulnerability and unboundedness' of others may be regarded as 'weakness' or 'deviance' and thus 'terrifying' (ibid.). Certainly, there is still a sense of fear among patients attending the hospice for the first time, fear of what they might find, and a strong sense that the hospice as a place is 'different' and 'dangerous', fearing that once they have crossed the threshold they will never get out alive.

My first experience of visiting a hospice was as an art therapy student; I had been given palliative care as my second-year placement, and I resisted this strongly as it had never been my intention to work with this client group. I tried everything to get the placement changed, but was told in the end that if I could not 'face death' I couldn't be an art therapist. I remember sitting in the car park shaking with anxiety, afraid to get out of the car and cross the threshold into that liminal space and face 'death'. Of course, what I found was not 'death' but 'life', and more joy and laughter than there was 'fear' and 'sadness'; however, hospices *are* liminal spaces *for* liminal people, and conversely it is often the one place where liminal people say they can feel *safe* and *understood*.

## The challenge of depicting a person's subjectivity

When I was researching the portrayal of *subjectivity* (van Alphen 1997), my supervisor recommended reading a book called *Family Snaps* edited by Jo Spence and Patricia Holland (1991), within which I found a chapter called 'I Have Begun the Process of Dying' by Barbara Rosenblum. Within this moving and eloquent chapter, Rosenblum (in the final stage of terminal cancer) questions whether it's possible to portray another person's subjectivity through visual, audio or written word. As Rosenblum said, 'The question for me is: can subjectivity ever be made visible or given a material form by a person who is not me?' (Rosenblum 1991, p.241). This therefore became an important question to consider when developing portrait therapy.

Subjectivity is a central philosophical concept and is subtly different from, but also a part of, self-identity. 'Subjects', as opposed to 'objects', are conscious beings with their own personal views of reality, feelings and perspectives, with their own agency or capacity to act. Subjectivity encompasses one's own specific personal interpretations of any aspect of experience, and also the unique way we as individuals experience the world. Subjectivity is often used as the opposite of 'objectivity' or 'objective' (meaning a view of the world or reality that is free from personal influence or bias). Whether objectivity is possible is debated, as even if you think you are being 'objective', you are probably being unconsciously influenced by something, e.g. your upbringing, culture, advertising.

Within Roland Barthes' (1985, p.102) seminal text on photography *Camera Lucida*, he describes searching for a photograph of his late mother in which he could recognise her 'air' or subjectivity, something he describes as *more* than a likeness (ibid., p.107). However, Barthes describes his search as turning up photographs which were 'like so many masks...I never recognized her except in fragments' he says (ibid.). Then finally Barthes finds an image of his mother as a young girl, and says all the masks dropped away when he saw that photograph. Within this one photograph of his mother, Barthes says, 'there remained a soul, ageless but not timeless, since this "air" was the person I used to see, consubstantial with her face, each day of her long life' (ibid., pp.109–10). Barthes refused to publish this one illuminating picture of his mother, saying that its meaning would be lost on anyone else (Freeland 2007, p.106).

This brings us back to the question...can someone capture through portraiture another person's subjectivity? It seems that it can be captured, but fleetingly, and portraits have historically, and are today, attributed as capable of showing a person's 'unique essence'; however, the question remains...can this be achieved through the powers of observation, or is it through the interaction, through the stories told and the relationship built over many sittings, that 'subjectivity' is found?

I visit the BP portrait exhibition every year, looking for that distinct 'air' or 'subjectivity to shine through the paintings, but I seldom find it. Often photorealist or hyperrealist portraits leave me feeling 'cold', or shut out, and I end up looking at the portrait, not as a painting of a 'subject' but as a painting of an 'object'. This may be because photorealist artists work from photographs, and make every effort to remove their own presence or subjectivity from the work, i.e. no brush mark remains to indicate the artist's presence. I therefore believe that it is the 'presence' of the artist within the portrait, combined with the intersubjective relationship with the sitter, that enables the portrayal of subjectivity. Yet Rosenblum talks very specifically about her need to 'shut everything and everyone out' in order to find her own subjectivity:

> The rapid oscillation of my interior emotional life does not easily yield to expression and representation. ... How can you convey the awful helplessness I experience when I must take medicine because of nausea or pain? How can I tell you about the shyness I've always had about my body and the especial shyness I feel now, now that my hair is patchy and short, now that my figure has been altered by the effects of chemotherapy? The camera, by its very nature, demands exposure, that I open to it. Subjectivity, by its nature, demands that I shut everything and everyone out, so I can hear myself. I find myself placed squarely in a contradiction between the objectifying nature of representation and the requirement of quiet and solitude in order successfully to stay alive to the subjectivity in myself. (Rosenblum in Spence and Holland 1991, p.242)

My search for portraits which portray the subjectivity of people living with *illness* has been an interesting one, as historically, portraits of illness have been depicted, either in a way which 'pathologises and objectifies the patient', or in a way which 'romanticises' the ill person, as in Victorian depictions of people with tuberculosis (Sontag 1991, p.29). However, contemporary artists are more likely to depict illness and even death in a way that confronts, and challenges, this romantic view. In what she calls a *devotional study*, entitled *Last Portrait of Mother* (see Figure 2.1), former president of the Royal Society of Portrait

Painters (1994–2000) Daphne Todd paints her 100-year-old mother Annie Mary Todd, laid out in the 'cool room' of an undertaker, during the three days following her death (Jones 2010). This portrait was the winner of the BP Portrait Prize in 2010, and painted by Todd as part of a series of portraits depicting her mother at different stages in her life. Seen in this context the final work seems to be a natural conclusion to the series.

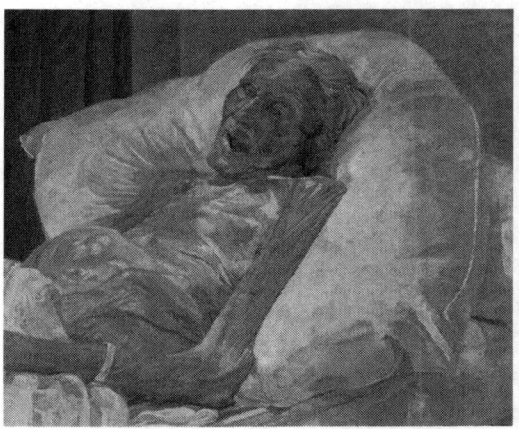

Figure 2.1 *Last Portrait of Mother* by Daphne Todd © 2009
(see also Coloured Plate vii).

It seems that painting death could be described as an attempt to paint the *absence* of subjectivity, as agency and opinions are lost in death. However, I wonder if portraying the absence of subjectivity is as difficult as capturing it? Todd describes being called to the hospital when her mother's condition deteriorated, but arriving too late (Brown 2010). Her three-day vigil could be seen as a self-imposed penance or conversely the curious artistic eye, painting her mother's decaying body? Susan Sontag in her book *Regarding the Pain of Others* (2003, p.75) quotes Leonardo de Vinci as suggesting that 'the artist's gaze be, literally, pitiless. The image should appal, and in that *terribilità* lies a challenging kind of beauty.' Todd describes painting the portrait as 'therapeutic', giving her a reason to be with her mother, and time to come to terms with her death (Brown 2010). One may question whether Todd's mother wanted to be remembered this way – naked and vulnerable with waxing, yellowing skin, but seen in the context of all the other portraits Todd painted of her mother, it was a final ritual, a final 'making special' that Todd was able do for her. After all, portraiture is a relational activity, and by studying the person before them, the artist gets to know each curve and contour of the person's body (Brown 2010). For Todd to do this for her mother was a unique acknowledgement of their relationship, a performance of the last rites that only a portrait artist could perform, and a final way of *seeing* and *knowing* her mother with love and compassion (Jones 2010).

Visual artist Juliet Chenery-Robson – in her photographic series *Kingdoms of the Sick* – portrays young people, including her daughter Emilia, living with ME (Myalgic Encephalopathy), and explores ways to make this invisible illness visible. Through photography Chenery-Robson attempts to freeze a moment and capture the isolation, stillness and immobility of the subject. Each portrait depicts the subject in their bedroom or own personal space, surrounded by their belongings and holding a favourite soft toy. In the photograph entitled *Lucy's Kingdom* (see Figure 2.2), Lucy appears calm and stoical on the surface, and to look at her you would not know that she is ill. However, then you realise that these 'rooms', that are their 'kingdoms', are also their 'prisons' for long periods of time, perhaps many years, just as the body becomes a prison for their subjectivity. There is a 'silence' and 'stillness' in these photographs that reflects these 'kingdoms' as isolated liminal spaces, cut off from the outside world.

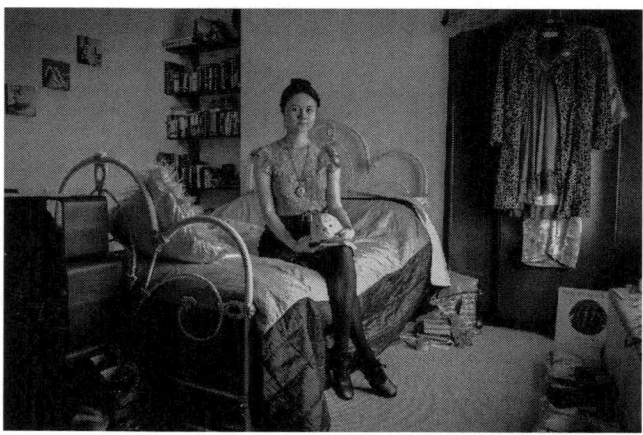

Figure 2.2 *Lucy's Kingdom* by Juliet Chenery-Robson © 2010.

Chenery-Robson's intention was to challenge the disbelief and misconceptions surrounding this invisible illness – invisible in the sense that people diagnosed with ME have no 'wounds' with which to 'authenticate' their suffering (Bell 2002, p.24).

In another participatory project called *Portrait of an Invisible Illness* (2016), Chenery-Robson employs metaphor and portrait photography, to explore collaboratively, with people living with ME, the multi-layered nature of the disease. Chenery-Robson shows, through a series of photographic portraits, that by doubting the genuineness of their disease and therefore their subjective lived experience, the medical profession is 'objectifying' these patients. Within each head and shoulder portrait the person depicted sits with their eyes closed, shutting out the world and hiding their subjectivity, just as the world shuts them out and denies their lived experience (Figure 2.3).

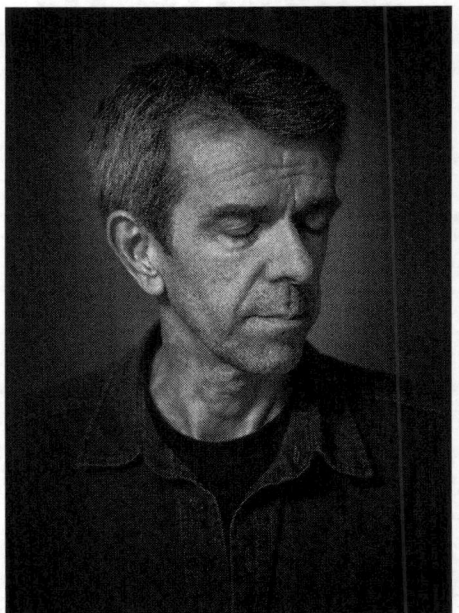

Figure 2.3 *Portrait of Philip* by Juliet Chenery-Robson © 2016.

Both these projects are reflected within a photograph by Jo Spence and Tim Sheard called *Included* (see Figure 2.4), from their series 'Narratives of Disease', where Spence is depicted as a newly diagnosed cancer patient, naked, expressing her vulnerability, eyes closed, holding a teddy bear – evoking images of the frightened child needing to be comforted.

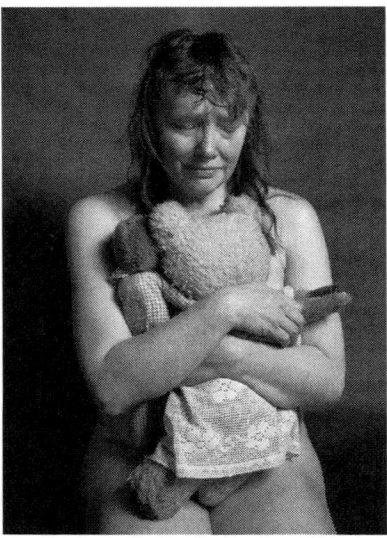

Figure 2.4 *Jo Spence, from Narratives of Disease (Included)* by Jo Spence and Tim Sheard © 1990.

Spence talks from her lived experience, saying: 'I want to show you what I think happens to a cancer patient when they go into hospital. I displayed to him what I felt – literally I was a tearful child holding her teddy bear...' (Spence quoted in Chambers 2009, p.6).

Curiously, photographic images of suffering can send mixed messages, as Sontag says: 'Stop this! ...it urges. But it also exclaims, what a spectacle!' (Sontag 2003, p.77). Images can also be dangerous, where a few seconds on the retina can leave a lifetime of unwanted flashbacks in the mind's eye of its viewers. James Elkins, in his book *The Object Stares Back*, talks about this phenomenon:

> Some pictures affect me for a few minutes, and others make permanent alterations in what I am. If you spend time in front of a painted portrait, the figure's mood will begin to change the way you feel. (Elkins 1996, p.41)

Within an illness narrative a painted portrait offers a unique mirroring device and validation of the sitter's subjectivity or self-identity, providing a visual demonstration that they have been *seen* and their story *heard*. However, when attempting to paint another person's subjectivity, particularly when they are seriously ill, it brings forth a dilemma for the artist. The portrait becomes an attempt to record not only the subjectivity of the person being painted but also the gradual loss of that subjectivity. When depicting this, it seems probable that artists replace this loss with their own subjectivity and the painting thus becomes a 'fusion' of subjectivity, combining the depicted and the depicter in an image which speaks about the continuation of the artist's life in relation to the disappearing life before them. This is eloquently portrayed by Daphne Todd's image of her dead mother, overriding individual subjectivity when it becomes weakened and vulnerable through the devastation of illness and death, with a universal human intersubjectivity.

## The challenge of problematised bodies and gender

An embodied approach to the description of illness recognises the *central role of the body* in all aspects of perception, consciousness and human experience (Merleau-Ponty 2002), and the human body has historically been 'informed and inscribed by many political, social and cultural discourses' (Cancienne and Snowber 2009, p.199), as have self-identities. It is therefore important to view the body and self-identity from different perspectives including aspects of sociology and philosophy which have influenced knowledge in this area (ibid.). In Western society, the body is increasingly problematised and objectified, with the drive to 'improve' health and body-image feeding the consumerist campaign to sell new products (Evans 2005b, pp.44–5). This consumerist propaganda has led to the belief that we can change who we are by changing our bodies or external props (e.g. hair colour, breast size, clothes), and historically there has been a human propensity to 'experiment with impersonation, to become momentarily someone or something else' (ibid.). This links into Irvin Goffman's (1959) thesis whereby people present their 'selves' theatrically to one another through different guises (using props and costume) depending upon their 'audience' and influenced by whether this takes place in a 'front stage' (public) or 'back stage' (private) situation. Charmaz and Rosenfeld (2006, p.38) claim that people who attempt to conceal their illness or disabilities utilise 'a range of Goffmanian/dramaturgical techniques to produce a publicly and privately valued self, e.g. deference, physical grace, and props that signal healthy bodies'. Goffman's (1963) ideas on 'stigma' are also important, particularly in relation to the diseased body and attempts to use 'information control' around their illness as a way to manage what is *seen* or *not seen*, and so avoid social stigma.

The pressure to conform to the 'sick role' within caring institutions, and the medicalised objectification of the body, indicates the subtle institutionalised reconstruction of a person's social self-identity, characterised not by individuality, choice or control, but by depersonalisation and powerlessness (Evans 2005b, p.39). On the one hand the body is idealised and worshipped and on the other it is a focus of self-hatred, anxiety and depression, characterised by the two extremes of eating disorder: anorexia nervosa and obesity (ibid., p.43). The body is further problematised by cancer treatments known as 'slash, burn and poison' (i.e. surgery, radiation, chemotherapy) (Sibbett 2005b, p.59), as patients often feel their illness is a *punishment* for some past misdemeanour, which is logical when one considers how the body has historically been used for punishment and discipline.

In an intervention focused on portraying self-identity it is important to be aware of how cultural constructs such as *gender* (Holmes 2011) influence self-identity in life-threatening and chronic illnesses, and the role the portraits may play, overtly or covertly, within this (for a detailed overview of gender issues from an art therapy perspective, see Hogan 2003). As soon as we are born our bodies are ascribed cultural meanings, or are 'encultured' purely on the basis of what sex we are, and while we cannot totally escape cultural influence, we can learn to question the process of normalisation within socially constructed institutions (Hogan 2003, p.14). As philosopher and gender theorist, Judith Butler (2004a, p.21) says:

> Constituted as a social phenomenon in the public sphere, my body is and is not mine. Given over from the start to the world of others, it bears their imprint, is formed within the crucible of social life; only later, and with some uncertainty, do I lay claim to my body as my own, if, in fact, I ever do.

When engaging in portrait therapy with patients it is important to understand how social and cultural representations of gender can limit individuals, and play a key role in how people think about themselves (Hogan 2003, p.12), how people are treated within society, and the opportunities or difficulties they may encounter (Hogan 1997). It is also important to avoid imposing 'preconceived or universalised ideas' about what constitutes 'gender norms' (Hogan 2003, p.21).

Since the Renaissance, portraiture has been an integral part of wealthy patriarchal societies and as such has also been a key part of gender identity construction (Pointon 2013, p.14). When working collaboratively with the patients portrayed within this book, gender issues did manifest as an underlying tension in some of the portraits and collages, highlighting the covert pressures patients suffer in trying to maintain roles and expectations around gender in the face of life-threatening and chronic illnesses.

## The challenge of de-personalised care

The fragmented nature of our society, and our lack of connectedness to each other, results in a loss of *identity-affirming* opportunities (i.e. mirroring and attuning opportunities) through intersubjective relationships. The impact of this on mental and physical health cannot be underestimated. This is highlighted within 'instrumental reason' (Levinas quoted in Taylor 1991, p.4), which is 'the kind of rationality we draw on when we calculate the most economical application of means to a given end. Maximum efficiency, the best cost-output ratio, is its measure of success' (Taylor 1991, p.4). Taylor (1991, p.105) described the effect of 'instrumental reason' as:

> ...the medical practice that forgets the patient as a person, that take no account of how the treatment relates to his or her story and thus of the determinants of hope and despair, that neglects the essential rapport between caregiver and patient...

My interest in instrumental reason, as a driving force in contemporary society, is the impact that this has on the relational aspects of caring in our national health service and also in hospices, with the development of a 'technological approach' to medicine and the implication it has for patients' experience. This has ramifications for the way that increasingly patients are not treated as whole persons with a life story (Benner 2003; Benner and Wrubel 1989). Science, and therefore a healthcare system dominated by science, ignores the embodied lived experience of illness and suffering, and the human need to *make meaning* out of such experiences; science has no way to explain or alleviate suffering and does not look for or provide *meaning*.

Researching portrait therapy has highlighted the need patients have for intersubjective 'I-thou' (Buber 2004 [1937]) mirroring and attuning encounters that enable self-identity formation and validation. This involves healthcare professionals being able to identify when the biomedical disease model is ineffectual in understanding suffering and supporting primary care (Reeve *et al.* 2010, p.16). Care giving also needs to be recognised as *central* to the discourse in healthcare, rather than secondary to a focus on political and economic dimensions, or 'something that is hollowed of its humanity and moral value' (Kleinman 2012, p.1551). This present system does not recognise individuality, or the need people facing end of life have for continued personal growth and development as a way to find 'health' within illness (Carel 2008, p.16). There also needs to be a recognition of the *harm* that can be done by healthcare professionals who do not recognise their own power to 'affirm or demean' the self-identities of patients, within the medical or clinical encounter (Kinsella 2006, p.25).

Listening to the stories of patients, and mirroring their self-identities through portrait therapy, challenges the way knowledge is created around illness and highlights that health*care* and *therapeutic care* is a human intersubjective endeavour. People are not robots, and real healing cannot be found purely in identifying and treating the mechanics of an illness, but is found in human connections that involve the emotional, psychological and spiritual realms.

Traumatic experiences are often non-transferrable into language, so the voices of the sick and injured remain unheard. This is a problem when healthcare is defined by discourses with no access to the lived experience of the patients they are treating. As Eisner says:

> It is to the artistic to which we must turn, not as a rejection of the scientific, but because with both we can achieve binocular vision. Looking through one eye never did provide much depth of field. (2005, p.74)

## The challenge of meaninglessness and ontological *in*security

One of the consequences of identity disruption for people living with life-threatening and chronic illness is the way it impacts on a person's sense of 'ontological security' (Giddens 1991, p.38), which is where a sense of meaning, continuity and worthwhileness of a person's life is called into question (Watts 2009, p.3). Sociologist Anthony Giddens defines ontological security as a basic sense of trust and security in the world and other people, a sense of continuity of being, a sense of protection against threats and dangers, and the sustaining of courage and hope in the face of adversity (Giddens 1991, pp.38–9). Notwithstanding Giddens' suggestion that *narrative* is the key to a coherent self-identity, Giddens (1984, p.45) identifies 'practical consciousness' (a non-verbal form of knowledge) as essential for the maintenance of ontological security.

Postmodern society can perhaps be characterised by an increasing sense of *isolation* and *fragmentation*, a falling away of traditional values, and a loss of confidence in what has been called 'the grand narratives of the past', but also by a search for belonging and relationship. People anxiously scan their mobile phones, email, Facebook, Twitter, for 'shreds of evidence that someone somewhere may need or want' them (Bauman 2004, p.25). This highlights a need to 'keep in touch' without the inconvenience and 'discomforts that actual "touching" may hold in store' (ibid., p.69). The effect of 'globalisation' has meant the breakdown of the 'protective framework of the small community', where people were traditionally shielded through their relational ties, and lived within protective boundaries (Giddens 1991) – in other words, where they were *known*. These frameworks have now been replaced for the most part by large impersonal organisations, and the individual person is left feeling 'bereft and alone in a world in which she or he lacks the psychological support and the sense of security provided by more traditional settings' (Giddens 1991, p.33). Modern society is therefore characterised by its 'implicit anonymity and alienation' (Kinnvall 2004, p.744) and this is compounded by the restrictions caused by illness and disability, leaving patients vulnerable to feelings of ontological insecurity and without that comforting feeling of *being known*.

A threat to an individual's ontological security can be described as the experiencing of events that are not consistent with a person's own life meanings, therefore causing a sense of 'cognitive dissonance' (Pinker 2002, p.265), resulting in *confusion* and *disorientation*. My understanding therefore of what it means to be ontologically *secure* is: to have an understanding of one's place in the world, from which a sense of direction, self-worth and security are generated (Watts 2009, p.3), which is something that must be 'routinely created and renewed and sustained in the activities of the individual' (ibid.).

Within the case-study chapters of this book, I will therefore present the case for portrait therapy being an opportunity for patients to 'create and renew' a sense of *meaning*, and *homelike-being-in-the-world* (Svenaeus 2011), thus supporting a person's sense of *ontological security*.

## The challenge of 'being-towards-death' (Heidegger 1962)

I remember visiting a patient called Reggie on the in-patient unit; we had a very strong therapeutic relationship developed over several years and I knew he was dying and wanted to visit him before he died. When I arrived at his bedside Reggie was lying with his eyes shut propped up in bed and his wife was holding his hand. 'Reggie!' said his wife, rubbing his arm, 'Susan has come to see you'. As she said this, Reggie's eyes opened and as quick as a flash he reached out and grabbed my hand. 'Susan, am I dying?' he said earnestly, looking me directly in the eye. Reggie had expressed his fear of death to me many times, and yet I was taken aback by his directness… 'Hmm…I don't know,' I said, '…only God knows that, Reggie…but I'm afraid you are very poorly…' Reggie nodded and closed his eyes, his wife smiled at me sympathetically, perhaps he asked all his visitors that? I don't know if it was the right thing to say or not but it seemed Reggie was satisfied with that…and he didn't die…not that day or the next… in fact he went home and died there a week later. But I have always worried that I was in the 'denial' camp that day by avoiding a direct answer to Reggie's question (Becker 1997).

The inevitability of death and the fear of dying is a frequent (if not always overt) presence within palliative care. Heidegger suggests that in order to understand our 'being-in-the-world' we need to recognise ourselves and our lives as finite; he called this 'being-towards-death', which is a recognition of the temporal nature of human existence, which propels us forward through time to our eventual death or non-existence (Heidegger 1962, pp.276–7). Conversely Heidegger is not interested in the *experience* of death, as he claims it cannot be experienced; his focus is on the ways people are affected by the anticipation of death, hence the emphasis is 'being *towards* death'. This does not mean that Heidegger dismisses the losses surrounding death, as he says:

> Death does indeed reveal itself as a loss, but a loss such as experienced by those who remain. In suffering this loss, however, we have no way of access to the loss-of-being as such which the dying man 'suffers'. (Heidegger 1962, p.282)

For Heidegger, it is necessary to understand our 'finiteness', so that we can lead what he calls an 'authentic life' (Heidegger 1962), something that involves 'perspicuity', which is having a 'clear overview of one's life' (Carel 2008, p.99). Carel suggests this is achieved by having a 'coherent grasp of one's full temporal existence – past (birth), present, and future (death)' (ibid.). Responding in an *inauthentic way* means ignoring or denying death, therefore we cannot escape from having one or the other attitude, meaning we are 'bound by death' (ibid.).

Portrait therapy supports the aims of the Dying Matters Coalition, which endeavours to change the current thinking and behaviours around death, dying and bereavement, and through this to make *living and dying well* the norm; it also embraces Elizabeth Kubler-Ross' focus on death as 'the final stage of growth' (1975, p.145).

## The challenge of aesthetics within art therapy: An uneasy relationship

> The effect in sickness of beautiful objects, and especially of brilliancy of colour is hardly appreciated at all. … People say the effect is only on the mind. It is no such thing. The effect is on the body, too. As little as we know about the way in which we are affected by form, by colour and light, we do know this, that they have an actual physical effect. … Variety of form and brilliance of colour in the objects presented to the patients is an actual means of recovery. (Florence Nightingale, 1860, quoted in Harms 1975, p.241)

The capacity for 'beauty' or aesthetics, to move and heal people (both mentally and physically), seems to be largely ignored within contemporary art and art therapy, and yet was understood by Florence Nightingale over 150 years ago, as well as by pioneer art therapists Adrian Hill (1945, 1951) and Edith Kramer (1971, 1986). The 'beauty' revealed to Eileen in the portrait of herself as a child (Figure 1.3) initiated a thought process within me about the uneasy relationship between aesthetics and art therapy. Certainly, within my art therapy training the 'art' in art therapy was purged from any associations with aesthetic value or technique, and this was underlined by the basic, kindergarten quality of art materials we were offered with which to express our 'selves'.

Perhaps because of this training art therapists generally have steered clear of aesthetics, as an attempt to create distance between themselves and the 'elitist, judgemental perspective of the art world', concentrating instead on the 'process' rather than the final product (Moon 2002, p.139). Some art therapists do attempt an integration of aesthetics into therapeutic art making, acknowledging however that there are differences between art created in therapy and other types of art (Henley 1997; Moon 2002, p.139). Moon suggests developing a 'new aesthetic' for art therapy, 'one that is inclusive rather than elitist and that is based in an ethic of care' (Moon 2002, p.139).

Art therapist David Maclagan (1989, 1998, 2001) has written extensively about art therapy and aesthetics, and my understanding of aesthetics is similar to his own:

> By 'aesthetic' I do not intend to refer only to a picture's 'beautiful' or 'good' qualities, or to the philosophical criteria for making such judgements; but to a more phenomenological approach, which would include the entire spectrum of aesthetic experience, from its riches to its most impoverished forms. (Maclagan 1998, p.49)

My interpretation of 'beauty' within portrait therapy is similar to that found in Japanese *Wabi Sabi*, which is described as:

> A beauty of things imperfect, impermanent, and incomplete. It is a beauty of things modest and humble. It is a beauty of things unconventional. (Koren 1998, p.7)

Beauty can also be described as a process where we become aware of the 'essential qualities of a person, object, or experience', which allows a shift from 'judging the relative merits of a phenomena to the ability of a person to perceive distinctive features' (McNiff 2004, p.58). McNiff says that art therapists have, with the influence of the medical model, concentrated on 'expressions of pain and trauma' and have not given sufficient attention to how 'beauty nourishes, balms, and restores the soul' (2004, p.59). It seems therefore that 'the uplifting effects of beauty have much to offer people wanting to assuage these and other forms of pain and suffering' (ibid., pp.59–60). Whilst I do not argue against the focus on pain and suffering within the many approaches to art therapy, I believe that ignoring the potential power of aesthetics to transform ugliness and pain is misguided, as it limits the tools art therapists have at their disposal and the potential healing that a focus on aesthetics might provide (McNiff 2004, p.60).

Expressive arts therapist Paolo Knill (1995) outlines an 'aesthetic response' within arts therapy, saying that aesthetics, in particular the notion of 'beauty' within therapeutic artwork, has been a 'taboo' subject based upon the fear of 'judging' a client's work, and that 'in suppressing our aesthetic sense, we have thrown out the baby with the bath water…wasting one of our most valuable talents for engaging the healing power of the arts and for reaching depth in the psychotherapeutic relationship' (p.1). Knill warns however that the aesthetic 'must radiate from the work itself or the therapeutic relationship' in order to succeed (Knill 1995, p.7).

Roger Scruton (2012), in his BBC documentary entitled *Why Beauty Matters*, suggests that in the Western world between 1750 and 1930, the aim of poetry, art or music was 'beauty', which was recognised as and valued as much as 'truth' and 'goodness'. Scruton claims that during the 20th century, at about the same time that religion began to lose its dominance, beauty was dropped from the art agenda, and art and architecture developed into a cult of ugliness and alienation. Scruton says he is afraid that we are losing 'beauty', and with it the meaning of life, the meaning that shapes our world into a 'home' and ourselves as 'spiritual beings'. Scruton believes that beauty is not just a subjective phenomenon, it is a universal need of human beings, which if ignored leads us to a place devoid of spirituality, whereas beauty in the work of art consoles those who are grieving and affirms those who are full of joy, thereby acting as a force for redemption, through beauty (ibid.).

Scruton (2012) points to the advent of Surrealism and Marcel Duchamp with his ready-made urinal signed with the fictitious 'R. Mutt' as the perpetrator of the decline. The ready-mades are perhaps the precursors of *conceptual art*, which, Scruton says, is bound entirely by words and description, and the 'art' and 'creativity' have been left out. It is interesting to note that some of the early pioneers of art therapy were followers of Surrealism, perhaps, as Hogan (2001) says, discovering a link between André Breton's concept of 'automatic writing' and Freud's 'free association' in psychoanalysis.

This association perhaps explains art therapy's *dis*sociation from aesthetics and 'beauty', and conversely, through this *dissociation* effectively *aligns* itself with the elite art world, the very thing it wished to *detach* its self from! Contemporary and conceptual artists have, for the most part, detached themselves so overwhelmingly from any sense of beauty or aesthetic quality in their work, that now to engage in art that embraces beauty is to be the most *radical* of artists!

## A phenomenological approach to art therapy and illness

As painting a person's subjectivity is about portraying the *lived experience* of the sitter it was important to embrace a phenomenological approach to portrait therapy and its analysis. Phenomenology is a 'poetizing project; it tries an incantative, evocative speaking, a primal telling', it is a language that engages voices to 'sing the world' (Merleau-Ponty quoted in van Manen 1990, p.13). Phenomenology can be described as 'the attentive practice of thoughtfulness' or 'a caring attunement' (van Manen 1990, p.12; Heidegger 1962), within the search for the *essence* of human experience. There is a recognition within portrait therapy that life-threatening and chronic illnesses impact on a person's 'entire' life/world, and this therefore requires a phenomenological approach encompassing a description of the *lived experience* or *life/world* of the patients (van Manen 1990, p.9).

Phenomenology is not one distinct philosophical approach, there are many threads to phenomenology, but these approaches can be broadly divided into two ideologies: those with a concentration on the *pre-reflective* purely *descriptive* consciousness of the lived world, as in Husserl's (1970 [first published in 1954]); (1977 [first published in 1929]) *transcendental* phenomenology; and those embracing a *reflective interpretative* consciousness, as in Heidegger's (1962 [first published in 1927]) *hermeneutic* phenomenology. Husserlian *transcendental* phenomenology concentrates on the pre-reflective experience or a 'return to the things themselves', and aims to develop a deeper understanding of that experience and its meanings as they are presented to consciousness. Transcendental phenomenology does not seek to explain *theoretically*; rather it seeks to gain insightful *descriptions* of that experience. Hermeneutic or reflective-interpretative phenomenology aims to find 'universal meaning' from lived experience (van Manen 1990, p.19), it is a search for the 'fullness of living' and takes into account the sociocultural traditions that give meaning to the *life/world* (van Manen 1990, p.12). I believe both aspects of phenomenology are important and therefore combine the two approaches within the life/world phenomenological analysis I used to analyse portrait therapy.

Historically it is the artists, philosophers, poets and writers who have instinctively used a phenomenological approach to their work, in order to '(re)unite them with the ground of their lived experience' (van Manen 1990, p.9) and through this develop new knowledge. There are a growing number of art therapists who have used a phenomenological approach in their research (Bell 2008; Craig 2009; Lazarus-Leff 1998; Persons 2009; Quail and Peavy 1994; Reynolds and Prior 2003; Rossetto 2012; Rostron 2010; Tjasink 2010; Van Lith 2008), and those who support its use within art therapy (Betensky 1995; Skaife 2001). Phenomenology can be applied effectively to the many different theoretical approaches within art therapy and is particularly relevant in describing 'the relationship between seeing, making art, relating with others and "becoming" in a social context', and promotes a greater 'prominence for art in art therapy theory' (Skaife 2001, p.49). Tjansink (2010, p.76) claims that a phenomenological approach within art therapy enables an exploration and transformation of what self-identity 'was, is and can be' whilst understanding the other as an 'equal subject' (Tjansink 2010, p.76).

Within a phenomenological approach to art therapy the therapist seeks to develop an authentic, intersubjective and collaborative relationship with clients, becoming a 'mutual subject' who remains 'authentically present while being aware that the space is for the other' (Tjansink 2010, p.78). Becoming a 'mutual subject' highlights the danger that a therapist may *unconsciously* direct clients to explore aspects of the therapist's own issues. Attending regular supervision sessions with a trained therapist and developing a *reflexive* approach (Etherington 2004a, 2004b, 2004c) is therefore important in order to create transparency (Hiles 2008) and to acknowledge our own subjective responses and theoretical or cultural constructs (Etherington 2004b, p.46). However, as ethnographer Sarah Pink (2007, p.23) says, a 'reflexive' approach does not suggest that 'subjectivity' could or should be erased from the creative process; rather, she advises, 'subjectivity should be engaged with as a central aspect of ethnographic knowledge, interpretation and representation'. It is therefore important to acknowledge our reflexive resonances and then 'bracket them out' in the phenomenological manner within the case-studies. I refer to these 'bracketed out statements' as *statements of reflexive resonance*, and they contain my own subjective experience, so that I know what belongs to the patient and what belongs to me (this will be explained further in Chapter 9, Table 9.1).

There are a number of authors who have explored the lived experience of *illness* from a phenomenological perspective (Carel 2007, 2008, 2011, 2012, 2013; Kirkengen and Ulvestad 2007; Svenaeus 2000, 2001, 2011, 2012; Toombs 1988, 1990, 1992, 2001). Carel (2008, p.16) advocates a phenomenological approach to illness research, saying:

> A phenomenological approach enables the expression of these experiences in order to give a more complete description of the altered relationship of the ill person to her world and a better understanding of her experience.

A phenomenological approach allows a focus on the experiences of illness *as lived* by the ill person, encompassing 'physical, psychological and social' experiences, as well as a focus on the changes that define illness (Carel 2008, p.11), whereas traditional methods, such as the 'naturalistic' and 'normative' approaches of scientific research, often obscure the voice of the ill person (ibid.). This refocus on the individual's lived experience can be seen as liberating:

> …a focus on the individual (as the site of suffering and distress) liberates art therapy from developing an over-reliance on, and rigid adherence to, set theories and a priori categories of meaning inherent in theoretical orthodoxy, which can obscure as much as illuminate human suffering. (Hogan 1997, p.37)

Through using a phenomenological approach to portrait therapy the aim is for a fuller understanding of illness experiences, and an intervention which addresses the need identified by patients, rather than those assumed by others, and a focus on improving quality of life. After all, the improvement of the patients' quality of life is central to the ethos of palliative care, and it is important to demonstrate that portrait therapy contributes to this aim (Bell 2008, p.354).

— Chapter 3 —

# SELECTING THE MEDIUM

*Portraiture as a Therapeutic Tool*

In 1998 art therapist Michele Wood wrote an inspirational paper about a patient dying from AIDS who, in an art therapy session, used his own body intuitively as a 'portrait' (Wood 1998). Wood said that at the beginning of the session the patient asked for a large piece of paper to be placed on the floor; he then, with difficulty, lay down upon it (ibid., p.142). Wood suggested that the patient's presence, lying there on the paper, seemed to be saying 'here I am, see me', asking for a witness to his embodied illness story (ibid., p.145). Wood reflected on this session, saying, 'I was guided by thoughts of invisibility, of his being "lost" to the patient role and his battle to preserve his identity' (ibid., p.144). The description of how this patient instinctively combined the embodiment of his illness, within self-portraiture, added further weight to my conviction that portraiture could be used as an intervention for people who experience their illness as a disruption to their self-identity.

Painted portraiture in North America and Europe has traditionally occupied a 'default position as the art form of capitalist societies' (Pointon 2013, p.9) and thus indelibly associated with power and wealth (ibid.). What we understand as 'naturalistic conventions' in portraiture derive mainly from Rome's classical period and have persisted up to the present day within commissioned portraits of individuals for large institutions and multinational businesses (Pointon 2013, p.13). During the Renaissance, portrait artists employed the use of symbols and accessories to show character, personality, status and identity (Pointon 2013, p.15) and the focus was on portraits of divinity. This underlines the connection between portraiture and immortality, as well as the portrayal of people worthy of emulation, such as great leaders and warriors. The emphasis on emulation suggests the beginnings of a modern sense of self-identity as a 'manipulable, artful process' (Pointon 2013, p.60) and the power to control others perceptions of one's self-identity (ibid., p.61).

Postmodernism, with its methodologies derived from anthropology, social history, psychoanalysis and semiotics, transformed how portraiture was addressed, leaving it 'poised between resemblance and transfiguration, between objectification and psycho-social concepts such as identity' (Pointon 2013, p.62). Portraiture has traditionally been viewed by academic art theorists as inferior to 'fine art' (ibid., p.18); however, it has continued to flourish, with competitions such as the BP Portrait Prize receiving thousands of entries every year, and portraiture as a genre has been the subject of many conferences, exhibitions, books and articles (ibid., p.21). During the past 30 years, portraiture, as a focus of research, has gained popularity, as it offers a way to gain insight and understanding of historic and contemporary societies, and features as central to historical narrative as 'artefact, image and metaphor' (ibid., p.11). The importance afforded portraits is ingrained in our society; with faces used in most cultures as markers of identity (ibid., p.7). However, our self-identity is thought to encompass much more than our physiognomy, and portrait artists invariably attempt to portray something of the character and 'essence' of the sitter, creating a visual narrative of who they are.

## Portraits as visual portrayals of self-identity

Although narrative is used within the response art collages and prose poems in portrait therapy, I suggest that the *visual* qualities within portraiture have the power to 'extend' the narrative view and acknowledge the *primacy of the body* within illness (Carel 2008). As Wright says: 'discursive language, and arguably the language of interpretation, will generally lack the capacity of imagery to evoke and hold experience' (2009, p.190). Moving away from textual narrative and biography towards the visual allows a reconnection to a more direct 'sensual and intuitive' way of understanding ourselves (Moon 2002, p.50). As Freeland (2010, p.157) said regarding self-portraiture, 'the artist presents his or her embodied self to the world in a way that is simply *not narrative*', therefore *narrative* could never be the 'whole story' in self-identity portrayal, as it can never fully express the body (Freeland 2010, p.192). A portrait gives an illusion of life and presence, and also a physicality and materiality that is absent in text, meaning they can be used as objects within rites and ritual. Portraits are, however, also about 'absence' (Pointon 2013, pp.226–7), as a portrait sets up an 'expectation of human presence that is immediately denied by the very plasticity and materiality of the portrait' and that it is this 'gap between the sign and the referent, that makes portraiture so compelling' (ibid.).

There is no doubt that portraiture is imbibed with its own visual narrative, one that is often employed by curators and writers, alongside other fragments of data, to *authenticate* identities. As Pointon (2013, p.15) claims, 'Biography and portraiture (and autobiography and self-portraiture) are often seen as contiguous disciplines, useful to each other, and both serving in the creation of an authentic likeness.' However, both biography and portraits require subjective choices and interpretation by authors and writers, meaning that an 'authentic likeness' can only be 'relative' and 'approximate' (ibid.). Portraits therefore may be understood as 'imaginative documents that also bear a complex relationship to history as actuality' (ibid., p.22), and may include 'fictive' elements, meaning it is problematic to consider a portrait as an authentic record of a person's likeness (ibid., p.26). Despite this, historians have often tried to link a portrait to a particular individual to support their historical hypotheses (ibid.).

In visual anthropology, the relationships which images have 'iconographically' with each other are surpassed by a focus on the way individuals interact '*with*' images and the 'interactions which individuals form with each other *through* images' (Canals 2011, p.228 [original emphasis]). I see self-identity formation as intrinsically relational, and these different ways of knowing the self are indicated in the portraits that patients *needed to see themselves* and those *they needed others to see* (this is discussed further in Chapter 6).

Visual portraits are part of a complex tradition of human representation and display, where a portrait or self-portrait performs something important about being human, acknowledging the fact that we continuously 'present ourselves visually' to others and that 'there is something different about what we say in constituting ourselves and what we actually do when we go out and show ourselves to others in the world' (Freeland 2010, pp.190–1). I suggest that this difference is characterised by the way visual art utilises a specific kind of symbolism and metaphor (Lakoff and Johnson 1980), which work in a different way to narrative, with images having a more direct and immediate impact on our consciousness (Freeland 2010, p.189; Kramer 2006). This can include an intuitive sense of liking or disliking an image and not knowing why or how to explain it. Knowledge that cannot be articulated adequately by verbal means is called 'tacit knowledge', something which can only be known indirectly through symbolism and metaphor (Jongeward 2009, p.241). In images ambiguity is possible, meaning that interpretation is fluid and adaptable:

> Art by its very nature has the deviant potential for ambiguity. It has the capacity for holding many notions, many angles, many colours and places, in a way that the written or spoken word rarely allows. (Jones 2003, p.98)

Within art therapy one of the functions of the art therapist is the capacity to metaphorically 'hold' the experiences or affect offered by the client, and when a client creates an image around those experiences, the artwork is said to 'hold' those experiences, as they are separated from the client and can be looked at as separate. The same is true of portrait therapy with the success of the portraits being in part due to their ability to hold contradictory truths such as *fact* and *fiction* (Inckle 2010), as well as aspects of realism (Brown 2008a, p.23), and communicate these in a direct and sensory way allowing connections to be made to historical and contemporary symbols (Mullins 2006, p.7).

## Art therapy, portraiture and palliative care

Although the use of portraiture in art therapy is an area of practice that is largely unexamined or researched, several art therapists have written about the way painting portraits of their clients helped to build therapeutic relationships and a strong empathic connection between themselves and their clients (Costello-Du Bois 1989; Franklin 1990, 2010; Jones 1983, 2006; Kramer 1971; B. Moon 1990; C. Moon 2002). While working in an American hospital for the mentally ill, Don Jones (1983, 2006) painted portraits of patients as a way to connect empathically with them. Catherine Moon (2002, p.214) suggests that portraiture is one of the most direct ways that art therapists can 'witness' their clients, and through the portraits clients see themselves as she has seen them, which may promote feelings of being *acknowledged* rather than *judged*, and that 'taking the time to do someone's portrait is perceived as taking the time to notice and, at some level, to care' (2002, p.215). As mentioned earlier Kramer also drew portraits of her child clients as a way to 'reassure them and strengthen their feelings of identity' (Kramer 1971, p.40). The experiences of these art therapists are significant because of the connections they make between portraits and self-identity, and the power portraits possess to witness, acknowledge and care for clients.

It was the British art therapy pioneer Adrian Hill (1945, 1951) who coined the term 'art therapy' and made the initial connection between medicine and art therapy in this country, through a recognition that art making was helpful in his own personal recovery from tuberculosis (Hogan 2001, p.143). Michele Wood (Wood 1990, 1998, 2005; Wood *et al.* 2011, 2013), a more recent pioneer in this field, has written extensively on the subject. Wood, along with Mandy Pratt, co-edited the first academic book on art therapy in palliative care (Pratt and Wood 1998), which explored how art therapy approaches could be adapted to working in this area, something they claimed could 'precipitate a profound exploration of personal issues which positively affects the individual's health and quality of life' (ibid., p.viiii).

Research into art therapy and life-threatening and chronic illnesses is in its infancy and in Wood *et al.*'s (2011) survey into art therapy research in cancer care, they found only 11 published research studies worldwide, only one being from the UK. However, extensive anecdotal evidence does exist in the form of academic journal articles, describing a diverse range of individual therapeutic encounters and a general understanding of how art therapy may benefit patients living with life-threatening and chronic illnesses (e.g. Arnheim 1986, 1990; Connell 1998; Fenton 2008; Hardy 2001, 2005, 2013; Lerner 2005; Luzzatto 2005; Malchiodi 2007; Matho 2005; McGraw 1999; Minar 1999; Reynolds 2003a, 2003b; Reynolds and Lim 2007; Waller 2002).

The general themes covered in this literature include: facing death and dying, a search for meaning, hopelessness, and the effects of illness and treatment on self-identity, body-image, agency, and relationships with others. Wood (2005, p.96) says that within art therapy and cancer care there are two main recurrent themes found in patients' artwork; these are an existential search for meaning and 'making adjustments to one's self-image in order to survive the threat posed by illness'. For Sibbett (2005b, p.22) common themes in her work with cancer patients were issues relating to power and control, with one client saying they felt 'helplessness and no control over what the doctor will decide'. Luzzatto (2005) talks of 'musing with death' within art therapy groups; sometimes death is discussed covertly through symbolic images (Isserow 2013), making it more acceptable, or contained.

Other art therapists who have published on art therapy and palliative care include: Camilla Connell (1992, 1998); Mandy Pratt and Gill Thomas (2002); Sally Skaife (1993); and Diane Waller and Caryl Sibbett (2005). These and other publications have explored the diversities and issues of practice, and the potential benefits for patients, mostly through descriptions of single case-studies. Matho (2005, p.102) talks about how art therapy is able to 'fortify identity' in patients or help them 'come to terms' with a new identity after it has been 'devastated by illness and loss'. Lerner (2005, pp.163–71) claims that art therapy helps people find a voice to express their self-identity. An important finding in Sibbett's (2005c, p.50) study was the *embodiment of experience* in cancer and art therapy, suggesting the importance of paying attention to the body (Corbin 2003), as well as gender and cultural influences, for those living with life-threatening and chronic illnesses. Sibbett also talks about art therapy being a valuable place to express previously unknown or unvoiced aspects of the illness experience, describing some aspects as being 'unspeakable' and other's 'unhearable' (ibid.).

Within Hogan and Warren's 2012 study, which included four individual projects using innovative visual and participatory research methods including 'art elicitation, photo diaries, film booths, and phototherapy' (ibid., p.329), they used innovative and diverse therapeutic techniques to enable older women to create alternative visual representations of aging. Phototherapist Rosy Martin also contributed to the project and describes a process whereby participants worked in pairs to *perform* their stories, choosing clothes and props to aid representation, with the partner/photographer 'there for' the other, 'as witness advocate and nurturer' (Rosy Martin quoted in Hogan and Warren 2012). Hogan and Warren (2012, p.329) suggest that their project challenges the 'biomedical model of aging' and that representations of aging are of particular importance, because women's experiences of aging are profoundly rooted in their appearance.

Hogan and Warren's (2012) project embraces an interdisciplinary and innovative multi-method approach, focusing on the empowerment of the individual clients through a collaborative design. Hogan and Warren suggest that using a multi-method approach enables data to be 'contrasted and juxtaposed' in order to produce a 'collage' of the investigated areas (ibid., p.344); they also use participatory research methods to help mitigate power differentials felt by participants in research processes (ibid., p.345). In a similar way to portrait therapy, their work challenges the power structures and assumptions of therapeutic interventions, exploring boundaries around client confidentiality, encouraging choice, individuality and the opportunity to challenge and direct others. This means that artwork created in such projects can be used by the clients involved as politicised statements, highlighting inequalities and normative stigmatising social constructs, which often define vulnerable people in constricting and derogatory ways. Hogan and Warren's work highlights the need to look beyond the surface of media images of older adults and those living with life-threatening and chronic illnesses, and to give clients/patients the opportunity to portray *who they are*, often in surprising and innovative ways, e.g. see the portrait of *Hermi* (Hogan and Martin 2011; Hogan and Warren 2012, p.339).

Suggestions have been made that art therapy helps to 'maintain the individual's sense of identity in the face of illness' (Wood 1998, p.30); however, when researching portrait therapy, I was unable to find any published studies specifically researching this theory, although the use of art therapy to help restore a sense of self-identity is mentioned. For example, Wood *et al.* (2011) suggest that art therapy can help people suffering from cancer to 'recalibrate' their identity (ibid., p.144), saying that through 'strengthening the person (by the fortification of the self) and providing a means of adjusting aspects of self-image, art therapy may be used to achieve stability and improve psychological and social functioning' (ibid., p.141). Matho (2005, p.116) says that patients approaching end-of-life require an 'extra strengthening of their inner resources in order to affirm their sense of humanity and own a self-identity that is larger than the name of their illness' and that enabling the mobilisation of creativity at this time 'fortifies' a person's 'life-giving inner resources'.

## Artists who have painted people living with life-threatening and chronic illnesses

When researching portrait therapy, I found only one published research study involving portraiture and life-threatening and chronic illnesses; this was carried out in Canada by Aita, Lydiatt and Gilbert (2010) and was called *Portraits of Care: Medical Research through Portraiture*. In this study Aita *et al.* used the creation of drawn and painted portraits to study the relationship between patients and their carers. Portrait artist Mark Gilbert was engaged to draw or paint the portraits of a participant sample consisting of patients, carers and health professionals, 46 in all. This study was designed in two phases, the artistic component (painting the portraits) and an exhibition of the portraits, where attendees were asked to complete a survey. This survey was then used to confirm or discredit the findings from the first 'artistic' phase of the study. Interestingly, in designing the portraits, Gilbert made personal stylistic and compositional choices to 'jettison anything that felt extraneous or irrelevant' (Aita *et al.* 2010, p.6) in the paintings, so most participants are posed within a blank space, with little in the way of personal reference which might indicate clues to 'identity' (see Figures 3.1 and 3.2). There were two exceptions where patients were painted with medical appliances such as a naso-gastric tube and a wheelchair, although Aita *et al.* said that these were painted in the early stages of the project before the methodological approach was fully developed (ibid., p.6).

Within their analysis of the portraits drawn or painted by Gilbert, Aita *et al.* (2010) noted 'a sense of ongoing identity formation especially during transitions in health status' (ibid., pp.7–8). This is significant as it suggests it is possible to portray *identity formation* through portraiture; however, they do not discuss whether this *identity formation* could be attributed to the process of being painted. Aita *et al.* (2010) claim that each session gave the artist and sitter 'time to build a relationship over the period it took to work on the images', and this was considered an essential part of the artistic process by Gilbert, which '…mirrored relationships that develop between patients and caregivers'. However, there are no suggestions that a similar amount of time was given to each participant, but rather that Gilbert chose who he wanted to *draw* (perhaps in one session) and who he wanted to *paint* perhaps posing 'multiple times' (ibid., p.6). Also, although the focus of their project was 'care givers and care giving' there was no suggestion that the 'care giving' inherent in the painting of the portraits by Gilbert was recognised or evaluated. Whilst Aita *et al.* (2010, p.9) say that patient subjects 'responded positively' to their experiences of being drawn/painted and that the experience 'appears to have a therapeutic effect' particularly for those involved in the project for longer periods, they also question whether portraiture can be viewed as *therapeutic* for either the viewer or sitter. They say, the fact that 'these portraits and this project were *moving* for the subjects and viewers appears inescapable, but their actual role as a *therapeutic intervention* is less clear. This important question...clearly requires further study and analysis' (Aita *et al.* 2010, p.11 [my emphasis]).

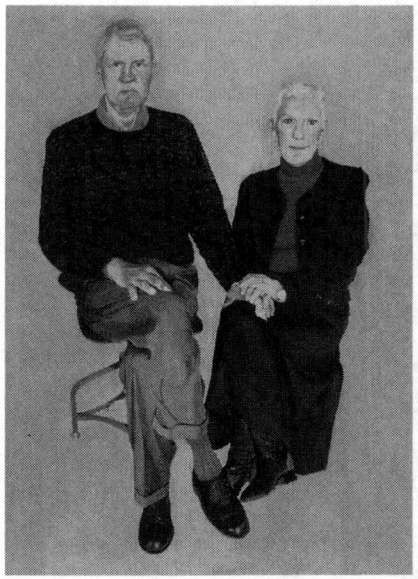

Figure 3.1 *Robin and Mardi* by Mark Gilbert © 2007
(*Portraits of Care* Project) (see also Coloured Plate viii).

Some of Aita *et al.*'s reported outcomes were: the development of new perspectives on health and illness, and in a reciprocal sense – 'helping others who will see the portraits recognise the strength in patients despite illness' (Aita *et al.* 2010, p.9). One patient reported that when attending portrait sittings at the hospital she had a change in feelings towards visiting the hospital, saying that instead of dreading the visits she found herself dressing up and 'putting on makeup for the first time since undergoing multiple surgeries on her face' (Aita *et al.* 2010). Aita *et al.* also make suggestions regarding the use of arts-based methodology in medical research, saying that the study 'yielded a wealth of insight...and helped investigators better understand how portraiture can be used to benefit patient care' (ibid.). They also suggest that as a research model, their study (i.e. painted or drawn portraiture and its exhibition) could be applied to examine other aspects of health and illness (Aita *et al.* 2010, p.12).

In their analysis Aita *et al.* noted that the portraits portrayed the 'interior' of the participants' experiences, communicating through 'non-verbal facial and bodily expression', which enabled patients to be seen as 'whole people', rather than people 'fragmented by diagnosis' (2010, p.8). They said that the portraits emphasised the way patients were 'living through their illness', portraying them 'remarkably *present* and functionally more *healthy* than might be expected given their illnesses' (ibid.). However, as there is no suggestion that the patients or care givers collaborated in the portrait design, it begs the question as to whether these were the characteristics which Gilbert 'chose' to depict, rather than a reflection of the patient and carers' lived experience. However, 'Roger' (a patient) is quoted as saying 'Mark captured the essence of what I feel in his work' and another patient 'Glenna' said the study enabled her to 'see myself as others see me. It helped me to accept the way I look' (ibid., p.8). Aita *et al.* stated they aimed to discover, through exhibiting the paintings, whether the portraits aroused empathy in the viewers; however, they found conflicting evidence saying that sometimes 'the subject did not feel as viewers had imagined' (ibid., p.11). They concluded that:

> ...the essence of care is what assists a person physically and emotionally during a transition in identity brought about by a change in health status. Care is like the wind, seen only by its effects in one's eyes, corporeal presence, emotional strength and sense of identity. The effect of giving care mirrors the same qualities as seen in the one(s) for whom one cares. (Aita *et al.* 2010, p.12)

Aita *et al.* (2010) call for further research in this area, saying that the role of contemporary art in healthcare is a 'necessity' for those in the health professions to access a 'better intellectual and affective understanding of what is critical' and that art can enable healthcare to overcome some of its 'narrowness of vision' (ibid., p.12).

In an earlier research project carried out between 1999 and 2000 entitled 'Saving Faces' (Hutchison, Gilbert and Farrand 2000), artist Mark Gilbert was commissioned by surgeon Iain Hutchison to paint portraits of patients before, during and after facial surgery. This resulted in an exhibition of 30 portraits called *Saving Faces*, which was exhibited nationally and internationally. It was claimed that the patients found the experience 'cathartic', developing a close relationship with Gilbert, enabling them to confide in him 'details of their lives which they shared with no one else' (Farrand 2000). Gilbert used the same stylistic and compositional choices in this earlier study as he used in the later (Aita *et al.* 2010) study, e.g. in his painting of *Barry C* (see Figure 3.2), *Barry* is painted *on* rather than *in* a flat pink background, the only prop being a video game console. By using a personal stylistic choice, Gilbert may have prevented his subjects from adding their own design suggestions and personal input, as well as metaphorical and symbolic content to the portraits, which may have limited their therapeutic value.

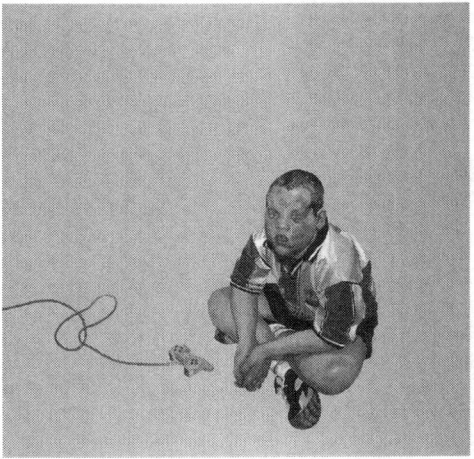

Figure 3.2 *Barry C* by Mark Gilbert © 1999 (*Saving Faces* Project).

Medical Psychologist Paul Farrand (2000) likened the *Saving Faces* project to *art therapy*, with a reversal of roles; however, he also warned that as an intervention portraiture would prove 'far too time-consuming for the patients and too expensive to be of widespread clinical benefit'. However, I have found that portrait therapy, as a 'third hand' art therapy intervention, does not necessarily take any longer than other person-centred art therapy interventions. Also, I suggest that, within the intersubjective therapeutic relationship, *time* and *attention* is a fundamental necessity for patients, in order to re-vision self-identity. However, Farrand (2000) does not dispute the potential of portraiture as a therapy:

> ...in an age where science is seen as offering the best and only way through which to treat patients, the widespread benefits derived from the portraiture suggest that along with scientific advances, art, in its many guises, can also make a significant contribution. (ibid.)

It has to be recognised that Mark Gilbert is a *portrait artist* rather than an *art therapist*, and although art therapists and artists may share similar interests and backgrounds (particularly the understanding of liminality), the relationship between them has not always been easy (Wood 2005, p.83; Learmonth 2002), with art therapists sometimes believing that artists without therapeutic training should not work with vulnerable people (Bolton 2004, p.79). However, in some hospices (e.g. St Christopher's Hospice and Trinity Hospice, in London), artists and arts therapists often work together, alongside, and with patients (Wood 2005, p.84; Hartley and Payne 2008).

Heath Rosselli is a portrait artist who began painting portraits of people recovering from, or living with, cancer and other illnesses in 1997. Rosselli's most well-known work is her painting entitled *Evelyn* (see Figure 3.3), depicted nude, seated and smiling confidently at the viewer, the symmetry of the painting is contrasted by the asymmetry of her breasts, a single diagonal mastectomy scar revealing Evelyn's fight against cancer. The painting has been exhibited in many exhibitions, including the Louvre, Paris, alongside Rembrandt's *Bathsheba*, Raphael's *La Fornaria* and Rubens's *The Three Graces* (Grice 2009b). However, because the painting attracted negative as well as positive responses from the public, it was eventually displayed behind protective glass, as it was feared that the portrait might be defaced in some way (Grice 2009a). Perhaps the painting provoked a negative response in some of the viewers because *Evelyn* displays that which people generally avoid seeing, and through the portrait *Evelyn* refuses to 'live silently' with the pain of her disease (Radley 2002, p.5). In 2009, I visited Rosselli in her studio and interviewed her about her portrait process, and she gave me valuable advice about the practical elements of painting portraits of people living with illness. According to Rosselli (2009) painting portraits involves a 'subconscious interaction' between the painter and the sitter, and that 'what comes out [in the painting] is the message'. Rosselli's portrait of *Evelyn* sought to show what is usually hidden from public view – Evelyn's mastectomy scar, revealed like a medal of honour on her chest, declaring her an inhabitant of the liminal world of illness – and yet through celebrating five years clear of cancer, the painting demonstrates that there is life after cancer and Evelyn's physical beauty had not been diminished by it.

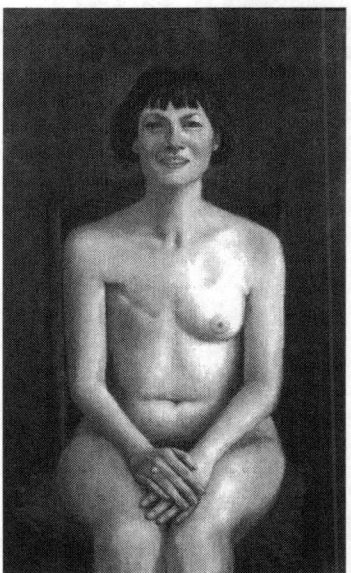

Figure 3.3 *Evelyn* by Heath Rosselli © 1997 (see also Coloured Plate ix).

Another artist who paints portraits of people living with life-threatening and chronic illnesses is Antonia Rolls (2013, 2014a, 2014b), who was moved to paint a series of portraits of her partner Steve when he became terminally ill, painting him right up to the day he died, as a way to cope with the distress of his illness and the prospect of losing him (see Figure 3.4). Rolls (2014a) says, 'I began to paint him and found that his vulnerability, his beauty, his soul, was as wonderful in this state of dying as they were when he was well.' Rolls has since painted many people living with life-threatening and chronic illnesses (Figure 3.5) and also their partners/carers, and has exhibited these works in a touring exhibition called 'A Graceful Death', which she says opens up a discussion on what it means to die.

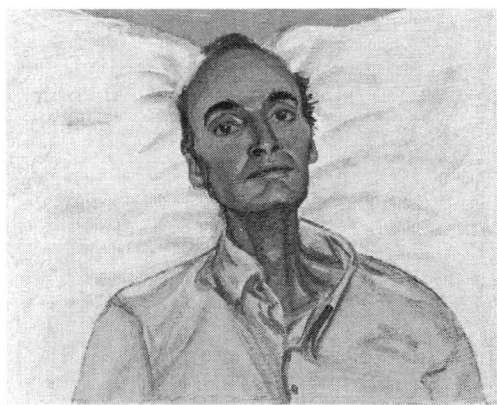

Figure 3.4 *Steve* by Antonia Rolls © 2007 (see also Coloured Plate x).

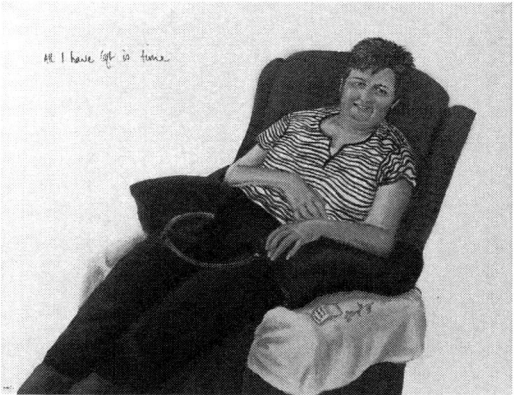

Figure 3.5 *Julia* by Antonia Rolls © 2013.

Rolls (2013) talks about the time it takes to build relationships with people who are dying, but also about how sometimes these relationships become deep and meaningful very quickly, facilitating profound conversations about life and death. There is a strong focus within Rolls' portraits on self-identity and Rolls says, 'I want to know, now that their life is coming to an end, who they are and what they want to say' within their portraits (ibid.). This process includes 'acknowledging' the person and seeing them 'without fear or prejudice' and giving their 'voice and presence an audience' allowing their 'truth' to come out (ibid.). Rolls talks about how sometimes the most important relationship she has when painting a portrait is with the family or partner, as she sometimes paints retrospective portraits after a person has died, or when the person has become too ill to take an active role. Rolls also uses poetry and words alongside her portraits and includes a 'wall of words' in her exhibitions, including poems provided by exhibition visitors and attendees to poetry workshops run alongside the exhibition. Rolls says, 'It seems that art and poetry can touch places which people have kept locked for a long time' (ibid.). Rolls sees the portrait process as a way to give patients a voice, to affirm their sense of self-identity, to access places and memories people have kept locked up for a long time, and for mourning and bereavement.

Brilliant (1991, p.11) says that portraits 'exist at the interface between art and social life', which means that in their composition there is a pressure to conform to the present sociological value system, which may result in artists 'idealising' their sitters as in the private portraits that resemble funeral eulogies, i.e. portrayed in formulaically positive ways. David Fisher's (2009) painting *Dead Man Posing, Portrait of Philip Ledbury* (see Figure 3.6) perhaps gravitates towards this, in the easy smiling and relaxed attitude, complete with cigarette, adopted within it, the title being the only suggestion that Philip is suffering from leukaemia, a life-threatening disease.

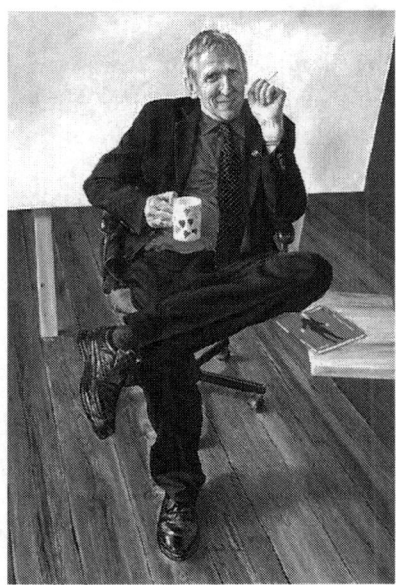

Figure 3.6 *Dead Man Posing, Portrait of Philip Ledbury* by David Fisher © 2009 (see also Coloured Plate xi).

This positivity may however be more indicative of the attitude which Ledbury has adopted throughout his illness, and his enjoyment of the portrait process. The contemporary focus in popular culture on 'celebrity' as a state to be desired also affects the way portraits such as this signify, as well as the historical position that portraiture in North America and Europe has traditionally occupied, as an art form indicative of 'capitalist societies' (Pointon 2013, p.9), and thus indelibly associated with power and wealth (ibid.). Using Goffmanian ideas portraits could also be considered 'performances' making the subjects 'actors' in their own life story, and as actors say, 'if no one is watching you, you don't exist'. I was privileged to meet both Ledbury and Fisher in 2009, after *Dead Man Posing* won the Holburne portrait prize and was exhibited at the Royal West of England open exhibition 2009. When I asked Ledbury about the experience of being painted he talked initially about the relational aspect of portraiture, of becoming close friends with the artist David Fisher through the sittings, before citing the importance of being immortalised:

> I am extremely honoured and flattered to be immortalised in oil paint, this portrait could be around for hundreds of years. The whole experience has been good... (Ledbury 2009, p.1)

The research studies discussed within this section, along with the anecdotal evidence supplied by artists working in the field, demonstrate that the potential for portraiture, as a communicative, therapeutic and identity-forming intervention, has previously been recognised by others, but not developed, until now, into a recognised therapeutic intervention, practised by art therapists.

## Portraiture, photography, and life-threatening and chronic illnesses

Although I acknowledge that there are important differences between photographic and painted portraiture, I explore in this section examples of some of the photography artists who have over the past 30 years used self-portraiture as a way to interrogate death and dying and the effect of disease on the body. I also briefly outline some of the ways that these two mediums differ, both in the way they portray self-identity and also in the way they signify presence.

Pointon (2013, p.17) claims that photographic portraiture requires similar choices to be made regarding composition, lighting, etc., as portraits produced through the use of art materials; however, she later acknowledges that photography focuses on 'surface and physiognomy...on the materiality of the subject as object'. I suggest therefore that there are important differences between photographic and painted portraits, the most important of which is that a camera can only ever make a *copy of reality* (of course it can be manipulated later on a computer); however, in a painted portrait the portrait is something *wholly*, and *humanly created*, and may include imaginative additions to 'reality'. In portraiture, the human mind of the artist constantly analyses and interprets the sitter and the environment, and makes decisions on how to portray them, whereas the camera captures only a 'snapshot' of 'reality'. The painted portrait therefore becomes a physical and analytical creative expression of the sitter and the artist, developed through an intersubjective relationship, captured over time.

### *Phototherapy and autopathographic self-portraiture*

This project builds on the work of photographic artists Jo Spence and Rosy Martin who developed a therapeutic intervention they called *phototherapy* (Martin 2009; Spence 1986), which is a way of using photography, in particular portrait photography, to promote healing, as well as confront social issues. As a photographer, Spence was obviously acutely aware of the viewer as 'audience' to her images, and therefore portrayed her 'self' in relation to that 'audience' (Bell 2002, p.23). Tembeck (2008, p.87) argues that autopathographic images contain 'tactical rhetorical devices', which attempt to influence the way they are received by the general public and raise important ethical questions about the response of viewers and their 'responsibilities in the face of images of suffering'.

In her photographic series *The Picture of Health?* (1982–1991), Jo Spence represented her own journey through treatment for breast cancer, using photographic self-portraiture as personal therapy, and as a way to ask questions about *ownership* of the body in a medical context (Chambers 2009). Spence said of this practice: 'I still oscillate between going subject and object/victim, but am no longer "stuck" and have begun to live in my own totality' (Spence 2005, p.374). Similarly, Martin notes:

> By creating a wide range of images, I have been able to examine many different aspects of myself and my past history and to integrate these into a whole. By acknowledging aspects of myself and my past, which I might otherwise hide, or see as my shadow side, I have freed myself from internalised restrictions and oppressions and have come to accept myself as I am, complete with all the contradictions that have formed me. Phototherapy is photographic feelings in all their rawness. (Martin 1986, p.174)

Hannah Wilke is another artist who used autopathographic images to document first her mother's terminal illness in the exhibitions *So Help Me Hannah* (1978) and *Support Foundation Comfort* (1984); and then, tragically, her own in *Intra-Venus* (1992–1993).

Clearly there is a dual aspect to autopathographic works, a restorative and therapeutic one, but also a confrontation, a demand to be seen, invoking a 'silent scream' in the viewer (Radley 2002, p.5). These images are a stark reminder of our human mortality and the inevitability of suffering; however, they go beyond this, as Tembeck says: 'Witness the fact that you are powerless before *my pain*, which is also *your pain*' (2008, p.99 [my emphasis]). Photographs of 'wounds' could also be seen as an 'authentication' of suffering, a legitimisation or proof, which demands belief from its audience (Bell 2002, p.24).

The photographic works of Spence and Wilke give 'voice' to an unspeakable suffering, and it is arguably this metamorphosis into *visible symbolic form* which brings about some amelioration from suffering. Through depicting their bodies in 'deep illness' (Frank 2000), they were able to regain control over how their 'body-selves' were depicted, and therefore recover a sense of an autonomous person, or 'self'. The mirror-like qualities of the self-portrait speak of both the symbolic 'capturing' of a moment and the curtailing of time, attesting to the 'tensions and contradictions' inherent in the experiences of illness and impending death (Tembeck 2008, p.99).

Despite photographic images becoming increasingly subject to manipulation, photographs have been imbued with what Foucault refers to as the 'truth effect' (Foucault quoted in Pointon 2013, p.128), whereby the viewer is convinced that they have access, through the image, to historical facts (Pointon 2013, p.128). This may have affected how images such as those created by Spence and Wilke signify, in that they are proclaiming their personal experience as 'the truth'. It could be argued that painted portraits also invoke the 'truth effect', through the recognition of a sitter's likeness; however, as Alfred Stieglitz (1864–1964) claimed, an artist (in this case a painter of portraits) is someone who depicts 'the spirit of the truth' (Stieglitz 2000 [1922], p.229), rather than the *copy of reality* gained through photography.

The portraits discussed in this chapter, both painted and photographed, have offered glimpses into the private worlds and bodies of the artists and their sitters, demonstrating how for some people painted and photographed portraits can unlock hidden pain and feelings, and transform them into something tangible, beautiful, confrontational and meaningful, adding evidence to support the concept of portraiture as a therapeutic intervention.

― PART II ―

# COLLABORATIVE CASE-STUDIES

— Chapter 4 —

# PORTRAIT THERAPY AS A COLLABORATIVE INTERVENTION

*Paint Me This Way!*

Here I will introduce the patients whose case-studies will be drawn upon in the following three chapters. I then will outline the ethical considerations for portrait therapy and 'third hand' interventions in general, as well as the possible effects of embodied counter-transference on the therapist. In order to explain the findings from the research study, I will bring in elements from the different forms of data generated, using extracts from patients' case-studies, end of project interviews, painted portraits, collages and 'essence statements', as evidence within the discussion. In order to ensure the patients' voices are fully heard, as far as possible I have used the patients' dialogue within the discussion translated verbatim from their end of project interviews. However, to improve readability I have sometimes made minor changes, removing word repetitions, etc. I have indicated missing material by using bracketed dotted lines […], and where I have added material to explain what a patient is referring to, this is indicated within square brackets [e.g.]. Dotted lines without brackets e.g. … indicate a pause or a break mid-sentence.

## Selecting the patients for the study

The patients were recruited from the 36+ patients already attending the day-hospice where I worked as an art therapist. I recognised that this posed potential risks involving research with a 'captive' patient group (Lee and Kristjanson 2003), so measures were taken to ensure that potential patients were aware that their participation was entirely voluntary and would in no way affect their attendance at day-hospice, or the treatment they received there. Criteria for referral to the day-hospice was that it is for: men and women over the age of 18 who are living with a life-threatening and chronic illness, usually with a prognosis of less than one year. Careful purposive selection was used to help maintain boundaries around the study. A maximum number of eight participants (four male and four female), their involvement spread over two years, was decided upon with my supervisors, after consideration of the time and resources available and the minimum number of participants required to create a valid cross section of patients attending the day-hospice. Smith *et al.* (2009) suggest that between four and ten participants for doctoral phenomenological research studies is generally sufficient.

The selection of potential patients was carried out within the day-hospice multi-disciplinary team meetings (MDT) (comprising of: a state registered nurse, an occupational therapist, an art therapist [myself], a rehabilitation assistant and a chaplain, all with relevant palliative care experience). The aim was to select up to ten patients who met the criteria for inclusion in the sample (it is through this meeting that patients are referred for other therapies, including art therapy, within day-hospice). It was thought necessary that the selection process took place within the MDT, to mitigate against any biases I may have through knowing the client group in my capacity as art therapist within the day-hospice.

The criteria for *inclusion* was to recruit people who were:

- able to give informed consent (either written, verbal or through sign language)
- identified as having experienced some disruption to their self-identities
- identified as likely to benefit from involvement in the project
- not currently in the 'terminal stage' of their disease (last weeks of life)
- not currently undergoing invasive treatment
- likely to live long enough to be involved for the length of the intervention.

The criteria for *exclusion* was to exclude people who were identified as:

- without the mental capacity to give their consent
- in the 'terminal' stage of their disease (last few weeks)
- undergoing active treatment (e.g. chemotherapy, radiotherapy, surgery)
- involved in any other research project
- attending any other psychological therapy.

Over a 24-month period, eight patients, four men and four women, were offered portrait therapy; seven agreed and engaged for the duration of the intervention, and one (gentleman) declined after receiving the initial letter and information pack. These seven patients were living with a broad range of life-threatening and chronic illnesses, including three diagnosed with different types of cancer, two with chronic obstructive pulmonary disorder (COPD), one with motor neuron disease (MND) and one with brittle asthma, heart failure and arthritis. The signing of consent forms took place within the normal day-hospice setting and was facilitated by the day-hospice team lead. All patients were assured that they could withdraw from the project at any time and for any reason with no questions asked.

The patients' involvement varied, demonstrating the flexibility of the intervention. On average individual involvement was spread over six months, but sometimes with several weeks/months in between where no work could be carried out because of illness or treatment constraints. A sense of continuity did not seem to be affected by these 'breaks', with patients eager to resume as soon as possible, to discover how far their portraits had progressed during this time. On average patients attended 13 portrait sessions, lasting 1–2 hours each.

The flexible nature of this design recognised that there would be some weeks when patients might not feel well enough for sessions to take place, therefore reassuring them that a *missed* session did not mean a *lost* session, and that, within reason, they would still be able to complete the intervention no matter how many sessions they missed. This avoided the patients feeling 'guilty' about missing a session, or 'forcing' themselves to attend a session when they felt unwell. This may also have contributed to a zero drop-out rate by patients.

## Introducing the patient-researchers

The names used for the patients are those they elected to be known by and may or may not represent their 'given' first name. The following are descriptions taken from those offered by patients about their self-identities during the initial portrait sessions. The participants in this study were all white British citizens, which reflected the demographic of the hospice. This demographic does limit the findings and it would have been useful to include people from other ethnic backgrounds had that been possible. The patients (three men and four women aged between 49 and 92) were all from different social and economic backgrounds, and living with a diverse range of life-threatening and chronic illnesses, therefore offering further sample diversity. The ages given are the ages the patients were when we began working together.

## — ROSE —

Rose, a 61-year-old lady, was diagnosed with motor neuron disease (MND) (a progressive neurological disease for which there is limited treatment and no cure) over 20 years previously, and therefore has what she described as a 'slow onset' form of MND. MND has primarily affected Rose's speech, swallowing and the muscles in her face. Rose has a facial palsy and her lower lip falls open unless she holds it closed, which she tends to do when she speaks and eats. Rose is unable to smile or make any other facial expression and her speech is severely affected, with communication therefore difficult. Rose was an only child and her father died when she was 15 years old, and Rose said she did not 'get on' with her mother, who had died several years previously. Rose lives in a small flat which she rents from the borough council; she has been married and divorced twice, and has three children from her first marriage, as well as a grandson and granddaughter. Rose's family life is characterised by estrangement and loss; however, Rose sees her grandson and granddaughter frequently; they are in their early twenties. Rose had worked in various shops and factories prior to, during and after bringing up her children (for the most part) alone. Together Rose and I co-designed three portraits, and ten collages and prose poems.

## — HILARY —

Hilary, a 64-year-old lady, was diagnosed with cancer six years prior to our work together. Hilary is married with three grown-up children and several grandchildren, ranging in ages from 6 months to 11 years. Hilary is the youngest of three children, and has a strong Christian faith. Hilary describes herself as non-academic at school, saying her siblings were both 'cleverer' than her. Hilary said her mother and sister were 'gregarious' whilst she has always been the 'shy' one. Hilary has a keen interest in genealogy and ancestry, particularly of her father's family. Hilary has red hair, whilst her family and siblings are all dark haired, although one of her grandchildren has inherited her red hair. Hilary is primarily affected by her disease through suffering pain, fatigue and sickness, and can only eat a limited diet. Hilary has undergone extensive treatment for her disease including several operations, chemotherapy and radiotherapy. Together Hilary and I co-designed three portraits and ten collages and prose poems.

## — PETER (AND MARK) —

Peter is a 69-year-old gentleman, diagnosed with chronic obstructive pulmonary disease (COPD) (a progressive lung disease for which there is limited treatment and no cure). Peter is married with four grown-up sons (one of whom, called Mark, died six months prior to our working together, aged 47 at the same hospice Peter is now attending). Peter has several grandchildren between the ages of 5 and 16. Peter's parents divorced when he was 11 years old, and Peter became estranged from his father. Peter's mother remarried and a half-brother was born a few years later. Peter's family ran a florist shop and Peter remembers driving up to Covent Garden with his father to buy flowers, and making up posies of violets at a young age. Peter joined the army at the age of 16 and was transferred to Kenya, where he took up flyweight boxing. Peter was involved in a fatal accident whilst in Kenya, when the lorry he was travelling in went over a cliff. Peter's first child Mark was born in Kenya. Peter has worked in various occupations, including working in the family florist shop, and later became a fruit and veg wholesaler, and then an insurance salesman. Peter's illness has severely compromised his lifestyle as he struggles to breathe most of the time, needing to use oxygen frequently. Peter engaged with portrait therapy wholeheartedly despite his recent bereavement and together Peter (and by default Mark) and I co-designed six portraits (including two of Mark, two of Peter and Mark, and two of Peter), and 12 collages and prose poems.

## — BILL —

Bill is a 91-year-old gentleman and was diagnosed with cancer a few years prior to our working together. Bill was born in London and had two sisters, now deceased. Bill's father ran a butcher's shop, where Bill worked on leaving school. Bill's mother died suddenly of a heart attack when Bill was still a young man and his father never remarried. Despite working in a profession where he was exempt from being 'called up', Bill joined the army during WWII, volunteering for the army flying corps. Bill trained as a glider pilot and gained the rank of staff sergeant. Bill was involved in flying missions during D-Day, Pegasus Bridge and Arnhem. Bill met his wife whilst he was undergoing flying training; however, they were not married until two years after the war ended, as Bill was sent to a sanatorium to recover from his (untreated) wounds. After they were married Bill joined his father-in-law's painting and decorating business, and his two children, a girl and a boy, were born. Bill now lives alone and has to rely on his family and carers to support him with his basic needs as his mobility has been severely affected by his illness, and he is no longer able to walk. Bill engaged in portrait therapy enthusiastically, and together we co-designed four portraits and 16 collages and prose poems, as well as appearing on ITVs *Tonight* programme together (05/07/2012) talking about the portraits.

## — SUSAN —

Susan is a 62-year-old lady who was diagnosed with cancer several years prior to our working together, and although her disease is 'inoperable' has undergone radio and chemotherapy treatments. Susan described her childhood and teenage years as 'miserable', saying her father had an unpredictable temper, and she described him as 'a brute' who she lived in fear of. Susan has one half-brother from her father's previous marriage – although she was essentially an only child as her half-brother did not live with the family and she seldom saw him. As a teenager Susan experienced feelings of acute depression, anxiety and suicidal ideation, and used self-harming as a way to cope with and contain her difficult feelings. Susan kept all this to herself, feeling unable to talk to anyone about it. On leaving school Susan worked for an accountancy firm. Susan married young, and had two children; however, the marriage ended in divorce and a few years later her ex-husband died. Susan met and married her present husband several years later. After Susan's children left home she returned to studying and gained her BA, MA and PhD degrees, beginning an academic career at a university, and gaining recognition for her academic writing in the field of children's literature. Before Susan's diagnosis she was physically fit, and enjoyed travelling, walking and playing golf. Unfortunately, these pursuits are no longer possible, as Susan's disease and treatment have severely affected her mobility meaning she is only able to walk short distances with crutches, and mainly uses a wheelchair or motorised scooter. Susan engaged creatively with portrait therapy and was an insightful and enthusiastic co-researcher. Susan and I co-designed four portraits, five portrait-sculptures and ten collages and prose poems. Susan also wrote one of the poems 'The Rainbow Snake' in its entirety (see page 197).

## — NORMA —

Norma is a 59-year-old lady who has suffered ill health throughout her life, and has been diagnosed with brittle asthma, heart failure and arthritis. Norma has also suffered from several strokes recently that left her with a weakness down her left side. Norma said she was born in Aberdeen and was abandoned by her mother when she was three days old. Norma lived in an orphanage run by nuns until she was three years old, when she was then placed with various foster families. A year or so later she was adopted; however, there were already two male siblings in the family who she said did not accept her as their sister. Norma said that when she was first adopted she was very withdrawn and frightened and would not do anything without being told to. Norma underwent heart surgery when she was seven years old and was absent from school for about a year. Norma left school when she was 14 and worked in a 'fish factory' in Aberdeen. Norma met and married her husband when she was 18 years old and suffered many miscarriages and stillbirths, losing seven babies over the years including a two-year-old son who died of cancer. Norma has two surviving sons and several grandchildren. Recently Norma has embraced the North American Indian spirituality and has been adopted into a Native American Indian tribe, where she is known as 'North Bear'. Norma engaged enthusiastically with portrait therapy and together we co-designed four portraits, nine collages and prose poems and co-created one portrait-sculpture.

## —— PAUL ——

Paul, a 49-year-old single gentleman, was diagnosed with chronic obstructive pulmonary disease (COPD) (a progressive lung disease for which there is limited treatment and no cure), three years prior to our working together. Paul's COPD has developed to the stage where he is dependent upon oxygen during the day and a Bi-pap machine (which breathes for him) during the night. The slightest exertion leaves Paul fighting for breath and extremely fatigued. Being unable to work or care for himself, Paul has been forced to give up his independence, returning to live with his mother. Paul's early family life was characterised by estrangement and isolation, stemming from his parent's divorce when he was a young child. For Paul, this resulted in suppressing his negative feelings, isolating himself from others, poor self-care and self-image, as well as depression and anxiety attacks. Paul was anxious about leaving the house alone, and consequently he had not been out alone for many months, only leaving his room to attend day-hospice and hospital appointments. Paul described a disruption to his sense of autonomy and of being 'unable to be' the *Paul* he used to be, talking about feeling 'low, helpless, hopeless, trapped and frustrated'. I was surprised by Paul's enthusiastic engagement with portrait therapy, as he had previously refused all offers of psychological or emotional support, including art therapy. This suggests that the 'third hand' aspect of the project attracted Paul, for whom just breathing was an effort. Together Paul and I co-designed four portraits, ten collages and prose poems and one portrait-sculpture.

## **Collaboration as a therapeutic tool**

The collaborative nature and third hand aspect of portrait therapy was something that developed directly out of the initial focus groups that

I held with patients attending day-hospice (as discussed in Chapter 1). This focus group ensured that portrait therapy as an intervention was something developed *with* patients, *for* patients, and I believe that this collaboration was the key to its success.

There is certainly great potential for user collaboration within the many different theoretical bases of art therapy, and this facilitates embracing the subjective and collective insider/outsider experience as an important part of knowledge generation (Gilroy 2006, p.110). The research behind portrait therapy brought into focus the necessity for a collaborative therapeutic and research process as evidenced by recent experience-based co-design (EBCD) practices (Springham and Woods 2014). In counselling psychology research, Rennie (1994) suggests that researcher-participation should be promoted in all areas of a project, and that this collaboration is potentially therapeutic and can lead to greater insight (see e.g. Carr and Hancock 2017). Hart and Crawford-Wright (1999, p.211) warn, however, that true collaboration in research can only occur where both researcher and participant will benefit in the publication of findings. This is difficult to achieve; however, the thought that their publication will help others is very often enough, and to see their words in print is confirmation that they have been *seen* and *heard* and taken seriously.

When asked how she found the collaborative design process, (patient) Susan said:

> That was probably the most important part of it. [...] I think it is good, because [...] you have ideas triggered by things I said. I like the way it develops, it's more kind of organic development [...], because everything else to do with the illness is rigid, 'you take this medicine' or 'you have this treatment'. It's very prescriptive, whereas something grows out of this in a much better way. I feel really comfortable about saying what I like or what I feel could be different. (Quoted from Susan's end of project interview 18/10/2012)

The co-designing of the portraits offers an intersubjective and collaborative way of working, and directing the art therapist helps patients retain their own 'expert' status and goes some way towards equalising the power structures in art therapy. Together the patients and I created a 'third space' within the portraits, one in which *relational meaning* was developed, something necessary for self-identity construction and revisioning.

## Ethical considerations for portrait therapy

On 7 October 2010, ethical approval was granted by the National Research and Ethics Service (NRES) to begin researching portrait therapy, and I began working with the first patient, Rose, on 2 November 2010. Gaining ethical approval from NRES involved writing a detailed protocol for portrait therapy, which was a lengthy and complex process; however, it enabled the development of an ethically based intervention, which identified, and therefore avoided, potential problems during research.

When developing portrait therapy, potential participants were engaged in all aspects of the research design, process and analysis; I was therefore able to incorporate hospice patients' insights into the design of the intervention, ethical issues and creative methods used. Strohm (2012, p.100) suggests that involving potential participants in the early stages of research planning is 'ethically conscious' research. I also used the British Association of Art Therapists (BAAT) ethical procedures as a guide, and to gain further insight into the ethical issues from an art therapy perspective, in 2009 I met with members of the art therapy palliative care special interest group called 'The Creative Response', to discuss the potential ethical issues of portrait therapy. The main ethical issues raised by my colleagues were: confidentiality, avoiding exploitation, dual-role conflict, and burden on patients near end of life (Clark 2010, 2012; Hart and Crawford-Wright 1999, p.213; Martin *et al.* 2007; Sinding *et al.* 2008; Springham 2008). These were therefore central considerations in the design of portrait therapy and inform the ethical considerations outlined below. This only reflects the use of portrait therapy as an intervention for patients within a palliative care setting; ethical considerations for the use of portrait therapy with other client groups would need to be evaluated on a case-by-case basis.

### *Confidentiality*

Guaranteeing confidentiality and anonymity is usually a prerequisite in art therapy (see point 10 in the *British Association of Art Therapists (BAAT) Code of Ethics and Principles of Practice*, available on the BAAT website); however, complete confidentiality was not possible in this project due to the identity-revealing nature of portraiture. All patients were therefore fully informed about the *limits to confidentiality* in this project and also my *duty of care* requirement to share information with relevant services should I believe that they, or a person they mention, are at risk of harm. The gaining of patients' informed consent, through their signing of an informed consent form, was of paramount importance (ibid., see point 10.2). None of the patients expressed concern that their portraits would be seen by others; on the contrary this was seen as an important part of the portraits' therapeutic value. I believe that despite the ethical considerations vulnerable groups such as those living with life-threatening and chronic illnesses should be invited to join research projects that offer a platform for their insights on the impact of illness on self-identity, as well as the opportunity for reciprocity (Spaniol 2005). Confidentiality issues for the use of portrait therapy with other client groups are not considered here and would need to be evaluated on a case-by-case basis.

## *Exploitation*

By involving the patients and their views in the development and research of portrait therapy, including the analysis of findings, I am reflecting a change from research carried out 'on' to research carried out 'with' participants, acknowledging their presence as valued co-researchers in this process (Springham and Woods 2014). This levelling of the traditional hierarchy of therapist/patient means that empathic understanding was increased (Vick 2000, p.217) and instead of a focus on being 'helped', clients felt empowered through taking on the role of *expert* (Moon 2002, p.290). However, it is important to be aware that patients may not want the things they said within the collaborative intersubjective context made public in another context (Pink 2001, p.43). It was important therefore for patients to be involved where possible, in a review of the case-studies and analysis themes, which ensured that they were able to revise statements made and recorded in different contexts, as well as suggest amendments to portraits, collages and prose poems. I included a question in the end of project interview asking the patients if they felt in any way exploited by their involvement in researching portrait therapy and all answered 'No', some suggesting that it was actually *the reverse* of exploitative.

Ultimately it is important to defend the right of palliative care patients to make their own decisions around being involved in research and to recognise our own obligation as therapists to carry out research that enables the voices of people with terminal illness to be heard (Reeve *et al.* 2010, p.183).

## *Dual-role conflict or 'insider' research*

The concerns expressed by my art therapy colleagues about the 'dual-role' (Martin *et al.* 2007; Finley and Knowles 1995) nature of my position as art therapist/researcher were important to consider, and the dual-role identified actually turned out to be a triadic one, with my researcher, art therapist and portrait artist identities all coming to the fore at different times. An awareness of these three aspects of my self-identity meant I was prepared for potential tensions and conflicts. A key aspect of the reflexive (Etherington 2004a) nature of portrait therapy therefore included the management of these three identities within the collaborative relationship. All three identities were however focused on the centrality of *an ethic of care* towards the patients and the establishment of a *collaborative intersubjective relationship* based upon *unconditional positive regard* (Petruska 2003, p.xxxiii; Rogers 1951, 1957) and the commitment to *do no harm* (Hippocrates). In attempting to reconcile ethical considerations with research aims, it was important to draw on my art therapy training (2002–2005) and experience of working in palliative care (2005–2017), and this is a positive aspect of doing 'insider' research (Mercer 2007).

## *Burden on patients*

Consideration was given to concerns regarding patients being upset by focusing on personal losses (Barnett 2001), and of research involvement taking up precious time at the end of life when people are easily fatigued (Addington-Hall 2002; Barnett 2001). However, instead of finding portrait therapy a burden time-wise, patients often wanted *more* time, expressing feelings of regret that a session and/or the project was ending. The positive effects of research involvement may also have given patients a sense of 'purpose' (Barnett 2001) and feelings of 'ownership' over the study, enabling reciprocity and reclamation of their 'caring' identity (Maiter *et al.* 2008; Wahrendorf *et al.* 2010). An inherent anxiety exists about raising painful issues with patients in palliative care, that they may not have the time or energy to resolve (Skaife 1993); however, through using the creative elicitation techniques patients self-selected the topics they wished to discuss. I was also careful not to 'pry' or 'question' where I sensed patients did not want conversations to go, and a collaborative approach to visual research can help to avoid harm to participants by allowing them to maintain control over the content of images, thereby reducing anxiety (Pink 2001, p.42).

All the patients expressed some anxiety and emotional affect at different times during the process; however, drawing from my experience of working in palliative care, I would say this was 'normal', as in this client group emotions are generally held very close to the surface, and patients often need to express these emotions with someone other than their family (McPherson *et al.* 2007). Flexibility built into the design of portrait therapy was important to accommodate the patients' need to take breaks from the therapy due to the contingencies of illness. Portrait therapy therefore offers further evidence for the importance of using a collaborative approach to art therapy research: design, application and evaluation. It is also a *non-pathologising, non-stigmatising* approach, liberating the patient from a focus on illness to a focus on their subjective experience of self-identity.

## *Body-centred counter-transference and vicarious traumatisation*

I have found that working with those who are dying does have a holistic impact physically, psychologically and emotionally on the art therapist, and portrait therapy is no exception. Whilst working collaboratively with patients I felt an increase in body-centred counter-transference (also called embodied vicarious-traumatisation) (McCann and Pearlman 1990; Pearlman and Saakvitne 1995). This can be described as physical manifestations (such as pain and discomfort), before, during or after working with a patient (Booth *et al.* 2010, p.285), combined sometimes with an experience of loss of meaning and hope (ibid., p.284). Over the 12 years working in palliative care I have come to realise, and treat with respect, the amount of pain, distress and suffering I am asked to witness in my role as art therapist. Therefore, I was not surprised that whilst practising portrait therapy I have felt increased tension in my neck, shoulders, throat and chest, as well as breathlessness, particularly during and after sessions with COPD sufferers such as Paul. This can be described as 'listening with the body' (Field 1989), and is part of my empathic reaction to, or unconscious mirroring of, patients. However, whilst painting the portraits I noticed a marked relief from these symptoms and I believe that creating images *for* the patient, enabled my body and mind to calm itself, to self-soothe (Fish 1989). I also feel that painting the portraits mitigated feelings of 'helplessness' and 'hopelessness' resulting from being unable to 'rescue' (Falk 2005, p.181).

— Chapter 5 —

# INCREASING THE PATIENTS' CREATIVE CAPACITY TO ADAPT TO ILLNESS

Improving a patient's creative capacity to adapt to illness is a key way that portrait therapy works and it is often through this that an improvement to their overall quality of life can be achieved. My understanding of *creative capacity* is that it enables people to develop 'adaptive behaviour through imaginative potential' (Higgs 2008, p.551), and that this can be used to adapt to illness. Adapting implies that 'the individual acknowledges impairment and alters life and self in socially and personally acceptable ways' (Charmaz 1995, p.657).

Within this chapter I will describe how portraiture increases feelings of control and autonomy, and enables the rediscovery of adaptive strategies used in pre-illness lives, resulting in increased self-care and agency.

## Adaption through transforming meanings and changing perspectives: Re-imagining self-identity

> Art offers a way for us to enter into this paradox, where imagination forms reality and fiction reveals truth. (Moon 2002, p.243)

Art therapist David Maclagan (2001, 2005, 2011) argues that 'art therapy is not just a therapy *with* imagination, but a therapy *of* imagination' and that imagination, within both ourselves as artists and the people we work with, needs to be 'restored and renewed' before therapeutic work can commence (2005, p.23 [my emphasis]). Maclagan sees imagination as fundamental to all aspects of our life:

'it colours our perceptions, it recreates our memories, it contributes to shaping and solving problems' as well as being 'the creative wellspring of art-works' and 'a principle means of responding to them' (ibid.). Eisner (2008, p.11) suggests that what we need is to unfetter our imaginations, to find new ways to see and understand the world, creating 'vivid realities that would otherwise go unknown', a way of utilising the creative imagination to expand worlds shrunk by illness. The neuroscience behind imagination has shown that when we imagine something, the activity shown in our brain resembles that associated with the real experience (Buckner and Carroll 2006), which suggests that our imagination has a very real impact upon how we feel, meaning that 'imagined phenomenon are not just *a figment of our imagination* they are part of our *embodied experience*' (Carr 2014, p.10).

In the end of project interviews several patients talked about how their involvement had enabled a change in perspectives and meanings, causing them to look at things *differently*:

SC:   Well…I have really enjoyed it…

R:    So have I, because…it's so…it makes you look at things quite differently.[1]

It is therefore this transformation of meaning or experience of *change*, in the way patients 'look at' and experience things, which I will identify here. Transformation of meaning may include changing patients' preoccupation from a dominant (often negative) story of self-identity, to a more positive story, which enables them to think of themselves *differently* and therefore *act* differently or *creatively* (Burt 2012, p.25). This is highlighted within Hilary's portraits (Figure 5.1 and Figure 5.2):

---

1   SC = Susan (Artist-Therapist-Researcher). R = 'Rose' (Patient-Researcher). End of project interview 22/03/2011.

# INCREASING THE PATIENTS' CREATIVE CAPACITY TO ADAPT TO ILLNESS

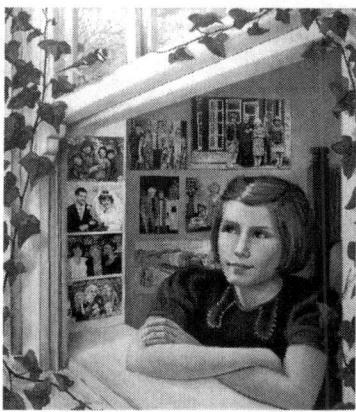

Figure 5.1 *The Window* by Susan Carr (co-designed by Hilary), 2011.

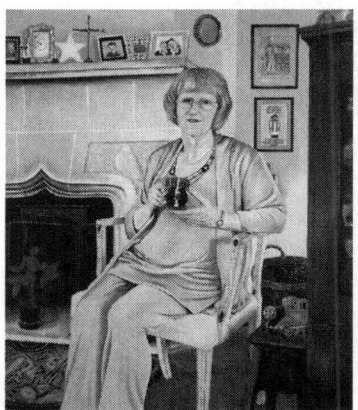

Figure 5.2 *The Heart of the Home* by Susan Carr (co-designed by Hilary), 2011.

Initially it seemed that these portraits were fairly straightforward depictions of past and present selves; however, within the analysis process unexpected themes emerged. In the *Statement of Emergent Knowing* created for *The Heart of the Home* portrait, it becomes clear that Hilary has used symbolism heavily within her portrait:

### Statement of Emergent Knowing: *The Heart of the Home*

Hilary smiles a welcome into the heart of her home, a place where children have played and grandchildren still play. A place where adults drink tea and talk and read, a fireguard protects, and a mantelpiece supports...precious memories. Hilary is relaxed and happy here, at ease in the place she loves – the stage for her most devoted roles of wife, mother and grandmother. Surrounded by so many reminders of others Hilary risks losing herself; however, she is held firmly in the chair which once held her father.

### Statement of Emergent Learning: *The Heart of the Home*

Through surrounding herself with so many possessions, Hilary risks losing herself. Hilary labels things so that her family will know what they are, where they have come from, and why they must not be thrown away. Perhaps this is a way of working out...' Where is Hilary in all of this?'

### Statement of Reflexive Resonance: *The Heart of the Home*

I have come to learn that amassing more and more 'things' makes us invisible...it is perhaps a way of hiding ourselves? Hilary was trying to put labels on things to itemise them, so that her family would know the significance of them, or perhaps it was a way of working out what was Hilary and what wasn't?

Therefore, when painting these portraits, and visiting Hilary, I became aware of a recurring question in my mind, which said...'where is Hilary in all of this?' The loss of self-identity for Hilary seemed to be profound, and was tied up with the loss of her matriarchal 'doing' and 'being' roles, which are a focus of her *The Heart of the Home* portrait (Figure 5.2).

The following collage (Figure 5.3) encapsulates the issues Hilary faced, losing her beloved self-identity as a 'proper grandma'.

This collage led to a discussion to identify what Hilary thought a 'proper' grandmother was, and whether her fixed ideas around what a 'proper' grandmother *does* could be extended creatively, to include, for example, sitting on the sofa and reading to her grandchild or playing a game together at a table. We also looked back at whether Hilary's own grandmothers had got down on the floor and played with her (which she said they hadn't, despite them still being 'proper' grandmothers in her eyes).

# INCREASING THE PATIENTS' CREATIVE CAPACITY TO ADAPT TO ILLNESS

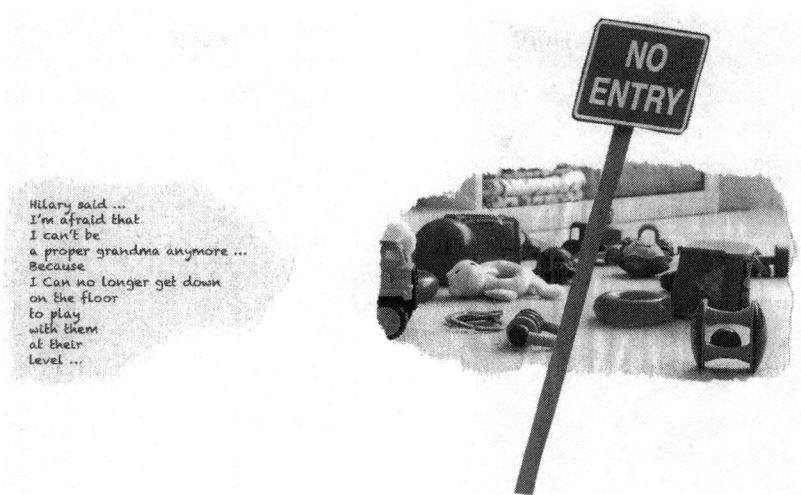

Figure 5.3 *A Proper Grandma* by Susan Carr, 2010.

When Hilary and I first began working together Hilary stated that she had 'no imagination', and a possible clue to Hilary's lack of confidence in her imaginative potential is highlighted within the *Statement of Emergent Knowing* for her *Heart of the Home* portrait, which says... 'Surrounded by so many reminders of others Hilary risks losing herself; however, she is held firmly in the chair which once held her father'. Hilary's choice to be painted in her father's chair indicates her feelings of solidarity with him and mourning his loss; however, her father had a prodigious imaginative talent, and as such may have overshadowed Hilary's belief in her own imaginative abilities.

As is often the case with the patients living with life-threatening and chronic illnesses, a sense of containment was often elusive for Hilary and the theme of needing to be 'held' came to the fore often. I reflected upon this in Hilary's active documentation sketchbook (ADS):

### Notes from Hilary's active documentation sketchbook 02/12/2010

I have been thinking today about Hilary and her need to be 'held'. In her *Heart of the Home* portrait Hilary chose to be painted seated in the chair which once belonged to, and therefore 'held' her father, who was a highly imaginative person (now deceased).

> I was wondering about this from the point of view of Hilary's own professed 'lack of imagination', and wonder if she had been 'held back' unconsciously by his success, and also by her religious upbringing, which may encourage 'black and white thinking' through the 'certainty' within its doctrine. Consequently the 'liminal' world of illness is not one Hilary has the tools to navigate and therefore she feels lost and alone. This means Hilary is perhaps looking for something *outside of herself* for support, or to 'be held', when imagination means *looking within herself*?

This 'holding back' and avoidance of existential questions is outlined in Hilary's end of project interview where she says 'not to dwell too much on *I wonder why?*'

## Listening for Contrapuntal Identity Voices

> 1. <u>Listening for Adaptive Matriarchal Hilary.</u>
>
> 2. *Listening for Religious, I believe in Angels Hilary.*
>
> 3. Listening for Souls and Shadows (Shy, could do better Hilary).
>
> 4. Listening for Ancestral Hilary (Where is Hilary in all of this?).
>
> H: Yes, yes… When you first explained it to me I didn't know how that [the portrait] would turn out… <u>but it's very telling really, very accurate.</u>
>
> SC: So, do you think that this kind of project helps to reinforce a sense of identity?
>
> H: <u>Yes. I think this probably helped in… I mean people say I am brave and strong</u>, I'm not really <u>but if that is how they see me,…I would say this has helped me in building that image</u>, having to think back and reflect. *Not to dwell too much on 'I wonder why'* <u>but to just carry on. If the hospitals can keep saving me then…</u> [laughs].[2]

---

2   SC = Susan (Artist-Therapist-Researcher). H = Hilary (Patient-Researcher). End of project interview 20/02/2012.

Within this section of Hilary's end of project interview, her 'adaptive matriarchal' voice of self-identity comes through strongly, over and above the other three, perhaps less adaptive self-identities. As the portrait therapy sessions continued I believe that Hilary's imaginative potential and therefore creative capacity developed. My thoughts around this are noted in the ADS:

### Notes from Hilary's active documentation sketchbook 18/02/2011

I was surprised today because when I went to see Hilary she had come up with a very imaginative idea for her third portrait. (I was surprised because Hilary professed to have 'no imagination' when we began working together.) 'Paint me being held by an Angel!' she said, 'I would like the angel to be in a garden, surrounded by animals and spring flowers. I have a picture by my bed that I've had since I was a young child, of Jesus surrounded by animals.' I told Hilary I would do some sketches and bring them in for her, together with a book by Edward Burne-Jones to show her next week, as Hilary said she liked more 'traditional' kinds of painting.

These are all revealed in the portrait *Held by an Angel* (Figure 5.4).

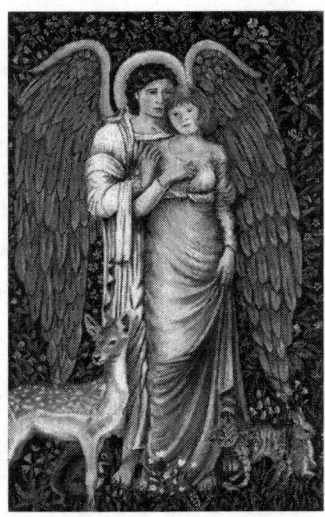

Figure 5.4 *Held by an Angel* by Susan Carr (co-designed by Hilary), 2011 (see also Coloured Plate i).

It seemed that Hilary's imaginative potential was inhibited at the beginning of the project, which may have affected her ability to adapt to illness, as in her fixed views regarding 'a proper grandma'. McNiff (2004, p.5) believes that the central premise of healing within art involves the 'cultivation and release of the creative imagination' and that once liberated the creative process will always find its way to what requires 'attention and transformation'.

Within this section I have shown how involvement in this project enabled Hilary to awaken her creative and imaginative potential, finding relief and comfort in a portrait of herself finally and eternally 'held'.

## Humour: An adaptive and imaginative way of being-in-the-world

One of the things that struck me particularly when I began working in palliative care was the use of humour by patients and staff as a way to 'lighten the atmosphere' in difficult situations, and how reciprocal laughter was a way to show both appreciation and gratitude, to each other (Weisfeld 1993). Humour has therefore been an important component of this project and is something that I see as intrinsically *adaptive* (Hellema 2011).

A 'ludic' defence mechanism (Turner 1982, p.27), such as humour or black humour, can help practitioners face and manage liminality; indeed in traumatic work humour can be liminal itself (Sibbett 2005c, p.240). The use of humour in palliative care has been acknowledged in its ability to 'build therapeutic relationships, relieve tension, and to protect dignity and a sense of worth'; it has also been found to be helpful in 'managing stressful situations and maintaining a sense of perspective' (Dean, Kinsman and Gregory 2004). Using humour is an *imaginative way of being* (Hellema 2011), in which a sense of intimacy is created, through the tacit intersubjective knowing required to understand personalised humour.

Humour is also a way of testing the intersubjective connection and asking 'Do you get it? Do you get me?' and also 'Do you *know* me?' By making humorous remarks about difficult subjects, a sense of emotional distance can also be created (Hellema 2011, p.163). However, humour is a 'complex, challenging, context-dependent' skill and one must be mindful of the danger of misinterpretation especially when communicating with 'disempowered patients who may be struggling to cope with illness' (McCreaddie and Wiggins 2007). This is contested by Dean, Kinsman and Gregory (2004) who say their findings support the view that humour and laughter are significant 'humanising dimensions' when caring for the terminally ill. I believe that humour must initially be patient-led, and when expressed needs to be appreciated and reflected sensitively by the therapist, until they know the patient sufficiently to understand the boundaries of their humour.

There were significant moments of humour within most portrait therapy sessions, with the male patients using humour most frequently. Bill (aged 91) would often joke about me being 'his girl' and was very clever at introducing a 'play on words'; this is highlighted by the exchange at the beginning of Bill's end of project interview:

SC: First question is…how have you found the experience of being painted and having paintings made of you?

B: Very proud I think, very proud and I've been made a celebrity in this local place! [laughs]

SC: Yes. [laughs]

B: I've enjoyed it, and a lovely girl paints me! So I mustn't grumble about that. *And I've never given her the brush off!* [laughs]

SC: No! [laughs] I've got to put this in my PhD! [both laugh] So have you enjoyed it then?

B: Yes, I have! [laughs][3]

This sharing of humour demonstrates the closeness of the intersubjective relationship built up between Bill and myself during the project and the deep connections that were made.

Similarly, Paul would make jokes during his portrait sessions, and humour seemed to be something that he *trusted*. I related the following in Paul's active documentation sketchbook after a session with Paul where we were looking for portrait design ideas within the portrait reference album:

---

3   SC = Susan (Artist-Therapist-Researcher). B = Bill (Patient-Researcher). End of project interview 24/04/2012.

## Notes from Paul's active documentation sketchbook 15/10/2012

When we looked through the portrait reference album Paul discovered the Frida Kahlo self-portrait 'Broken Column', exclaiming...'That's a bit naughty!' He later returned to it and said he liked it, because it showed Frida's 'pain' and he could identify with it. I wondered about the sense of 'naughtiness' within the painting, was it the fact that she was showing her breasts, or the fact that she was showing her 'insides'? I was surprised that Paul was 'taken' with it, but he said he thought we could design a portrait of him around the image. I think Paul meant the 'naughtiness' in a sort of 'ouch' way? I also wondered if he was ever able to be 'a bit naughty' in any real sense since his illness? Also, whether he wanted to 'shock' people with the portrait, and if this was because his illness was invisible to others, perhaps they did not recognise or acknowledge his inner pain?

This therefore resulted in the following *Statement of Intention*:

## Statement of Intention: *Broken Lungs*

Paul said 'Paint me like Frida Kahlo in *Broken Column*, cut down the middle, and instead of showing a broken vertebra you can show my broken lungs'.

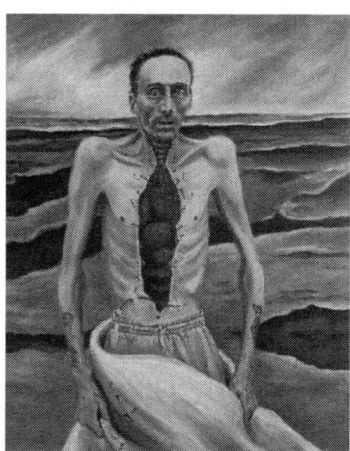

Figure 5.5 *Broken Lungs* by Susan Carr (co-designed by Paul), 2013 (see also Coloured Plate ii).

*Broken Column* (1944) by Mexican Surrealist artist Frida Kahlo is an iconic self-portrait of physical suffering and stoicism, an image Paul claimed never to have seen before. The portrait explores what it is to be 'embodied' (Latimer 2009, p.50) and reveals the pain and suffering Kahlo endured following her injuries in a serious bus accident aged 17 years. In *Broken Column* Kahlo depicts herself semi-naked in a barren landscape, her chest ripped open, a broken Ionic pillar replacing her vertebrae. Kahlo said her paintings reflect her lived experience or 'personal reality' and within *Broken Column* she portrays a divided, fragmented and leaky body-self, existing in the borderlands between object and subject (Latimer 2009, p.46). In Kahlo, Paul recognised a fellow inhabitant of the 'world of illness' (Radley 2009), or 'liminality' (Sibbett 2005a; Turner 1969) saying he chose Kahlo's painting because 'you can see that she's in pain…you know what she's going through'. Paul suggested that I paint him into the same barren landscape and instead of the cut-open chest revealing a 'broken column' Paul's portrait could show his 'broken lungs'.

The following week I arranged to visit Paul to take reference photographs for this portrait; I recorded the following exchange in the ADS:

### Notes from Paul's active documentation sketchbook 22/10/2012

I went to take reference photographs and make sketches of Paul today for the *Broken Lungs* portrait and when I arrived Paul said, 'Oh here she is, come to paint me naked!' and laughed. I laughed too, but was a little embarrassed by this and I think Paul enjoyed my discomfort. I replied laughing and saying… 'don't say that! Your Mother (who was in the kitchen getting us a cup of tea) will get the wrong impression!' We both laughed again and I wondered actually if this was what Paul wanted. I then said seriously, 'It is only naked from the waist up…and you really don't have to if you don't want to!' Paul was clearly making a joke out of it, perhaps to see if I would 'get' his humour, or even to see if I 'get' him. When Paul undressed, I was shocked by the level of his emaciation, and took the photographs quickly so that he could replace his shirt. It was an intimate moment, and I felt protective 'mother' instincts on seeing him semi-naked, wanting to 'feed him up'. I also felt that Paul had trusted me, by showing me the effect of illness on his body.

Reflecting on this I believe my discomfort was largely due to the recognition that it is generally only the medical profession or our life partners who have the privileged view of our naked or semi-bodies, and to Paul I was neither. I was also very aware of a discrepancy in power as I stood there with my camera preparing to photograph his emaciated body. However, I reminded myself that this was Paul's idea and his design, and as such I needed to trust he was co-designing the portrait *he needed to see*, and also, that which he *needed others to see*. As Sibbett says:

> ...art therapy rituals and symbols have particular value in metaphorising the body, thus enabling expression of emotions and bodily states including conscious and unconscious aspects otherwise deemed unspeakable, unhearable, unseeable and unthinkable. (Sibbett 2005a, pp.71–2)

In this section I have identified humour as an adaptive process, facilitated and developed within this project, which enabled patients to manage their experience of 'liminal' or 'unhomelike-being-in-the-world'. Containing elements of ritual, humour tests the intersubjective connection between patient and therapist, asking the important question 'do you *get it?*' or 'do you *get me?*' – highlighting humour as an important function of *being known*. Humour was also used to manage stressful situations and maintain a sense of perspective.

## Adaptive dualities: Creating emotional distance and connection

Art therapy works on the premise that through making the artwork clients are able to externalise a problem into an art form, and by effectively controlling that art form, the relationship of the client to the problem can be changed. However, results from this study indicate that the 'third hand' art therapy approach works well as an emotional distancing/connection technique, despite the artwork being created *at once removed*. Through the revisioning process and the manifestation of aspects of self-identity within *externalised objects*, hidden pain and suffering is brought into being in the present, so that they can be *held, contained, moved, worked on* and *reflected upon*. Susan talks of the importance of this in her end of project interview:

SC: I don't know what you think...but in a way, it's power of fear promotion, the way that it affects you, is different in an object.

S: Yes, I think when it's been put into a portrait or sculpture, fear doesn't have such a hold over you. I think also that you reflect on the effect on you, but when you see something like the *Pin Hole Camera* sculpture, you can see how you were vulnerable, that it was actually somebody else's issue and it affected you when you couldn't understand that. You know, you think about how you felt but it takes it outside and puts the issue with somebody else. It's something that I shouldn't have had to feel, but did, so yes, it contains it and puts it away, but understands it. It doesn't put it away by belittling the fear, it takes on board the fear in all its manifestations, I suppose, and contains it elsewhere.[4]

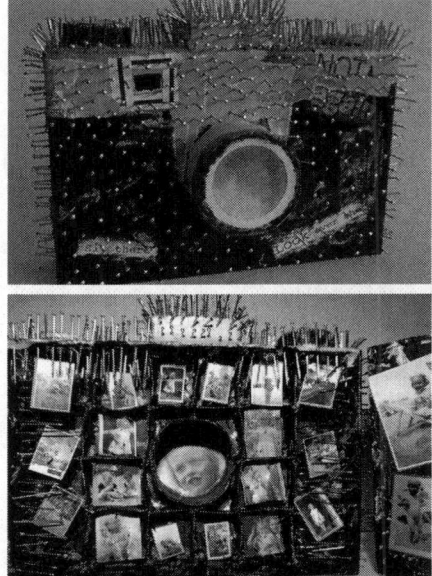

Figure 5.6 *Pin Hole Camera* by Susan Carr (co-designed by Susan), 2012.

This portrait-sculpture will be discussed further in the following sections.

---

4   SC = Susan (Artist-Therapist-Researcher). S = Susan (Patient-Researcher). End of project interview 18/10/2012.

Susan goes on to talk about the difference between emotional distance techniques in portrait therapy and those in 'talking' therapy. The attuning process highlights this difference, where I reflected back stories of self-identities through creating the artwork *for* patients:

> S: By creating the portraits *for* me you are *lending me your vision on my life*. There's a difference between you asking me specific things that relate to the portraits…it was easier for me to say what I felt than if you had simply said 'did you have a difficult childhood?' It was the catalyst that allowed me to let some of these things out. It's you taking things hidden inside my head and making them visible to me…and then I can see it made into something that expresses what I wanted to say in a way that *perhaps even I didn't realise*. This seems to be a much more effective way of dealing with hidden pain and giving someone who tends towards depression, the opportunity to recognise all the good parts of their lives that can be overshadowed.
>
> It's helped me to clarify how I felt and the connections that have arisen because of my illness, and *it's helped me to understand myself better, understand the way that I've responded to the illness.*[5]

Susan highlights the importance of *Pin Hole Camera* as a 'catalyst' to connect to and to 'let some of these things out', but also its ability to 'hold' difficult issues, saying 'it contains it and puts it away'. Susan also highlights the importance of my mirroring and attunement within the portraits, saying 'and then I can see it made into something that expresses what I wanted to say in a way that perhaps even I didn't realise'. Mirroring and attunement within the portraits will be discussed further in Chapter 6.

Within this section I have described Susan's experience of the portrait-sculpture as an externalised object, containing significant aspects of her self-identity, 'holding' and containing aspects of hidden pain and suffering, enabling both connection and emotional distancing to take place, and new meanings to be developed.

---

5   SC = Susan (Artist-Therapist-Researcher). S = Susan (Patient-Researcher). End of project interview 18/10/2012.

## Adaption through mourning losses: Learning to live with *being-towards-death*

Volkan (1997, p.36) argues that human beings are unable to accept change without mourning what has been lost and portraits have historically been linked to mourning (Hilliker 2006), with some of the earliest painted portraits of people being *funeral* portraits from the 1st century BC, discovered in Egypt's Fayum district. In Judith Butler's (2004b) book about the 9/11 attacks on the World Trade Center in New York, she examines the nature of mourning. We need to mourn, Butler suggests, as a way to acknowledge our 'ontological indebtedness' to each other:

> It is not as if an 'I' exists independently over here and then simply loses a 'you' over there, especially if the attachment to 'you' is part of what composes who 'I' am. If I lose you, under these conditions, then I not only mourn the loss, but I become inscrutable to myself. Who am 'I' without you? (Butler 2004b, p.22)

I suggest that Butler's quote also explains the relationship that patients have to lost aspects of their self-identity, meaning the question 'who am I without you?' becomes intensely *intra*subjective, and without mourning these losses patients become 'inscrutable' to themselves (ibid.). This offers an explanation as to why patients living with life-threatening and chronic illnesses often say, 'I don't know who I am any more.' However, I was surprised by the way patients used portrait therapy intuitively to mourn losses to their self-identity caused by the death of loved ones. This is exemplified in the work Peter and I designed together. Peter's son Mark had died at the same hospice he was now attending, six months prior to our working together, and it quickly became clear that if I was going to work with Peter, I would also have to work with his son Mark, or at least Peter's lost father-of-Mark identity. Klass, Silverman and Nickman (1996), in their theory of 'continuing bonds', recognise that for some people it is imperative to retain some sort of an ongoing relationship with a lost loved one after they have died.

The following account from Peter's active documentation sketchbook explains how we began working together:

### Notes from Peter's active documentation sketchbook 14/02/2011

I spent time talking with Peter today about the portrait therapy project and his focus was (quite naturally) on the loss of his son Mark. I am wondering about the combined impact that the loss of his 'father-of-Mark identity' and his illness has had upon him? Everything seems to be coloured by this loss and it seems impossible for me to work with Peter without working at-one-removed with Mark too, the two are so intricately entwined. Perhaps facing his son's death will help Peter face his own? Perhaps this is the main work that Peter needs to do through the portraits?

Focusing on the loss of Peter's *father of Mark* self-identity we co-designed portraits of Mark and Peter, including two portraits of the two of them together (see Figures 5.11 and 5.12).

Butler suggests that *who* we mourn, and *why*, tells us about which lives are seen as worthwhile. Mourning losses was particularly important for Peter and Norma as they had both lost children, and therefore were mourning, not only their child/children, but their 'mother of' and 'father of' self-identities.

When researching bereavement and loss I came across a quote by Rando (1991), who talks of a lady who was both a bereaved parent and a widow, who said, 'when you lose your spouse, it is like losing a limb; when you lose your child, it is like losing a lung'. As a COPD sufferer, Peter did focus on his breathing difficulties, and these were reflected within the collages (see Figure 5.7); however, Rando's quote seems to indicate that Peter had suffered a double blow where his breathing was concerned. In this collage (Figure 5.7), Peter talks of the inherent focus required by the body in deep illness.

This focus on revisiting Peter's 'father of Mark' identity through the portraits was not in the sense of 'denying' Mark's death, but as a way to contain and visibly mend this lost relationship; it was perhaps an attempt to reclaim a lost metaphoric 'lung'. The first portrait I painted of Mark *for* Peter was *Mark, Charlie & Rusty* (Figure 5.8).

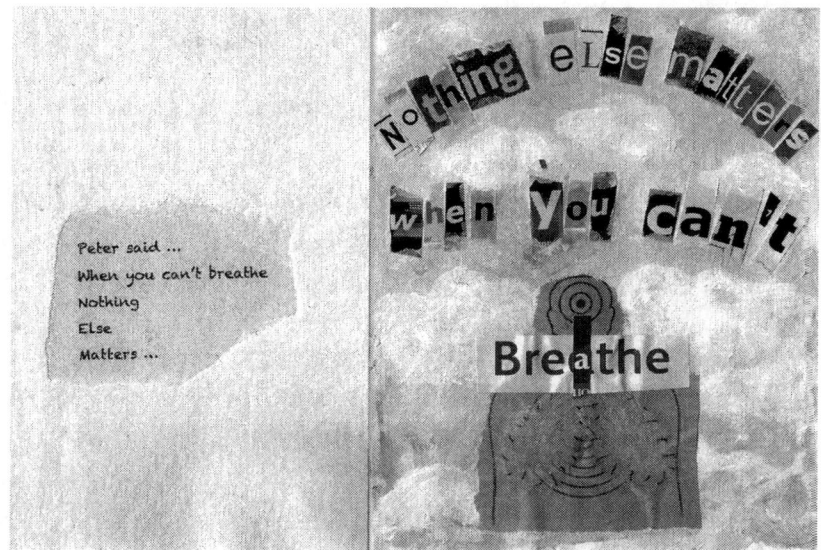

Figure 5.7 *Can't Breathe* collage by Susan Carr, 2011.

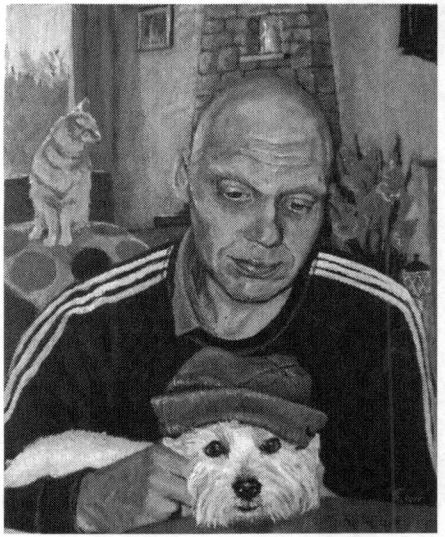

Figure 5.8 *Mark, Charlie & Rusty* by Susan Carr (co-designed by Peter), 2011.

It seemed important to Peter that Mark's love of animals and his humorous side was acknowledged, as well as honouring the family cat who had died the same day as Mark (Figure 5.9).

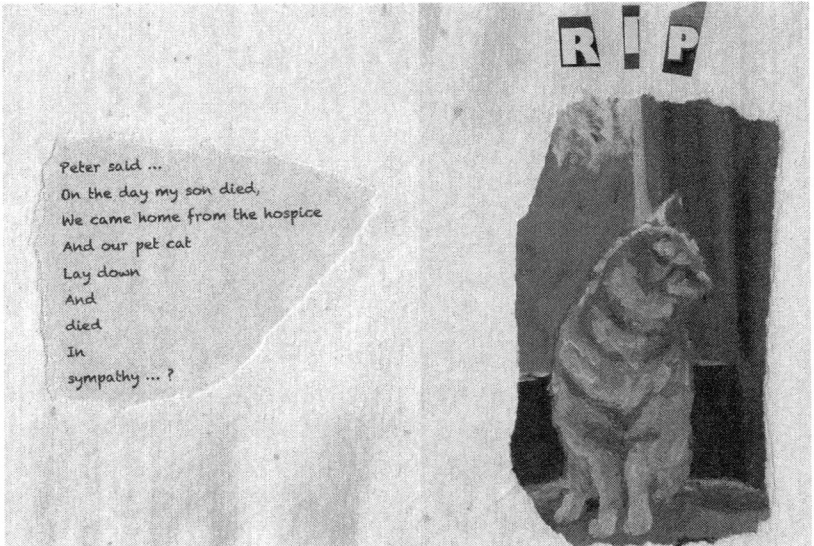

Figure 5.9 *RIP Mark & Rusty* collage by Susan Carr, 2011 (co-designed by Peter), 2011.

I had met 'Charlie' (Peter's west highland terrier) many times on my visits to see Peter, and Charlie's presence, held by Mark in the portrait, seemed to be a link between us all, and although I couldn't meet Mark in person, I wanted to learn all I could about him, so I encouraged Peter to tell me what kind of person Mark was. I also went to visit Mark's grave and I reflected on this in the active documentation sketchbook.

## Notes from Peter's active documentation sketchbook 25/02/2011

Today I went to visit Mark's grave, it seemed an important thing to do as I am unable to meet him in person, in fact it seems the 'least' I can do, especially as Peter is no longer able to climb the slope up to where the grave is situated. I think perhaps I am going more for Peter's sake than for my own or for Mark's, but I think that is ok. Peter described the position of the grave and I found it quite easily. It was in a lovely old-fashioned graveyard, overlooking the vale, with grass and well-tended graves all around. There were flowers on Mark's grave and I felt remiss at not bringing my own to place there. I sat for a while and thought about how to work with both Peter and Mark... most importantly I was then able to tell Peter that I had been...

As Peter told me stories of self-identity about both himself and Mark I began to put together a picture of Mark in my mind, and resolved to paint a double life-sized portrait to show the prominence of this relationship in Peter's life (see Figure 5.10). One of the things Peter would often say was 'there was *something about Mark...*' I used several photographs of Mark as reference for the portrait, and I was worried that because I had never met him, I would not be able to capture that 'air' or 'essence' that Barthes (1985) and Freeland (2010) talk about.

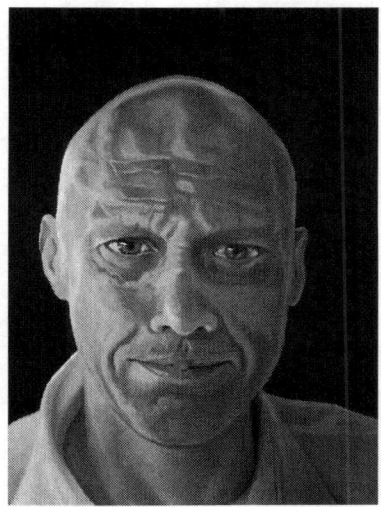

Figure 5.10 *There's Something About Mark, RIP* by Susan Carr (co-designed by Peter), 2011.

Whilst painting the portraits of Mark I was also painting portraits of Peter, and although he was deeply interested in these, it was clear that his main focus were the paintings of Mark. In his end of project interview Peter talked about how important this double life-sized portrait was to both him and his family:

SC: This is the portrait of Mark...

P: Oh, is this the big painting?

SC: Yes... [unwrapping *There's Something About Mark, RIP* to show Peter]

P: My word! ... What a lovely...oh my goodness gracious...that is superb, that is superb...goodness gracious me...you have really got it...oh my sons would love that. And to see it that size as well!

SC: Yes, I really loved doing that...his eyes are just so intense...

P: I wonder if my sons are around? They would love to see it... Do you mind if I give them a buzz...?[6]

As the portraits progressed I took photographs to our sessions to show Peter and to get his opinion about modifications, colours, etc. I also began two portraits of both of them together, one of Peter holding Mark as a baby in Kenya (see Figure 5.11) and the other called *At the Races* (see Figure 5.12) of them both at Cheltenham racecourse enjoying a day out together.

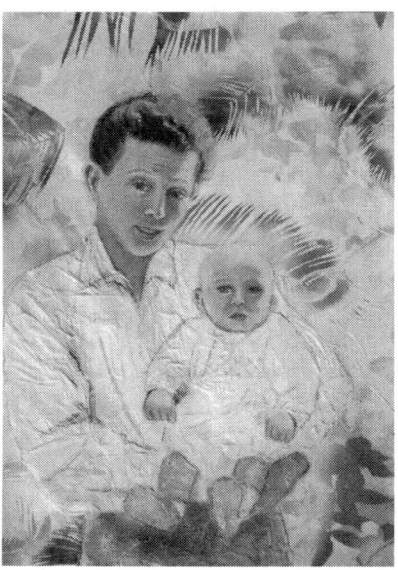

Figure 5.11 *Peter & Mark in Kenya* by Susan Carr (co-designed by Peter), 2011.

---

6  SC = Susan (Artist-Therapist-Researcher). P = Peter (Patient-Researcher). End of project interview 27/02/2012.

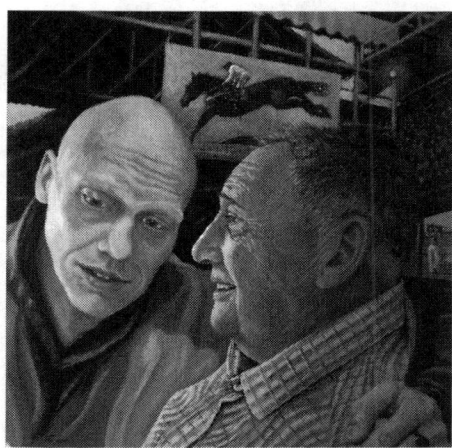

Figure 5.12 *At the Races* by Susan Carr (co-designed by Peter), 2011.

The *essence statements* derived from the *At the Races* portrait highlight the bond between a father and his first-born son.

> **Statement of Emergent Knowing:** *At the Races*
> 
> I tell a joke, you smile and laugh, we are there for the races, a small bet to place, not really for the winning but for being together and sharing our time, father and first born son, united, relaxed, no oxygen required, your presence mends my broken lungs...

> **Statement of Emergent Learning:** *At the Races*
> 
> Peter is happy in his treasured 'father of Mark' role, reunited in the painting, the relationship is remembered and validated, and together, without illness and pain, they rest in each other's enjoyment.

Through the portraits, collages and prose poems Peter was able to acknowledge the stories and events from his life that have shaped his self-identity, both those that have *made* and *un-made* him. The portraits of Mark enabled Peter to still *do* something for Mark and himself, to still *be* in that caring *'father of Mark'* role, whether through imaginative or prospective processes, not as a *denial* of Mark's death, but as an honouring of his life. Peter was therefore able to revisit that aspect of his self-identity, to talk actively and with a sense of agency and purpose, about how to portray himself and Mark within the portraits, and the artwork gave a focus to our discussion, enabling emotional distancing.

Peter's feeling of helplessness, loss, and guilt about outliving Mark were replaced with adaptive feelings of agency through his active role in co-designing the portraits, bringing in aspects of his *past, present* and *future* self-identities. The *past* aspect included the remembering of happy times at the races and being with Mark, the portrait was produced in the *present* as tangible results of our collaborative relationship involving action, agency and 'being held in mind', and the portrait also suggests that Peter and Mark will one day in the *future* be reunited in death. The portrait also exists in *present* time and will exist in the *future*, even after Peter has died. There was also a sense of the portraits being an acknowledgement that Mark's life was worthwhile and that he will be remembered.

Peter talked about how portrait therapy helped him 'accept the loss of Mark'; it was an acknowledgement of adaption and closure:

> SC: So is it important to you that your contribution to this project might help other people in a similar situation to you?
>
> P: Yes, and it's nice to be part of and *what it has done is help me to accept the loss of Mark.*
>
> SC: Has it? Oh good...
>
> P: *It's helped me in that respect, I don't know why but it has,* and I can talk about him now without filling up with tears, which I couldn't before...[7]

In a similar way to Peter, there was a sense of urgency within Norma to talk of the many personal losses in her life, and how these had impacted upon her sense of self-identity. The first such loss is reflected in the collage entitled *My Mother Walked Out and Left Me* (Figure 5.13).

This early abandonment and subsequent time in orphanages and foster care had a severe impact on Norma's sense of herself as a whole person, saying that she had spent her life searching for her self-identity. Norma also talked about ongoing ill health as a child and adult, and

---

7  SC = Susan (Artist-Therapist-Researcher). P = Peter (Patient-Researcher). End of project interview 27/02/2012.

the consequential loss of seven babies depicted in the *Seven Holes in My Heart* collage (Figure 5.14).

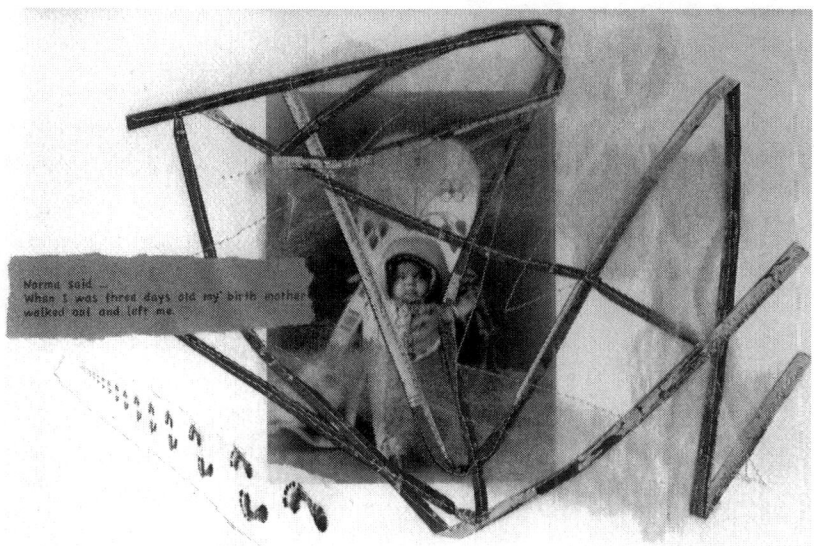

Figure 5.13 *My Mother Walked Out and Left Me* collage by Susan Carr, 2012.

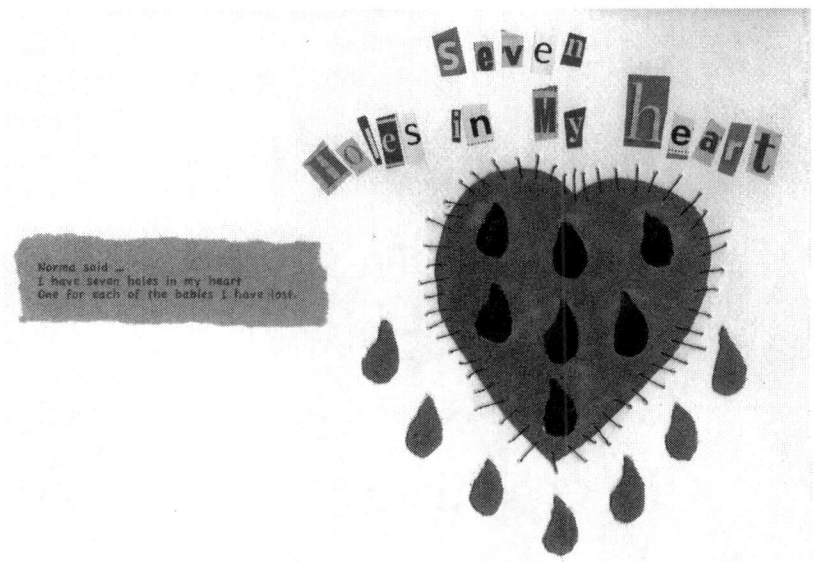

Figure 5.14 *Seven Holes in My Heart* collage by Susan Carr, 2012.

My reaction to Norma's stories of bereavement resonated with my own loss of a baby and I recorded this in Norma's active documentation sketchbook.

### Notes from Norma's active documentation sketchbook 22/08/2012

When Norma told me about the loss of her babies I immediately thought about the loss of my own baby halfway through my first pregnancy, and how I used art making to heal myself through postnatal depression. I thought about how I had created a baby and dress out of muslin as a kind of 'bereavement portrait'. I wrote a poem called 'unwelcome contradictions of death in birth' and embroidered it on the front of the dress. I thought about how sewing together the 'baby', and stitching the poem was therapeutic, as well as being able to 'hold' and dress the 'baby'. I wonder if it would be possible to replicate this in some way as a healing experience for Norma?

Remembering how important it was for me to actually 'hold and feel' the 'baby', I thought about making a portrait-sculpture for Norma, so I showed her a photograph of the 'baby' I had made to facilitate my own mourning process (Figure 5.15) and we discussed it together.

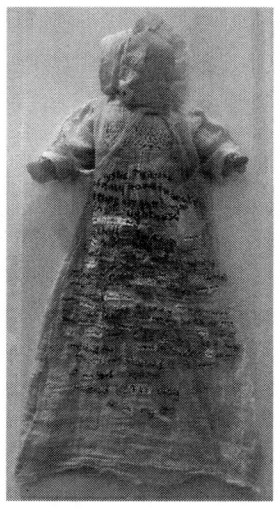

Figure 5.15 *Unwelcome Contradictions of Death in Birth* by Susan Carr, 1999.

The creation of bereavement portraits of babies and children was common in the 16th and 17th centuries (Mander and Marshall 2003), and with the advent of photography bereavement photographs became popular in the Victorian era. This practice has been brought back into maternity units, after a period (up to the mid 1970s) where stillbirths and miscarriages were seen as a 'non-event' and mourning rituals were not encouraged or facilitated (Rådestad et al. 1996, p.209). My own experience of losing a baby in the early 1980s fell into this 'non-event' category, with the baby taken away immediately, without me seeing or holding him, with no acknowledgement that his death (at 19 weeks) was a major event in my life, which required the healing processes of memories, ritual and meaning making.

I reflected on Norma's reactions to the idea of the 'baby' portrait-sculpture in the active documentation sketchbook.

### Notes from Norma's active documentation sketchbook 12/09/2012

I showed Norma the photograph of the 'baby' bereavement portrait I had made to mourn my own lost baby and she thought this idea might be something we could work with. I said that the baby would also represent her as a baby and that instead of being abandoned, this baby/self would be loved and looked after. Norma then said that it would have to be a Native American Indian baby and that she would make a cradleboard and special layette for the baby as this is what a Native American Indian mother would do. I was a bit worried about the burden of this, as it seemed she was taking on a lot of work – but then I remembered how therapeutic I had found making the baby dress and embroidering the poem on the front for my own baby. So, I realise the importance for Norma of being able 'to do' this for her 'baby' and herself.

Norma and I therefore co-designed and co-created the portrait-sculpture *My Baby/My Self* (see Figure 5.16). I made a full-sized Native American Indian new-born 'baby' from muslin, stretched and sized over a newborn baby doll 'mould', then removed and stitched together, and Norma made a Native American Indian cradleboard and layette for the 'baby'. The 'baby' represented a merging of Norma's lost babies, with her own self-identity as a previously abandoned baby now 'found'.

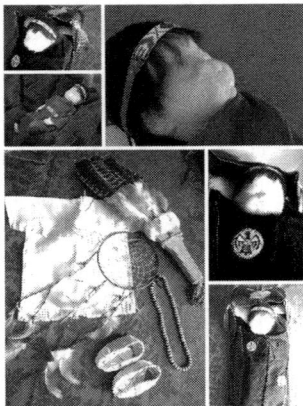

Figure 5.16 *My Baby/My Self* by Susan Carr and Norma, 2012.

Caring for bereaved mothers, offering emotional, psychological and spiritual support, now feature in interventions used within maternity hospitals, with a focus on 'creating memories' (Mallinson 1989) which may include *memento mori* such as photographs, wristbands, locks of hair, foot/hand prints, etc. (Rådestad *et al.* 1996). In a study looking at the bereavement interventions offered to a group of eight mothers, Moulder (1998) found that mourning photographs of their baby were an extremely important part of the grieving process for all the mothers interviewed.

In the end of project interview Norma talks about how the project had enabled healing for both herself and her husband, saying it had given her a sense of 'closure':

SC: So, how have you found the collaborative process? So, we've been talking about what we wanted to do...

N: Painful at times when I've had to go back and think about the past, because some of the past has been quite painful. *But, it's helped, because I've been able to put closure to some of it, which has been really helpful.* [...]

N: Losing seven children is not a pleasant thing to do. *It has healed both of us, there has been healing for both of us* [i.e. Norma and her husband].[8]

---

8  SC = Susan (Artist-Therapist-Researcher). N = Norma (Patient-Researcher). End of project interview 26/10/2012.

In this section I have used Butler's (2004b, p.22) quote to highlight the need for patients to mourn losses to self-identity caused by life-threatening and chronic illnesses, as a way to enable acceptance, and a process of adaption and change to begin. This study has shown that failure to engage in this process can result in people becoming 'inscrutable' to themselves. In their end of project interviews both Peter and Norma talked about finding a sense of 'closure' regarding important bereavements in their lives, bereavements that had stripped away part of their relational self-identities. The portraits therefore became an opportunity to engage in creative and adaptive rituals, enabling a process of *revisioning* or visible mending to occur.

## Adaption through increased flexibility and agency, and changes in perception of 'control'

Peter and Norma's experience of 'closure' and healing may also have been due to an increase in their lived experience of 'control', through their active involvement in the co-designing (and in Norma's case co-creating) process. This perception of control and autonomy mitigates the sense of helplessness, caused by uncontrollable losses such as bereavement and illness (Werner-Seidler and Moulds 2011).

Within Susan's post-diagnosis button task (Figure 5.17), she created a design that depicted the impact of illness on her self-identity (button tasks will be discussed further in Chapter 8). Within the design, Susan identifies her 'self' as the mermaid, 'trapped' within a metaphorical 'box' saying the small 'gap' left at the top was where 'memories could still get in' but which was too small to enable her to 'get out'.

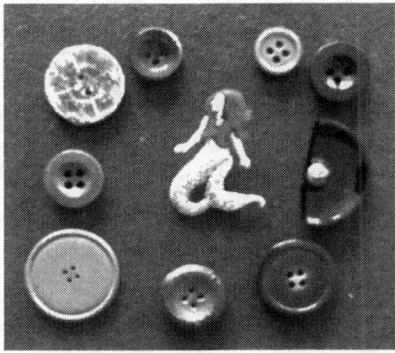

Figure 5.17 Susan's post-diagnosis button task, 2012.

Seeing the mermaid in the 'box' enabled Susan to see how 'boxed in' she felt and to link that to feeling over-protected/and under-protected as a child. This initial theme of the 'box' became one that recurred throughout Susan's involvement in the project, with Susan developing creative and adaptive strategies to 'get out of the box'.

The metaphor of 'being boxed in' is reflected within one of Susan's collages and prose poems (Figure 5.18); here the box becomes synonymous with being confined to a wheelchair and also Susan's dislike of being photographed.

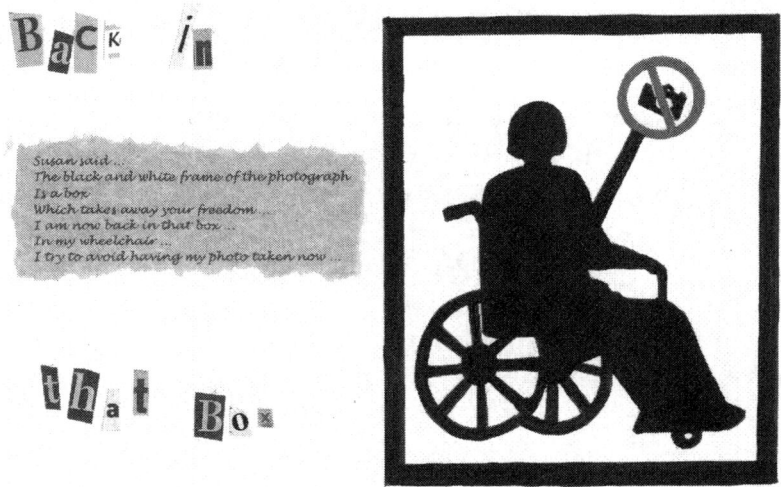

Figure 5.18 *Back in That Box* collage by Susan Carr, 2012.

This then led to a further development of the 'boxed in' metaphor into a 3D portrait-sculpture, *Pin Hole Camera* (see Figure 5.6) and the following exchange demonstrates the ongoing co-designing process:

SC: Ok then, about 'avoiding having your photo taken', about this thing, about 'being in a box', a black-and-white frame...

S: I quite like the idea of the camera. I don't know if you want to do something again but the camera there instead of the sea, I could be captured in it you know?

SC: Yes, almost like someone squashed into a very small space. A bit like Alice in Wonderland, where she becomes very big in a very small space.

S: Yes, just like that.[9]

Within this early co-designing phase, Susan and I were able to adapt ideas to fit Susan's thoughts and feelings and the *Pin Hole Camera* became symbolic of Susan's relationship with her father, a father she described as a 'brute' who she lived in fear of. One of the aspects Susan highlighted regarding her relationship with her father was his obsession with photographing her as a child, and this is reflected in: the prose poem which accompanied the portrait-sculpture, the essence statements from the analysis, and my reflections in Susan's active documentation sketchbook.

Susan said:
Throughout my childhood
My father was obsessed with photographing me…
I learned to dread the camera coming out…
And the orders to face the camera and smile
To face the sun and not squint
To please…
Albums and albums of photos remain
A testament to my father's persistence
And my stoic acceptance and attempts to keep the peace…

**Statement of Emergent Knowing:** *Pin Hole Camera*
I stand or sit doll-like, pretty in pink and bows, trapped by the lens, my coloured world converted into black and white. Each photograph a pin prick of discomfort, as my likeness is taken against my will, 'snapped' 'captured' 'caught', again and again and again.

**Statement of Emergent Learning:** *Pin Hole Camera*
Multiple images bear witness to a father objectifying his daughter in monochrome, and yet he captures only the surface, Susan complies to keep the peace, but only partially and retains her subjectivity within herself.

---

9   SC = Susan (Artist-Therapist-Researcher). S = Susan (Patient-Researcher). End of project interview 22/03/2011.

## Notes from Susan's active documentation sketchbook 27/01/2012

I have been reflecting upon Susan's *Pin Hole Camera* portrait-sculpture, and feel that the pins sticking into it are a reflection of the pain I felt tangibly between us as she spoke so eloquently about her fear of her father as a child, her desperate attempts to keep the peace, and her efforts to break the cycle and never allow such things to happen to her children. Each pin represents the discomfort of being photographed, but also represents each experience of her father's explosive temper, and Susan's own enforced suppression of her academic prowess. There was a contrast in Susan's upbringing, being over protected on the one hand and under protected on the other. Never allowed to ride a bicycle in case she fell off and hurt herself, her parents didn't trust that she could look after herself. Perhaps they were both acknowledging that neither could protect her from her father's temper. Pins, or needles, are used to 'repair the damage' even in health, such as acupuncture or injections, etc.

Within Susan's end of project interview, she reflects upon how exploring the theme of being 'boxed in' has changed her lived experience of agency:

> SC: I wonder whether you find that perhaps you are getting outside of *the box*...now.
>
> S: Yes, I think having recognised it, *I've recognised the steps that I need to take to change it.* I don't think when we set out on this that I would have, I don't think I was fully aware of that feeling. I think articulating it made it visible to me, I think. I think that's one of the reasons that I've got the crutches, partly because my back really hurts if I'm in the chair too long, but the crutches are a positive step out of that, I think. And, taking more care putting make-up on, nails, this kind of thing, is saying that I'm not going to be in *that box* if I can avoid it. So yes, *I think that has made a difference to stepping outside.*[10]

---

10 SC = Susan (Artist-Therapist-Researcher). S = Susan (Patient-Researcher). End of project interview 18/10/2012.

Susan and I also co-designed the *Swan Island Book* (see Figure 5.19), which depicted a positive mentalisation Susan employed when undergoing radiotherapy treatment. Susan describes how this reminded her of adaptive strategies she had used in the past:

SC: And that was a prototype for the book [*The Swan Island Book*]...

S: Yes, it's interesting to see that made visible. All of that went on in my mind at the time.

SC: Yes, that idea of the swan breathing fire and burning away... yes.

S: And then the soothing, being looked after, but not in a controlling way, in a gentle, positive way. In a safe place, a safe place to turn whenever you need. [...] *I suppose as well it kind of reminds me that I did have strategies that worked for me, as well, so some control over the illness. Probably a delusion but a good feeling.*

SC: No...I suppose that it's a self-healing strategy.

S: Yes.[11]

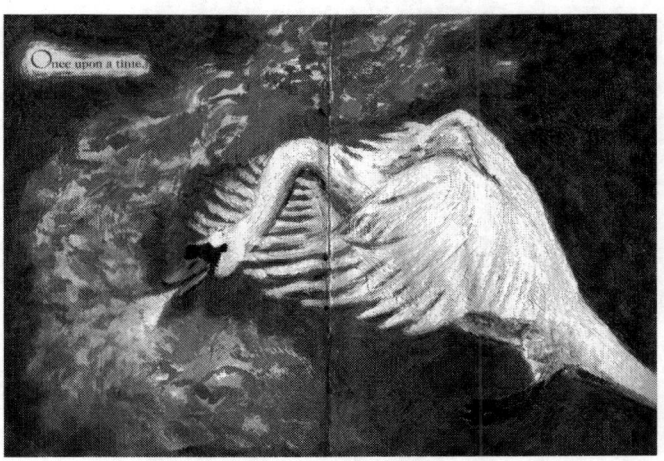

Figure 5.19 *The Swan Island Book* by Susan Carr (co-designed by patient Susan), 2012.

---

11 SC = Susan (Artist-Therapist-Researcher). S = Susan (Patient-Researcher). End of project interview 18/10/2012.

Increasing perceptions of control was another theme identified within the analysis and is utilised by Rose within her portraits as a way to 'control' her image and how people saw her. Charmaz and Rosenfeld (2006, p.37) talk about how 'embodiment complicates self and identity for people with chronic illness' and the tension between visibility and invisibility results in people attempting to control how they are portrayed, as indicated in the prose poem written to accompany Rose's *Paint Me Like a Picasso* portrait (see Figure 5.20).

> Rose said:
> Picasso painted in a quirky way…
> So, if you paint me
> like a Picasso,
> People won't notice
> My quirkiness…

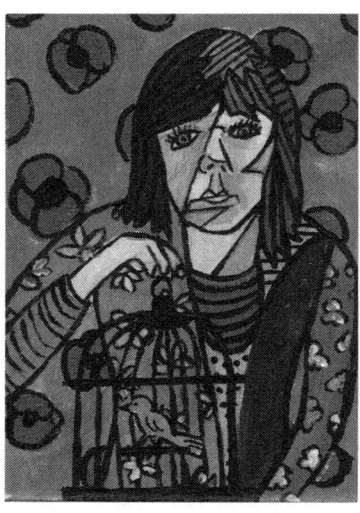

Figure 5.20 *Paint Me Like a Picasso* by Susan Carr (co-designed by Rose), 2011.

The following exchange recorded in Rose's end of project interview explains why a sense of control was important for Rose:

> SC: Hmm that's great. You also mentioned something interesting when we were talking about the *Paint Me like a Picasso* portrait. Because you were saying your friend asked you why you liked it, and you said it was because your face was 'not going to fall down in the painting, you don't need to worry…'

R: *Yeah, because in a photograph this* [indicating fallen lower lip/face] *people are going to look and notice. But in this* [indicating the painting] *they won't notice.*

SC: Do you feel that with that one as well? [indicating *Bohemian Rhapsody* portrait]

R: Yeah, because, although that is slightly down [indicating side of mouth] people won't notice. Because I won't have any more photos took because of that. You doing this…is, … because that's not going to happen.

SC: So, it's like you can control this more, so you can control your image and you can control how people see you?

R: Because, I know my face is like this [shows face fallen], but up here [points to brain] it's not, I still think of myself as… with the control in my face. Because when I look at people and I smile, that [points to mouth] doesn't smile, that [points to head/brain] *does*, I don't think of my face like this, so you doing that [indicating the portrait], *that's the thoughts*.[12]

Rose is indicating in this exchange that the portrait represents a melding of her inner and outer realities, and as such the processes employed within the *Paint Me Like a Picasso* portrait enabled the portrayal of a kind of *visible* mending, with a black line and blue triangular shadow below Rose's mouth outlining the place where her lower lip falls open and forward, acknowledging this as part of Rose's identity but 'controlling' it within the portrait. This brings the embodied reality back in-line with Rose's imagination and observation, '*that's the thoughts*'.

Towards the end of the project Rose demonstrated her new-found determination to challenge the restrictions placed on her through illness, in creative and adaptive ways (see Figure 5.21).

Rose said…
I'm going to walk 15 Kilometres for the hospice,
Dressed as a florescent fairy!
People say 'You can't do that!'
I say 'Maybe not, but I'll have a damned good try!'

---

12  SC = Susan (Artist/Therapist/Researcher). R = Rose (Patient-Researcher). End of project interview 22/03/2011.

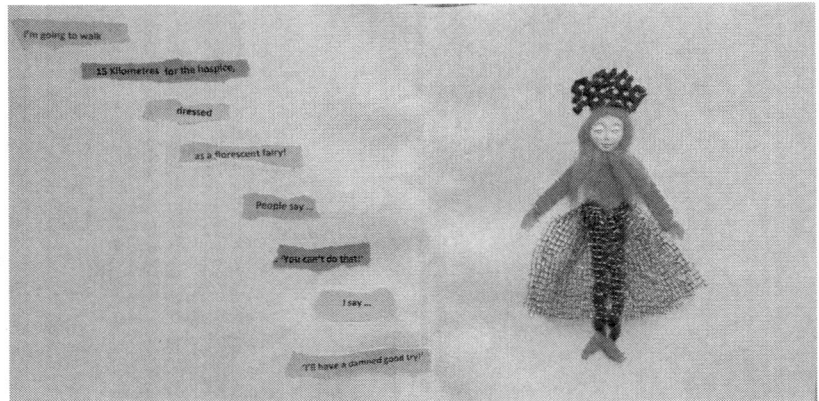

Figure 5.21 *I'll Give It A Damn Good Try*, collage by Susan Carr, 2010.

Rose also talks about this in her end of project interview. I have identified Rose's self-identity voices in different typefaces, to show how Rose's 'resilient, see me/hear me' self-identity voice dominates and has the last word:

## Listening for Contrapuntal Identity Voices:

### 1. Listening for 'Resilient, see me/hear me Rose'.

*2. Listening for 'Invisible, silenced Rose'.*

3.Listening for 'Earth-Spirit Warrior Child'.

4. Listening for 'Isolated City Child'.

R: **That's determined!** [indicating *Bohemian Rhapsody* portrait]

SC: And also, that sense of, you know, I'm here, yes, I have got this but I am going to carry on. It's almost like…'don't you stand in my way.' [laughs]

R: **It's like my t-shirt has got on it 'don't stop me now!' that's a Queen song. I've got a t-shirt with it on.**

SC: Yes…

R: I am determined to make the most of myself, so…

SC: Yes, I think it does...I think it has got a lot of courage in it. Courageous...

R: *Yes, because I could turn around and say I can't go shopping, because I can't ask for what I want, but I do go, I say to my son, 'I say it twice I don't give up...I say give us some paper and I will write it down', but I don't say to people come with me and ask [for me], I do it myself. I don't give up, I do still try.*

SC: Yes, I think that would be an inspiration to a lot of people, seeing that painting actually.

R: *On Facebook I said, 'Don't tell me I can't do it, watch me do it!'*, words to that effect. Like when I said I will do that walk. Friends of mine said but you can't do that. I said why? They said 'you can't walk that far'. I said 'well maybe not but I shall give it a good try!'. Why, just because it is a long way, why should it stop you trying? But I think I will do it because I will get myself to a steady pace and stick to it. I won't try to finish it in a rush...quickly. No...I shall set myself a pace. I shall do it.

SC: I am sure you will...

R: I shall do it. *By next day I may be on my hands and knees.* **But I think I can do it.** *I didn't think I could, I wouldn't try,* **but now I think...you can do it!**[13]

In her end of project interview Rose reflects upon her determination to overcome challenges and to maintain her independence, both of which are characteristic of an increase in *creative capacity* and the ability to find *health* within illness:

R: I think *this is a message*, well to me, *you're diagnosed with a terminal illness but that doesn't mean you gotta stop, you gotta keep going,* don't give in to it. Just because you have been given a life sentence, just because you have been told you are ill, told you are never

---

13 SC = Susan (Artist-Therapist-Researcher). R = Rose (Patient-Researcher). End of project interview 22/03/2011.

going to get better, doesn't mean to say you can't carry on, *I think that is what this has done for me.*[14]

In this section I have described the increase in feelings of agency, control and autonomy that patients have reported in their end of project interviews, mitigating feelings of helplessness caused by uncontrollable losses. This process enabled Susan to recognise the steps she needed to take to get 'outside the box', and allowed her to see the way illness had made her feel like a child again, 'captured' and helpless. I have also shown how portraits and portrait-sculptures become a way to rediscover and re-member adaptive strategies from the past, enabling patients to utilise these once more, increasing their perceptions of control. In this respect portraits effect a kind of visible mending which acknowledges both *brokenness* and *adaption*, highlighting experiences that have both 'made' and 'unmade' the patients' sense of self-identity.

---

14 SC = Susan (Artist/Therapist/Researcher). R = Rose (Patient-Researcher). End of project interview 22/03/2011.

— Chapter 6 —

# MIRRORING AND ATTUNEMENT THROUGH PORTRAITURE

*Intersubjective and Symbolic Ways of Knowing, Being and Relating*

In this chapter I describe the patients' experience of the *portraits* as visual channels for *mirroring* and *attunement* (Wright 2009), and how this process enables an awareness of previously unknown and 'untold' aspects of self-identity. I explain how for the patients, the portraits become a unique way of *being known*, both to themselves and others. I describe the *intra*subjective validation of self-identity that the portraits provide for patients through viewing portraits and collages that *they* needed to see, as well as the *inter*subjective validation provided by portraits that they needed *others* to see. I also describe a process of *aesthetic resonance* (Carr and Hancock 2017), which equates to adding meaning, complexity and coherence to the portraits, enabling patients to recapture a sense of themselves as *valuable* and *beautiful*.

Visual communication is relied on extensively by humans in their daily life, both in reading body language and facial expressions (Mandal and Ambady 2004, p.23), and in navigating their world. Arguably discursive language is less effective at expressing the 'quality, intensity and nuancing of emotion and affect' needed for diverse social circumstances, than is the face, with its myriad of expressions (ibid.). The preference for familiar faces defines the self throughout a person's life (Schore 2000), as Merleau-Ponty said, 'I live in the facial expressions of the other' (2002, p.146). James Elkins, in his book *The Object Stares Back* (1996), talks about a 'need to be seen by objects and by people;' a 'need to be caught in that intersection of gazes'. Elkins cites Lacan's emphasis regarding our equally important need to see ourselves in a mirror. He says 'by looking into the mirror each morning I check to make sure that I am the same person who went to bed last night – the person who dissolved into darkness and dreams' (Elkins 1996, p.70). The familiarity of a person's own face is therefore paramount to their self-identity; however, it is something which illness and invasive treatments can distort and change until people become unrecognisable to themselves and others. This highlights the importance of creating portraits that the patients recognise as a reflection of themselves.

## The role mirroring and attunement plays in the process of *revisioning* self-identities

As discussed in the literature review, within the design of this intervention I have extended Wright's (2009) relational model of mirroring and attunement, into a concept where the portrait becomes derivative of the (m)other's mirroring and attuning expressive face, and the therapist, as a 'good enough' (m)other/artist, validates their sense of self-identity. The mirroring and attuning process is, I have argued, dependent upon the therapist's own ability to *empathically engage* with the stories of self-identity presented by the patients. Wright (2005, p.534) describes *resonance* as a 'felt and immediate response', and as 'a feeling of being in the same state, the same place as the other' (ibid.). It is known that human beings have used art as a 'feeling form' (O'Neill 2008) to heal the body, mind and spirit, for at least the past 30,000 years; it is therefore the oldest healing resource in the world (Achterberg 1985). The portraits therefore become containers of self-identity, presented to others as relational, *inter*subjective 'feeling' in all its myriad forms:

> Humans have a self that is relational and that by its very nature involves self-presentation to others, with an awareness and concern about how one is seen, and this is part of what is rendered when an artist creates a portrait. (Freeland 2010, p.104)

However, the portraits are also presented to the self as *intra*subjective forms, which the patients themselves needed to see.

This intervention also offers patients, not only the visual aspects of self-identities, but also the opportunity to share aspects of themselves as told through stories of self-identity. This is facilitated by the button, LEGO® and photo elicitation tasks, which are then 'mirrored and attuned' (Wright 2009) within the narrative aspects of the portraits, collages and prose poems. At one stage or another all the patients involved in the study said they had told me stories of self-identity that they had *never told anyone else before*, and three repeated this within the end of project interview. This process of revealing the *self* enabled the patients to learn about themselves and how their illness had affected their perception of self-identity (Alea and Bluck 2003), and correlates with the observations made by Mark Gilbert in his 'Saving Faces' (Farrand 2000) portrait project (as discussed in Chapter 3), whereby Gilbert's sitters shared 'details of their lives which they shared with no one else' (ibid.). I therefore suggest that this sharing of previously untold stories of self-identity could indicate a unique *portrait effect* (Carr 2014), a distinctive quality of the relationship between subject and artist found within portraiture.

Susan describes this effect:

S: Yes, I felt perfectly free to say where I thought something didn't work or did work, so much freer, much more comfortable… Yes so, in fact there's a whole raft of things that I've never told anyone before, so there you go!

SC: A lot of people have said that!

S: In the portraits, you're turning negative memories around into something that's beautiful and lasting and giving them back as something that's not tainted by misery or pain or anything else.[1]

Paul outlines what he thinks it is about portraits that prompt sitters to tell stories of self-identity that they have never told anyone before:

SC: So, do you think this project has given you a stronger sense of self and identity? So, knowing who you are basically… looking back on your life.

---

1  SC = Susan (Artist-Therapist-Researcher). S = Susan (Patient-Researcher). End of project interview 18/10/2012.

P: Well I sort of already knew...I was quite a shy sort of person anyhow...but with you doing this I suppose it has opened me out a lot more than I would have with somebody else. To tell the truth, *I have told you quite a lot more things, that I wouldn't have told anyone else.*

SC: It's funny because everyone has said that.

P: You are my therapist! In a sense, I have put a lot of trust in you, haven't I?

SC: Yes...true.

P: Part of the family! [laughs]

SC: [laughs] I'll put me in the middle then shall I [indicating the *English Gothic* portrait].

P: Yeah [laughs].

SC: Yes, it is strange how everyone has said that...but it was one of the things I thought about portraits...that people talk and people tell you things that they haven't told anyone else before.

P: *I suppose it is because you want to see the person as they are* rather than just a photograph...

SC: Yes...get to the essence of the person.

P: Deep underneath what you are asking...*there is a heart* as such...[2]

Paul is saying in this exchange that he thinks sitters reveal secret stories of self-identity because they *recognise intuitively* that the portrait artist is attempting to depict not just the *outer likeness*, but the *inner essence* or *significance* of a person, and that this requires a *different kind of knowing*. This different kind of knowing requires the artist to see 'further' and deeper than others see (Taylor 1989, p.22). In order to show the inner heart of the person subtly within the portraits I have used metaphor and symbolism; as Paul says, they reveal that 'deep underneath what you are asking...*there is a heart* as such'. A successful portrait therefore

---

2   SC= Susan (Artist-Therapist-Researcher). P = Paul (Patient-Researcher). End of project interview 03/06/2013.

is capable of showing what is not ordinarily visible, a glimpse into a person's subjective inner world (Brough 2001, pp.43–4); this holding of dualities, e.g. *revealing* and *concealing*, is I suggest one of the key reasons why portraits are able to enhance a person's sense of self-identity *coherence*. Through this process, as patients see themselves and are seen, a sense of *re-cognition*, *re-integration* and *re-membering* is instigated. Through becoming aware of previously unknown or forgotten aspects of self-identity, they become *known* to themselves and others.

## *Intra*subjective validation of self-identity: Portraits patients needed to see

In this section I outline those portraits and collages that patients themselves *needed to see*, as a powerful way to validate and combine inner and outer realities, and the reflection and attunement of stories of self-identity that they had 'waited a lifetime to tell'.

An awareness and concern about how one is *seen*, both by the self and others, is one of the emergent themes within this project, highlighting the tension within illness between *being seen* and *not seen*, and the implications within that of risking anonymity, of not being heard or acknowledged, or facing social stigma. Being unable to conceal one's illness is therefore often a central concern, as Carel says:

> …intimate details become the first thing a stranger sees about you. Instead of being in charge of what you disclose about yourself, you become a passive vessel of information provided through your own betraying body, a body that cannot keep a secret. A stranger takes a cursory glance at you and already knows so much about what is sensitive, intimate and painful. (Carel 2008, p.58)

This concern about how the body-self is represented is therefore compounded by life-threatening and chronic illnesses, and our inability to depend on our bodies to 'look, behave, or move as they once did', which means that the image we believe others have of us changes in a negative way (Charmaz and Rosenfeld 2006, p.46), with 'judgements of character, ranging from saintly, courageous, dependent, or slothful to morally tainted…' (ibid., p.36) all being linked to stigma in illness. The embodiment of illness therefore 'complicates' self-identity for people living with life-threatening and chronic illnesses (ibid., p.37) and weakens 'boundaries of the self-concept', meaning they 'become vulnerable to redefinition – whether positive or negative' (ibid., p.47). One of the interesting things about portrait therapy is that patients are able to direct how they wish to appear in the portraits, and therefore harness art's *transformational* power to adjust or change meanings. As Eisner (2008, p.11) says:

> Art often creates such a powerful image that as a result we tend to see our world in terms of it, rather than it in terms of our world. Put another way, art does not always imitate life. Life often imitates art.

If as Eisner (2008) says life 'imitates art' it follows that patients may begin to 'imitate' their portraits, or at least begin to see themselves more clearly through the portraits so as to affect 'change' in themselves or their lives. A portrait that Paul *needed to see* was his *At Home* portrait (see Figure 6.2). As outlined in Chapter 4, Paul (at age 49) had been forced, by the deterioration of his lung condition, to give up his independence and live with his mother, and Paul said he spent almost all of his time (except for hospital appointments and hospice visits) alone in his bedroom. For Paul, connected almost constantly to an oxygen supply, the world had become a liminal, unhomelike, hostile and dangerous place, and Paul's sense of social isolation and frustration is reflected in the collage I made for Paul entitled *Hard to Leave the House* (Figure 6.1).

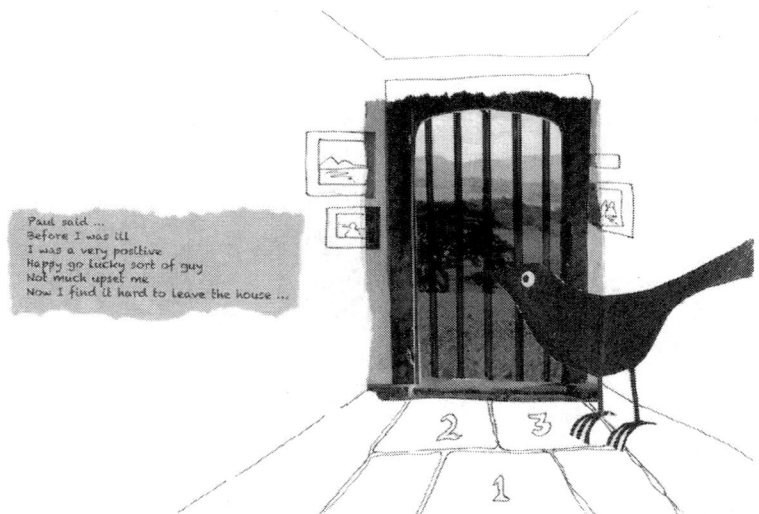

Figure 6.1 *Hard to Leave the House* collage by Susan Carr, 2013.

A portrait that Paul needed to see himself was his *Broken Lungs* portrait (Figure 5.5), as it enabled Paul to see how *thin* he had become:

> ### Notes from Paul's active documentation sketchbook 20/01/2013
>
> I took the *Broken Lung* portrait to show Paul today...I was a bit worried about showing him, because it seems quite shocking to me...and when Paul saw it he exclaimed...'I'm not that thin, am ? and I said, 'Yes I'm afraid you are'. 'I have always been thin,' said Paul, 'but not THAT thin!' 'Good God!' he said, 'I better try to eat more...the consultant says I can't be put on the heart/lung transplant register until I am at least 9 and ½ stone...but I have never been 9 and ½ stone in my life...I have always been thin. . but not that thin!' I felt disturbed that the portrait may have held up a mirror for Paul that he might not want to see...and yet there was also a feeling that perhaps he *needed* to see it...in order to take action, to try to eat and put on weight, so that he could have the hope of a transplant.

Paul's emaciation – whilst obvious to see even through his clothes – was for whatever reason *not seen* by Paul and his ambivalence to food highlighted this, usually refusing all offers of food at day-hospice. However, soon after this discussion Paul's attitude to eating changed (at least at day-hospice), where he began to eat a (small) meal each week with the other patients. I believe that for Paul, seeing himself mirrored through the eyes of another enabled him to see a more 'accurate' vision of himself, resulting in a renewed sense of agency.

Having already painted three portraits for Paul (i.e. *Broken Lungs*, *English Gothic* and *Virtual Paul*, see Figures 5.5, 7.11, 7.17), I had thought these were 'enough'; however when I sat down to review these portraits I was not so sure. I documented my thoughts in the ADS:

> ### Notes from Paul's active documentation sketchbook 14/05/2013
>
> I spent time today looking at Paul's portraits, collages and prose poems and I thought that the portraits didn't really reflect Paul's previously described 'happy go lucky', well, self-identity. I think

there needed to be more of a balance. I wonder if I should paint a further portrait that would do this. We did discuss painting a portrait of Paul in a bar, using the style of Edward Hopper, and the suave male loner figure that often feature in these paintings. I have not mentioned the portrait to Paul as I am not sure I will have time to complete it before the end of project interview. I realise I am taking a risk, since Paul will not get an opportunity to advise me of changes he might wish to make, however, I will focus on our initial discussions.

Following my intuition, I painted a final portrait for Paul and called it *At Home* (see Figure 6.2).

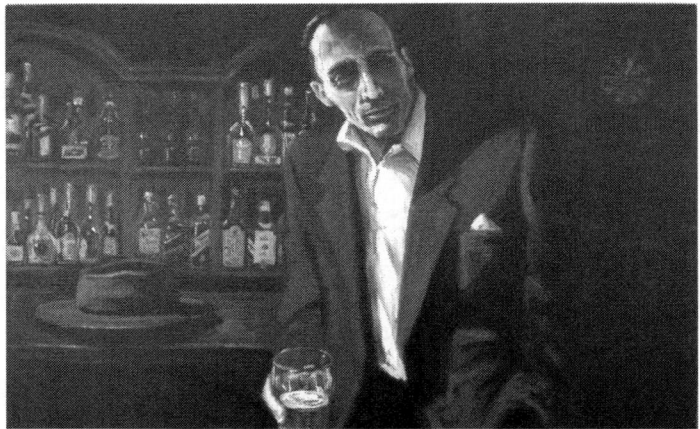

Figure 6.2 *At Home* by Susan Carr, 2013.

When I arrived for Paul's end of project interview I told him that I had another portrait to show him:

SC: [...] so, this one, you know we talked initially about doing a portrait of you in a bar, like an Edward Hopper painting, so I thought shall I do one? I didn't tell you about it because I thought I might not get time to do it, but anyway I did.

P: So, this is a surprise one, is it?

SC: This is supposed to be you in a bar with some drink and the...

P:    Gangster sort of thing isn't it.

SC:   Yes, in a way…but this idea of you being…

P:    *I look quite well there!*

SC:   I called it 'At Home' because you said you felt at home…

P:    Well considering I lived in a pub, pubs and what have you…

SC:   It's sort of like Humphrey Bogart, you know that kind of…

P:    Yeah…no *I like that actually!*

SC:   It's sort of a 'well Paul' kind of one…

P:    *It isn't far off actually…yeah, I like that one!*

SC:   It's good to have a balance with the paintings.

P:    *At one time, I always used to wear a suit jacket like that*, a brown pin striped thing.[3]

By saying 'I always used to wear a suit jacket like that', Paul is indicating his 'ownership' of the 'self' depicted within it, and goes on to acknowledge the adaptive change he may implement through *imitating* the portrait:

P:    Very good…*I do like that one…* [indicating the *At Home* portrait]…

SC:   That is the reason I wasn't here last week…trying to get it finished…

P:    *I will have to get a jacket now…go to the hospice like that!*[4]

Although this may seem a small thing to do, to buy a jacket, it implies a degree of self-worth and self-care, something that had been lacking in Paul's presentation of himself in day-hospice. In the portrait, Paul is extracted from his liminal space and placed where he feels a sense of home-like-being-in-the-world, something Paul says he would like to return to:

---

3   SC = Susan (Artist-Therapist-Researcher). P = Paul (Patient-Researcher). End of project interview 03/06/2013.

4   SC = Susan (Artist-Therapist-Researcher). P = Paul (Patient-Researcher). End of project interview 03/06/2013.

SC: And maybe a return to this one here [indicating the *At Home* painting]?

P: By the time I return to that I won't be able to afford a pint! [laughs] ... I would love to go out...even now *I would love to go to my local and have a pint...just walk in there...sort of thing*.[5]

I was worried when I painted *At Home* that Paul may see it as the embodiment of his 'lost' self; however, since the completion of our sessions together there were opportunities to catch up with Paul in the day-hospice and I noted further changes and developments in the ADS:

### Notes from Paul's active documentation sketchbook 09/06/2013

Since we completed the portrait therapy project I have noticed a change in Paul. He seems to be 'dressing up' to attend day-therapy now, wearing a smart shirt and jeans, and being clean shaven. This change in self-care is marked. And he has also been eating a small meal at lunch-time!

The difference between Paul in *Broken Lungs* and Paul in *At Home* is stark, and demonstrates why I felt it was important to paint the latter as a contrast, and it did seem to be the catalyst for positive changes in Paul's self-esteem and autonomy, and this continued and developed after the completion of the project. I recorded in Paul's sketchbook a conversation I had with him a few weeks later in the day-hospice:

### Notes from Paul's active documentation sketchbook 31/07/2013

After-note: Today Paul told me that during the previous week he had suddenly decided to go out...alone. He said he ordered a taxi and went to spend the afternoon at the local pub he had frequented before he became ill. Paul's face lit up as he talked about it, saying he walked in there (with his oxygen cylinder) and sat in his 'usual'

---

5   SC = Susan (Artist-Therapist-Researcher). P = Paul (Patient-Researcher). End of project interview 03/06/2013.

> place at the end of the bar. He said many people he used to know came to chat with him. The correlation with the *At Home* portrait is striking! I wonder if there is a sense that the portraits can be a template for a more positive self-identity that patients can adopt, meaning that in a way they 'become' their portraits? Or by seeing himself in a positive light in the portrait, did it give Paul the confidence or permission to fulfil that particular dream? This seems a significant step forward for Paul.

Perhaps for Paul, the experience of seeing his portraits enabled something to change or shift within him, giving him a sense of self-worth and agency. The local pub Paul went to visit was a place where he was known and welcomed, and the portrait encapsulates the sense of *being known* that is implied in being *At Home*. Art as a representational object perhaps enables a person to stop and confront life, allowing them to see it from a different perspective, and then change or modify their behaviour (Gormley 2002). The portraits have this capacity, in their ability to reflect that which patients *need to see*. This is highlighted in Norma's experience. We had decided I would paint a portrait of Norma using Frida Kahlo's *The Two Fridas* (1939) as reference, as the idea was to depict the two central aspects of Norma's self-identity, which she described as 'Scottish Catholic' born in Aberdeen, and also 'North Bear', her Native American Indian identity after being adopted into the Black Foot Tribe.

In *The Two Fridas*, Frida Kahlo paints the two halves of her self-identity, one wearing early 20th century European clothes, and the other a traditional Mexican Tehuana dress ripped at the chest to reveal a bleeding, broken heart. The two Fridas are sat on a bench holding hands, joined by an artery travelling between the two hearts, painted against a stormy sky. Within the portrait, Kahlo portrays her 'divided, unintegrated and uncontained fluidity' (Latimer 2009, p.51).

In *The Two Normas* (see Figure 6.3) the dual nature of Norma's self-identity is reunited and validated.

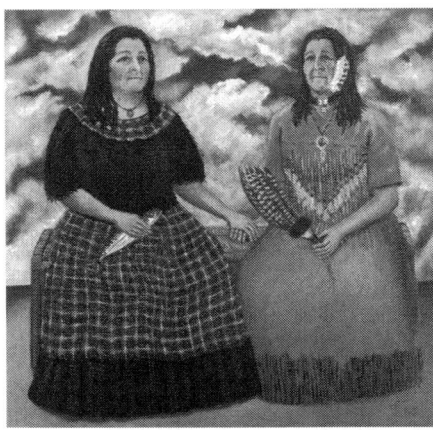

Figure 6.3 *The Two Normas* by Susan Carr (co-designed by Norma/North Bear) 2012 (after *The Two Fridas* by Frida Kahlo, 1939).

It was through this portrait that Norma was able to *see the difference* between the two sides of her self-identity for the first time:

SC: So, has this project helped to give you a stronger sense of yourself and your identity?

N: Yes.

S: And could you give me some examples of this?

N: It made me realise that I'm not the only child that was abandoned at a very early age, and it's made me realise that yes, I am probably a stronger person because of that. And, finding the Indian [NAI] side of myself, that has made a great difference in my life. I didn't realise how big a difference it had made until we first spoke. ... I knew it had made a difference, and everybody said that when I'm in my regalia, I'm North Bear, I'm not Norma. I'm a totally different person. *I didn't realise that until I just looked at that picture.* [indicating *The Two Normas*] *You can see there is a total difference.*[6]

Norma goes on to say how 'Norma' is supported by 'North Bear'. This new way of thinking about herself correlates with the analysis essences statements for *The Two Normas*:

---

6  SC = Susan (Artist-Therapist-Researcher). N = Norma (Patient-Researcher). End of project interview 26/09/2012.

> **Statement of Emergent Knowing:** *The Two Normas*
> Culturally diverse identical twins are linked in the holding of hands together, united in strength and compassion, two parts of a whole, supporting and nurturing each other.

> **Statement of Emergent Learning:** *The Two Normas*
> Norma acknowledges that North Bear supports her Scottish self, especially when she is anxious or ill. Norma is becoming aware of how different aspects of her self-identity can be called upon in times of need, which contributes to a creative and adaptive way of being.

In her end of project interview Norma clarifies how the different aspects of her identity support each other:

> SC: Again, it's unusual. I like that unusualness [referring to *The Two Normas*].
>
> N: It's different. The two sides of one person.
>
> SC: Sort of meeting and supporting each other.
>
> N: That's a good way of putting it because *North Bear does support Norma and Norma supports North Bear. And when Norma's not very well, she becomes North Bear, and North Bear comes through and carries her through it.* ...[7]

Norma realises that North Bear, as an aspect of her self-identity, can be relied upon not to abandon her in times of need. The dualities explored within this portrait are therefore characterised by hope and despair, of breathing and suffocation, of life and death, and the ability of the portraits to 'hold' these dualities is an important way in which they function, dissipating 'cognitive dissonance' (Festinger 1962). Norma summarises her experience of *revisioning* her self-identity through portraiture; going from a place where she felt 'worthless' to one of 'purpose'.

---

7  SC = Susan (Artist-Therapist-Researcher). N = Norma (Patient-Researcher). End of project interview 26/09/2012.

N: *I felt worthless and useless when we first started this project.* But by having to relive my life, by telling the story, I've realised that I've actually become stronger through the illness. The iller [*sic*] I've got, the stronger I've got. And that no, I'm not useless. *I've got a purpose in life and I'm fulfilling it!*[8]

Within this section I have described the *intra*subjective validation of self-identity that the portraits provided for these patients, using the portraits *At Home* (Figure 6.2) and *The Two Normas* (Figure 6.3) as examples. Paul found a renewed sense of agency after viewing his portrait, at least temporarily freeing him from his agoraphobic fears, and enabling him to make a final visit to a place he 'loved' and where he was *known*. In *The Two Normas* portrait Norma is able to *see the difference* between two important aspects of her self-identity and realise for the first time how they support each other. Norma says portrait therapy enabled her to move from a position where she saw herself as 'worthless and useless' to one where she says 'I have a purpose in life and I'm fulfilling it', equating in itself to a *homecoming* experience.

## *Inter*subjective validation of self-identity: portraits patients needed *others* to see

While personally viewing the individual portraits fulfilled different needs for the patients, as this project progressed it became clear that sometimes it was equally important for patients to know that their portraits were going to be *seen by others*. This is based on a view that portraits as objects hold significance, that they are 'made special', and as such act as *participants* in the world, able to influence and effect change in the views of people. As Freeland (2010, p.100) says:

> There is a further order of complexity in the fact that the *audience* adds an additional layer of interpretation to the artist's rendering of the original subject's presentation of a self. (original emphasis)

One of the prevailing themes identified within Rose's portraits (see Figure 6.4) is the tension between being seen and unseen. When analysing Rose's portraits, I noted a progression within them from 'invisibility' (Charmaz and Rosenfeld 2006) within *The Poppy Field*,

---

8   SC = Susan (Artist-Therapist-Researcher). N = Norma (Patient-Researcher). End of project interview 26/09/2012.

where Rose says, 'I lay down in a poppy field *where no one could see me*', to semi-invisibility in *Paint Me Like a Picasso* where she says, 'Picasso painted in a quirky way…so if you paint me like a Picasso, *people won't notice* my quirkiness…' Then in *Bohemian Rhapsody* Rose is finally *visible*, confronting the viewer with a defiant, strong and forthright look. As she says, 'Paint me like Freddie Mercury…strong and defiant!'

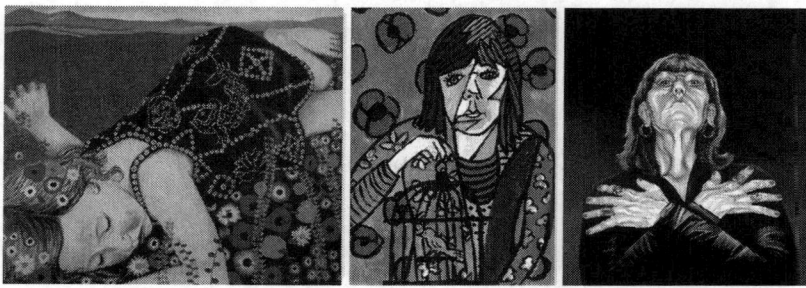

Figure 6.4 Montage of Rose's three portraits: *The Poppy Field, Paint Me Like a Picasso* and *Bohemian Rhapsody* by Susan Carr (co-designed by Rose), 2011.

Rose's sense of confrontation, and determination to be seen on her own terms, was highlighted in the *Statement of Emergent Knowing*:

> **Statement of Emergent Knowing:** *Bohemian Rhapsody*
> I take a risk and step out of the shadows into the light…through self-acceptance and strength…I look you in the eye…I will be seen and heard.

When viewing all three of Rose's portraits together, I noticed they all held an element of *performance* and *intentionality*, each with a distinct 'costume' and 'set'…which suggests that Rose may be playing a 'role' in each of them. This is poignant because autonomy, intentionality and the ability to 'be' who she chooses is something that may be lost to Rose if/when her illness progresses. The fear of this happening was highlighted within the collage and prose poems (Figure 6.5).

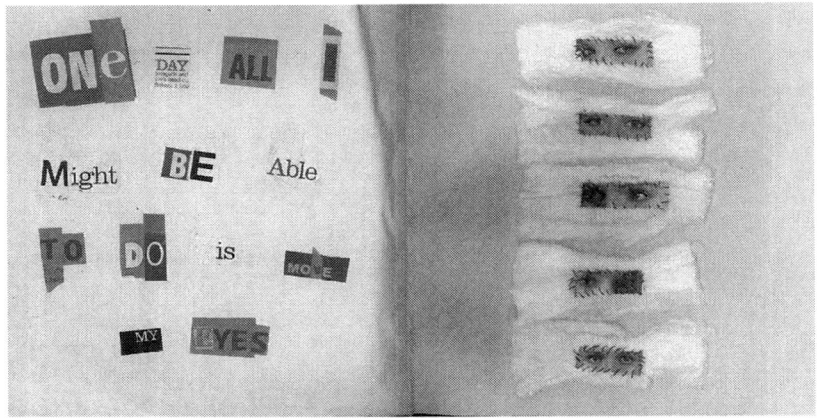

Figure 6.5 *All I Might Be Able To Do*, collage by Susan Carr, 2010.

In a similar way, Peter needed others to see the portraits of himself and Mark (see Figure 5.12 *At the Races*), and also himself as a fit and active young man climbing Mount Kilimanjaro (see Figure 6.7).

At the end of our time working together Peter asked for photographs of the portraits to keep in his wallet at all times, ready to show people he met. I observed Peter showing the images of the portraits regularly to other patients and staff at the day-hospice. For some reason, it seemed easier for Peter to show the portraits of his deceased son, rather than photographs, again bringing in a sense of emotional distance and yet connection inherent within the portraits. The fact that the portraits were painted by someone other than him seemed to give Peter 'permission' to show them and talk about his lost 'father of Mark' identity, as well as a sense of pride that he and Mark had been painted together. He would say to other patients, 'Look at these portraits that Susan has painted…that is my son Mark…who passed away last July…'

Peter spoke about the contrast or difference between himself prior to diagnosis and how illness had disrupted his self-identity. This contrast is captured in the collage in Figure 6.6.

When co-designing the portraits Peter's focus was also on portraying his autonomous, masculine self-identity, as he felt this had been most negatively disrupted by his illness. It seemed that Peter needed others to see what his illness had done to him – that he was still this fit young man inside, as shown in his *Climbing Mt Kilimanjaro* portrait (see Figure 6.7).

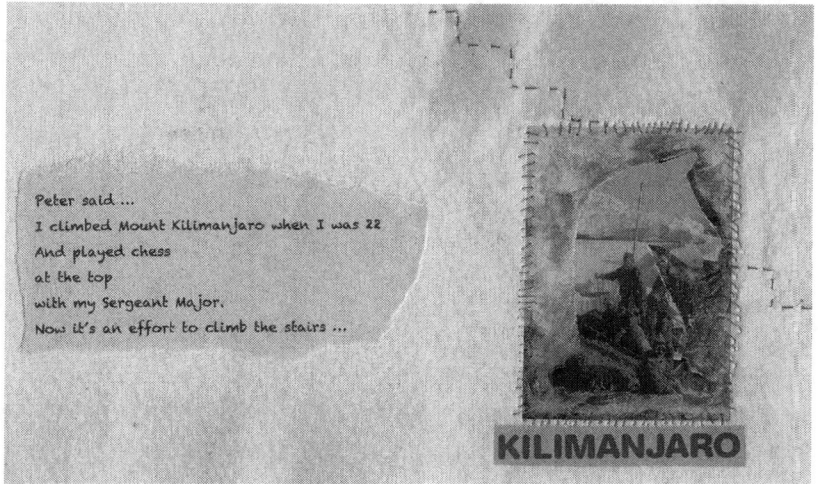

Figure 6.6 *I Climbed Mount Kilimanjaro* by Susan Carr, 2011.

## Statement of Intention: *Climbing Mt Kilimanjaro*

Peter said: 'Paint me as a young boy soldier climbing Mt Kilimanjaro, I climbed it so easily back then, I don't even remember getting breathless! No need for oxygen!' Peter chose an Impressionist style for this portrait and although he did not express a direct understanding of Impressionism as a school of painting, he did express a desire for me to 'capture the moment and the light'.

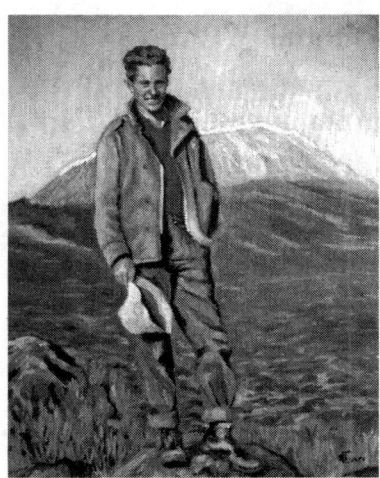

Figure 6.7 *Climbing Mt Kilimanjaro* by Susan Carr (co-designed by Peter), 2011.

## Statement of Emergent Knowing: *Climbing Mt Kilimanjaro*

A young man surveys the world, his mountain to climb and his life to live – a boy soldier, without a care in the world conquers nature, noticing only the beauty and majesty, confident in this harsh terrain, the boy soldier becomes a man.

For Peter this then became a reclamation and validation of his masculine, adventurous and autonomous self, something he feared he had lost due to his illness. Showing others this image enabled them also to see Peter in a new light, to look beyond his illness and disability to who he was…and still is…inside.

Paul needed *others* to see his *Broken Lungs* portrait (Figure 5.5), as a way to validate his inner reality and his invisible illness. Paul talks about how his mother reacted to the portrait:

P: Well it was actually, for no reason, like today…I was being pushed in a chair and just getting out of the chair into the car I just had to stop for five minutes just to catch my breath […] It just gets you now and then, it just gets you…it hits you really hard…it's weird.

SC: So, do you think that it reflects that…the *Broken Lungs* painting?

P: Yeah, yeah definitely.

SC: Yes…because people have said it is a very powerful painting… when I had it in that exhibition…

P: My mum hates it! [laughs].

SC: Well I can understand that…because she is your mum.

P: It is horrible I must admit…*but I tried to explain to her…that is me…I am damaged.*

SC: Yes.

P: *That is skinny though isn't it.* [laughs][9]

---

9   SC = Susan (Artist-Therapist-Researcher). P = Paul (Patient-Researcher). End of project interview 03/06/2013.

Paul's reflection that his mother 'hates' his *Broken Lungs* portrait may indicate a sense of denial or an inability to acknowledge or 'hold' Paul's feelings of despair and pain. However, through the portrait, Paul is able to talk to his mother about his illness, and about being 'damaged'. People whose expectations around their future lives have been challenged by a disrupted life course often 'engage in emotion work on and for their selves and on and for others' (Duncombe and Marsden 1998, quoted in Exley and Letherby 2001, p.115). The co-designing of portraits *for others to see* may therefore indicate a need for patients to help relatives and friends come to terms with their (the patient's) illness and mortality.

For different reasons Bill needed others to see his *Flying Ace* portrait (Figure 6.8) – to witness the young vital self that he had been willing to sacrifice for his country, something that many of his friends *did* sacrifice. The portrait was therefore a way of remembering and acknowledging their loss through bringing into being a self-identity hidden by the mask of time and illness, but still present within him. This was therefore a reflection of his past self-identity, but also a still present, internal self-identity landscape, which was made visible for others to see and validate.

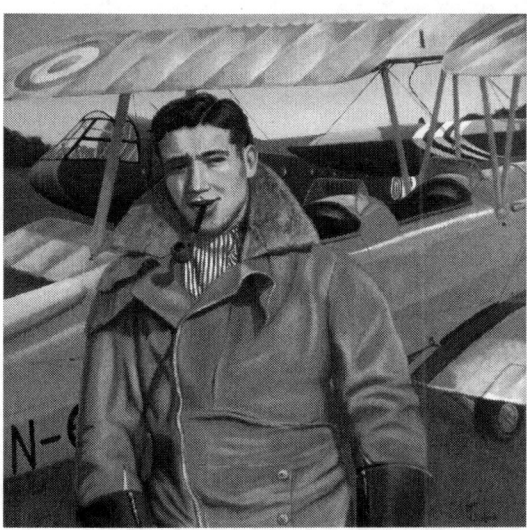

Figure 6.8 *Flying Ace* by Susan Carr, 2011 (co-designed by Bill), 2011 (see also Coloured Plate iii).

Within this section I have described the way Rose used the portraits to confront others with her intentionality and autonomy, with a gradual sense of determination *to be seen by others*, on her own terms. For Peter, it was important to keep images of the portraits with him at all times, in order to show others, the significance of his lost *father of Mark* identity, and as a way for others to witness the autonomous, adventurous masculine part of his self-identity, something he felt had been lost through the impact of illness. Paul needed his mother to see and hold the *Broken Lungs* portrait and this was the catalyst that enabled Paul to talk to her about his illness. Bill needed others to see his young and vital self within his *Flying Ace* portrait, something he had been willing to sacrifice for his country and it also served as a reminder of the many who made the ultimate sacrifice. It also drew back the scourge of time and illness to reveal an inner reality – an inner self that was...is Bill.

## Portraits, collages and prose poems as 'containers' of duality: *Holding hope and despair*

One of the ways portraits 'hold' dualities such as 'hope and despair' (Clayton *et al.* 2005, 2008) is through the use of metaphor and symbolism, which can also be seen as a way to reduce complex phenomena to 'essences'. These 'essences' can then be subtly changed through aesthetic or metaphoric attunement, and 'held' within the portraits. Being or feeling in touch with another person requires a kind of 'symbolic capability' in those who are interacting, in order to hold the experience in a symbolic form and therefore allow its realisation (Wright 2009, p.25). This 'symbolic capability' became highly developed between Rose and myself, and many of her collages and prose poems contained metaphor and symbolism (e.g. see Figure 6.9).

Rose said:
I collect Freddie Mercury Plates
On a display shelf
One day it slipped
And all my plates came crashing down...
I am still picking up the pieces.

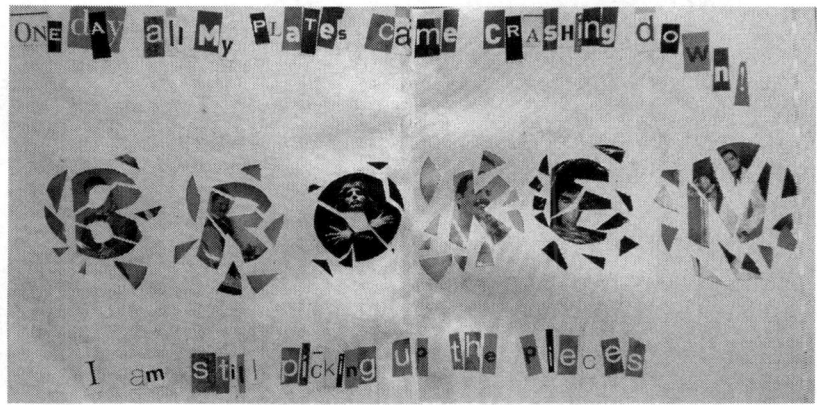

Figure 6.9 *All My Plates Came Crashing Down*, collage by Susan Carr, 2010.

Within this collage, the shelf of plates 'crashing down' becomes a metaphor for the moment when Rose was diagnosed with motor neuron disease (MND), highlighting the dualities of helplessness and agency through the 'sudden' catastrophic event and through Rose still 'picking up the pieces'.

Dualities are also held within Rose's *Paint Me Like a Picasso* portrait (see Figure 5.20). Within the portrait, Rose is wearing flamboyant colourful 'parts' of clothes or costumes, something that equates to a kind of 'camouflage'. The poppy motif returns in this portrait, and although a positive symbol for Rose (being her favourite flower), the metaphoric connotations of a poppy are of *remembrance, mourning* and *death*. Similarly, the canary in the cage was suggested by Rose to indicate that she had bred canaries for several years; however, the cage could also be seen as a metaphor for MND's propensity to 'lock' sufferers within their bodies. Although Rose's intentions for these motifs were positive at the time of designing the portrait they do hold dual meanings.

I became aware of a sense of 'holding' hope and despair for Rose within her *Paint Me Like a Picasso* portrait:

### Statement of Reflexive Resonance: *Paint Me Like a Picasso*

When painting this portrait, I felt unable to paint the door on the birdcage closed. This would, to me, have been a symbolic extinguishing of hope. I couldn't do it. So, the door remains open. The canary could therefore be seen as both *inside* and *outside* the cage.

Therefore, a sense of hope is reflected in the portrait through the 'open door' on the birdcage (Figure 6.10), allowing the possibility of 'escape'.

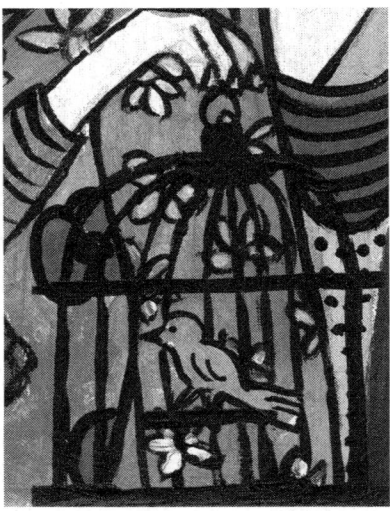

Figure 6.10 Detail of the canary in the cage, from *Paint Me Like a Picasso* by Susan Carr (co-designed by Rose), 2011.

In this portrait Rose physically 'presents' us with the canary in the cage, which also becomes a symbol of her ambivalence. For Rose, there is a sense of needing to be in control of what she reveals or conceals about her illness; she therefore reveals the canary – but at the same time presents it inside the cage, suggesting that Rose is 'hidden' within the portrait, a way of both *being seen* and *not seen*. This is outlined within the following essence statements:

### Statement of Emergent Knowing: *Paint Me Like a Picasso*

If I wear my identity brightly people may be blinded by the brightness, and they will not notice the darkness of my illness. I stand at the edge of the cage and ask, 'Can I still fly?'

**Statement of Emergent Learning:** *Paint Me Like a Picasso*
By choosing a Cubist style of painting, which breaks the surface into facets viewed from different angles, there is a sense of ambivalence in Rose revealing herself, and the opportunity for Rose to 'hide' herself within the brokenness of the image.

Ultimately the portrait becomes a container and holder of dualities for Rose, holding a sense of hope and despair about her illness.

When reviewing Susan's portraits, I became aware of how they also held complex dualities. During the initial stages of our work together Susan spoke about the early traumatic experiences in her life. Susan described her childhood as 'miserable', with a father she described as a 'brute' and a mother who was unable to protect her from him. Susan described how she was, on the one hand, idealised and over-protected, and on the other, unacceptable and unprotected, and faced with a father figure whose 'rages' she lived in fear of.

These issues were depicted within the collages I produced for Susan (see Figures 6.11, 6.12 and 6.13).

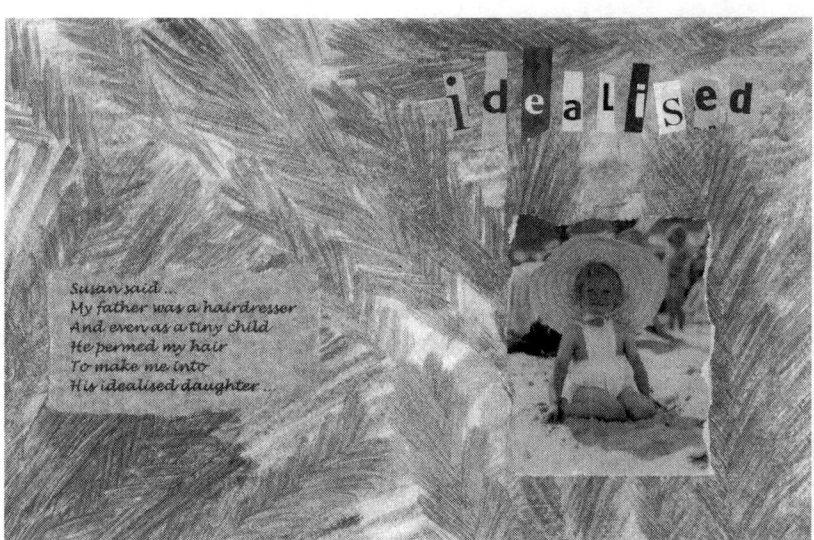

Figure 6.11 *Idealised*, collage by Susan Carr, 2012.

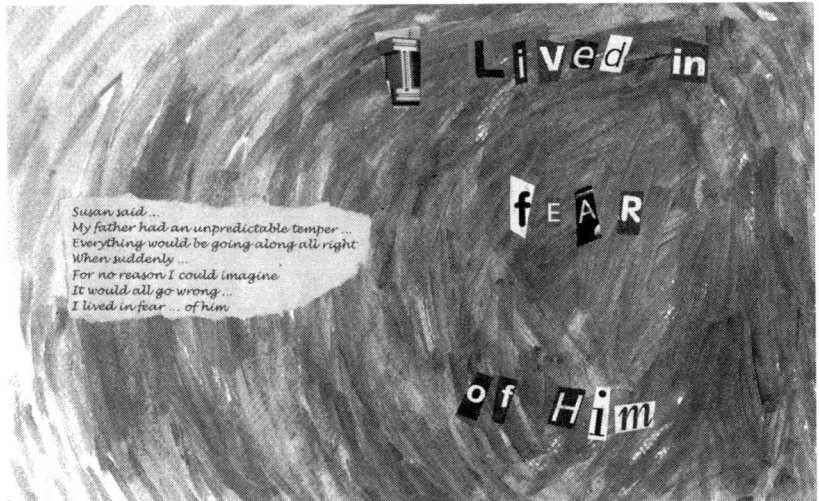

Figure 6.12 *I Lived in Fear of Him*, collage by Susan Carr, 2012.

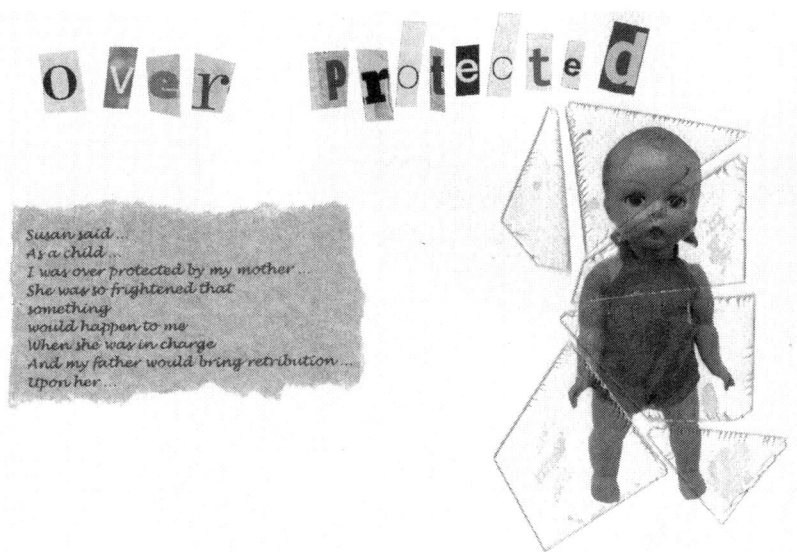

Figure 6.13 *Over Protected*, collage by Susan Carr, 2012.

These collages highlight the overt patriarchal domination within Susan's early life and the requirement to appear *feminine* and *submissive*. Within these collages and prose poems the dualities of being *over* and *under protected* came to the fore, and Susan's need to find a *balance* between a desire for protection, but also freedom.

During the photo-elicitation sessions, Susan said that as a child she was in a 'catch 22' situation with regards education and learning, with her father enraged if Susan showed signs of being an academic or 'too clever', and equally enraged if she was 'below average' in her school work. Susan said she had to hide her reading of academic and literary works from him, and could still 'taste the tears' and feel the anticipated fear of his fury if he found out. During our co-designing of Susan's *Catch 22* portrait-sculpture (see Figure 6.14) our initial idea was to depict Susan as a child walking across a tight rope; however, we also felt that there needed to be 'books' involved. The idea behind using a 'tight rope' was to portray Susan's attempt to find 'balance', therefore Susan is *balancing* books on her head, whilst also trying to *balance* on a giant book full of sharp pins. We reintroduced the pins used in *Pin Hole Camera* (see Figure 5.6) as a symbol for pain and discomfort, and to show the consequences for Susan if she 'over balanced' and fell onto the pins.

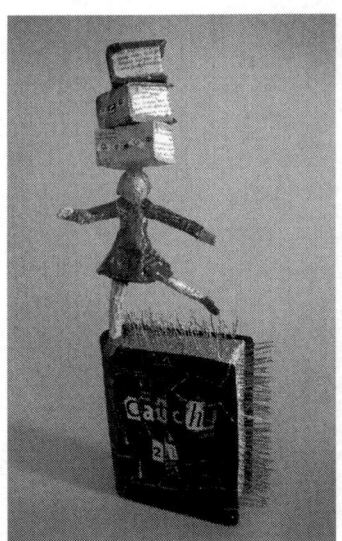

Figure 6.14 *Catch 22* by Susan Carr (co-designed by Susan), 2012.

### Statement of Emergent Knowing: *Catch 22*

A small faceless child attempts to 'balance the books', afraid to move, a heavy load on her young head, one slip and she is impaled on spikes of steel. And yet the child cannot help but fall?

### Statement of Emergent Learning: *Catch 22*

Susan is caught in a catch 22 situation, whereby she can only be acceptable to her father by denying herself. Susan's academic self is hidden to keep the peace. As her Father's daughter, Susan is not allowed to fail but also not allowed to be too clever. She must therefore maintain a perfect balance or face the fearful storm of tears and shame. As her Mother's daughter, Susan also hides her true self and colludes with her mother to maintain the façade of the idealised daughter, encouraged to placate her father to avoid them both being caught in the storm of his anger.

This portrait-sculpture demonstrates my mirroring and attunement of Susan's childhood distress, showing how impossible the task of 'keeping the peace' or 'balancing the books' was for such a small vulnerable child. As the project progressed the idea of 'balance' within the collages became something Susan focused on, making sure that there were an equal number of both positive and negative collages. We subsequently co-designed a portrait-sculpture that served to 'balance' the negatives in *Catch 22*; this was *The Cupboard of Imagination and Dreams* (Figure 6.15).

Susan said:
When I was a child
My parents had a locked cupboard with a
glass front full, of classic books.
One day I discovered where the key was hidden.
From that day on, I surreptitiously 'stole' the
key and read all the books one by one,
Risking my father's wrath
I discovered a world of freedom and adventure
In my cupboard of imagination and dreams.

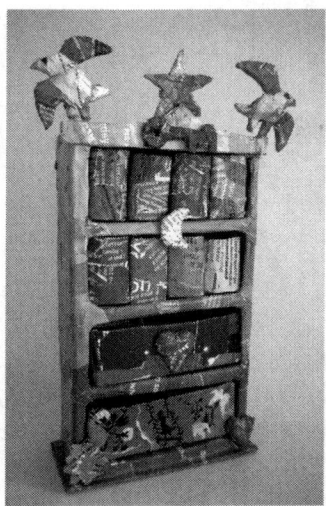

Figure 6.15 *The Cupboard of Imagination and Dreams* by Susan Carr (co-designed by Susan), 2012.

### Statement of Emergent Knowing: *Cupboard of Imagination and Dreams*

In the cupboard of imagination and dreams is a world where it is okay to take risks and explore, a land free from guilt and anger, a land where you can be yourself or an 'other', a land of magic, mystery and intrigue, a land without limits.

### Statement of Emergent Learning: *Cupboard of Imagination and Dreams*

Susan gains integrity in her love of learning. The cost of this is her idealised innocent self, which slips from the pedestal with each deception. Susan gains knowledge of the world and learns she must hide her deception and evolving self. Through this deception, Susan also comes to know her shadow self.

Susan 'slipped' a little from the idealised child pedestal with each deception; the portrait therefore holds dualities of truth and deception, and hope and fear. Susan reflects how the portraits helped her to find 'balance' in the collages and through this process find a coherent sense of self-identity:

SC: I suppose there is this idea that traumatic memories are perhaps…that they're stored in a part of the brain that is non-verbal…it's about images.

S: You probably do store it as images yes.

SC: So, it's probably difficult to talk about these things and you need a visual metaphor to describe some of these feelings?

S: It's certainly helped to bring up the positive parts of my childhood as well, because I probably would have… if somebody had put me on the spot and asked me about childhood, I probably would have remembered a lot of bad things, but not *how* they were bad, what made them so upsetting for me. I probably wouldn't have been able to consciously explore what it was about the things that I hated. And then, also to *counterbalance* them with things that were positive, more than I had thought would be there. *And I quite like this idea of me still being me despite everything.* So yes, I think it's been something that would have been a lot more difficult to achieve, with simply talking sessions.[10]

It is therefore *through* the *images*, and the reflective space created, that Susan finds a new understanding of herself (Lett 1998; O'Neill 2008), suggesting that through the mirroring and attunement inherent within them, a personal recognition of 'me still being me despite everything' is found.

The dualities of idealisation and vilification, of power and helplessness, of fear and courage, as well as her father's patriarchal views about femininity and education, were all depicted within Susan's *Being Pandora* portrait (Figure 6.16).

### Statement of Intention: *Being Pandora*

Susan said, 'I love the pastel painting of *Pandora* by Rossetti, which is in Buscot House, I cannot go and see it now as it is unreachable to me being upstairs and there is no lift.'

---

10 SC = Susan (Artist-Therapist-Researcher). S = Susan (Patient-Researcher). End of project interview 19/10/2012.

### Statement of Emergent Knowing: *Being Pandora*

Mysterious, mythical girl/woman is cast in the role of beautiful femme fatal, betrayed by her curiosity, she is blamed for releasing all ills into the world, yet she is also bountiful all-giver, peacemaker and holder of hope and grace.

### Statement of Emergent Learning: *Being Pandora*

Idealised uncapturable Susan, falls victim to her curiosity and opens the box, resulting in a loss of innocence, yet remains a romanticised, beautiful, 'all-giver', holder of hope and grace.

### Statement of Reflexive Resonance: *Being Pandora*

I have been to Buscot House many times to see Rossetti's version of this painting, and never tire of its powerful sense of mysterious, haunting womanhood, holding burdensome secrets and power. To paint Susan as 'Pandora' was risky, but I hoped that Susan's 'love' for the painting, would be transferred to a love for her 'self' in all her humanness.

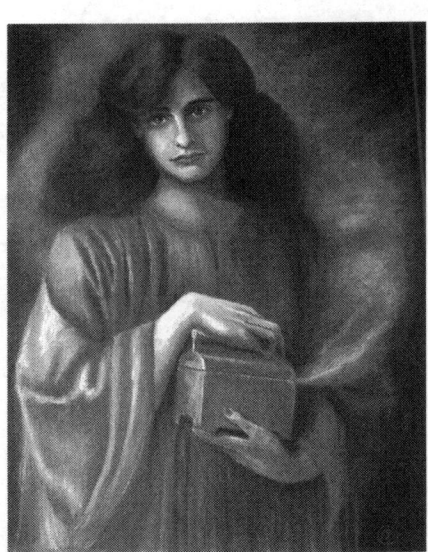

Figure 6.16 *Being Pandora* (after Rossetti, 1828–1882) by Susan Carr (co-designed by patient Susan), 2012.

This encapsulates the conflict of holding *idealisation* and *vilification*, but adds *aesthetic resonance* to mitigate this and leaves Susan literally 'holding hope' within the box. The idea of 'the box', explored earlier, is also revisited within this portrait – but this time Susan is outside of the box, holding the box, rather than the box 'holding' her.

In Paul's *Broken Lungs* portrait (Figure 5.5), the focus is on the dualities of inner and outer realities. Paul describes his intuitive 'drawing towards' Frida Kahlo's *Broken Column* self-portrait when he saw it for the first time in the portrait reference album:

SC: So how did you find the collaborative process…where we looked through the book of images…you chose the Frida Kahlo one and we talked about the American Gothic one, thinking of ideas…

P: I suppose we chose that [indicating *English Gothic* portrait] because it was more into my sort of life…that's why I chose them…to see them now is very good actually.

SC: They reflected…they obviously resonated with something…

P: Yeah, well…*you could understand what she* [Frida Kahlo in *Broken Column*] *was going through*, yeah, I found them quite good actually, those paintings.

SC: Yes, because if you have an illness that's invisible…

P: Yeah…like *you could tell that she was in pain* and all that…[11]

Images are able to convey physical pain in a way that is *inexpressible* in any other form (Padfield 2003; Toombs 1990, p.235), and Paul recognises this when he says '*you could tell that she was in pain*'. Paul is therefore choosing to reveal his inner pain and suffering through the portrait, and through this aligning his inner and outer landscapes or realities. This was highlighted within the knowing and learning essence statements:

---

11 S= Susan (Artist-Therapist-Researcher). P = Paul (Patient-Researcher). End of project interview 03/06/2013.

> **Statement of Emergent Knowing:** *Broken Lungs*
> You stand in naked isolation, chest ripped open, revealing your pierced lungs, a window onto invisible suffering, stripped back, laid bare, revealing your pain in a barren landscape. Is there anybody there…to see…me?

> **Statement of Emergent Learning:** *Broken Lungs*
> Portraying his body 'unbounded', Paul connects his inner and outer realities…it is hard to look at…but even harder to be…Paul. Holding his breath, he opens himself to hope, that by some stroke of luck someone may reach out and switch his faulty heart and lungs for some that work…allowing him to breathe…and love… life…once more…

Exposing the outside flesh and the inside organs of the body, Paul reveals his 'inner-self', within this portrait. It is a brave and risky thing for him to do. If the cut-open chest is not enough to indicate Paul's suffering, the nails driven into his flesh and lungs serve as emphasis. The portrait reveals how Paul's feeding tube punctures his abdomen wall and snakes its way up inside him to find his stomach. The 'unboundedness' (Lawton 1998, p.127) of the body evokes a sense of shock, as viewing the interior of our bodies is something that modern physicians normally protect us from (Sawday 1996 [1995], p.12). The 'unbounded body' refers to a body where the skin has been broken, allowing bodily fluids to escape (Lawton 1998, p.127). As Anzieu says, 'Bodily containment seems related to our sense of identity and self-containment' (1989, pp.98–108); however, within invisible illnesses the perfection and seamlessness of intact skin, as the ultimate container of a person, may contrast sharply with a person's inner reality (ibid.). By portraying himself with an unbounded body Paul reverses reality to acknowledge the 'unboundedness' of his inner self, and a recognition of his *being-towards-death*.

Paul often expressed feeling 'trapped' within his own body, therefore portraying himself with an unbounded body may also have been a way to express his hopes of *escape*. From my experience running art therapy groups with cancer patients, there is often a need to create images that focus on the negative, such as 'anger, fear and death, as a form of catharsis' (Luzzatto 2005, p.164). Although this portrait clearly contains painful and cathartic content, in the end of project interview I suggested to Paul that the *Broken Lungs* portrait may also be a *hopeful* painting, a way of visibly rehearsing the possibility of a heart lungs transplant:

> SC: Do you think it [the *Broken Lungs* portrait] is a hopeful portrait as well though…because there is this sense that you might have a heart-lung transplant…
>
> P: Well there is that in it…because there I am open…you can reach out and take them out and put some new ones in…as such… [laughs][12]

For Paul, even the background reflects his feelings of *unboundedness*. The barren landscape in which Paul stands is a replica of the background from Kahlo's *Broken Column* painting, and a barren landscape as a metaphor in paintings is indicative of feelings of depression, a lack of nourishment and social interaction (Thorne 2011, p.24), all characteristics of Paul's lived experience. The significance of the landscape in this portrait is not lost on Paul as he equates it to a war zone:

> P: That one [indicating *Broken Lungs* portrait], it looks like I am in one of those landscapes with bomb holes…[13]

Through the portrait, Paul literally 'lets us in' to his interior world of pain and suffering, uncharacteristically letting down his guard, and demonstrating vividly his vulnerability. By portraying himself with an open 'unbounded body' (Lawton 1998, p.127), Paul reverses reality to reveal the *unboundedness* of his inner self, and his closeness to death, acknowledging that he may suffer acute respiratory failure at any time. As such this portrait portrayed dualities of fear and courage. By combining the patient's 'inner' and 'outer' landscapes in one image, this allows for feelings of *integration* and identity *coherence* to develop (Ulman 1980, p.6). *Broken Lungs* was also a portrait that Paul needed others to see, perhaps as a way to help them understand the gravity of his illness and to demonstrate his need for love and acceptance and his connection to all humanity:

---

12 SC = Susan (Artist-Therapist-Researcher). P = Paul (Patient-Researcher). End of project interview 03/06/2013.
13 SC = Susan (Artist-Therapist-Researcher). P = Paul (Patient-Researcher). End of project interview 03/06/2013.

SC: Yes...get to the essence of the person...

P: *Deep underneath what you are asking...there is a heart as such.*

SC: Yes...I can see it... [laughs]

P: Yeah [laughs] ...in that one... [indicating the *Broken Lungs* portrait]

SC: We found it somewhere in there... [laughs]

P: Yeah...well *you know what I am saying...*

SC: *I know what you are saying...*[14]

In this exchange, Paul indicates his awareness of how much I *know* him, so much so that he assumes I can 'read between the lines' of his attempts to explain his feelings and I reflect that when I say '*I know what you are saying...*' I remember this as a poignant emotion filled moment within the end of project interview, filled with *I-thou* (Buber 2004) recognition and intersubjective *knowing*.

In this section I have described the way portraits are able to hold dualities such as hope and despair in all its myriad forms, that these were 'given' to me to hold and contain within the portraits. In her three portraits Rose explores *being seen* and *unseen*, as well as *imprisonment* and *freedom* and I am unable to close the door on the cage, as this seems to be a metaphor for hope. For Susan, the portrait-sculptures allowed her to see the impossible task she was given as a child, trying to 'balance the books' and 'keep the peace', and recognising the dualities of being *under* and *over* protected. In *Being Pandora*, good and evil, power and helplessness are explored and Susan is left holding *hope* in the box. In *Broken Lungs* Paul explores the dualities of *inside* and *outside* realities, and literally opens up and lets us into his inner world of pain and suffering. I suggested that the development of an intersubjective symbolic capability with each patient was crucial to this process, enabling them to unravel the layers of meaning within the portraits, and thereby developing a stronger sense of self-identity coherence through increased self-knowledge and understanding.

---

14 SC = Susan (Artist-Therapist-Researcher). P = Paul (Patient-Researcher). End of project interview 03/06/2013.

## Portraits of transformation: *Attaching aesthetic resonance*

I define *aesthetic resonance* as a process of adding beauty, complexity and coherence, through layered meanings and symbolism within the mirroring and attunement process.

This project has shown that within the *revisioning* process the patients needed to recapture a sense of themselves as valuable and beautiful, as Broyard (1992, p.134) says… 'with the tubes and the weight loss, *I have to recapture myself and my beauty*. I have to *reinvent* myself'.

I suggest that attaching *aesthetic resonance* or 'beauty' to portraits and collages dealing with difficult feelings and events, whilst not taking away their painful significance, lends them a sense of 'hope' mitigating against the sense of despair felt in life-threatening and chronic illnesses. As art therapist Lachman-Chapin (1983, p.21) says of response art she made for an art therapy client, 'where Bob saw beauty in my work – it may represent something of my ideals, spirit, and hope'. Beauty is also described as a 'universal need of human beings', which 'brings consolation in sorrow and affirmation in joy', showing human life to be 'worthwhile' (Scruton 2012). There is also a sense of meaning in aesthetics, adding 'coherence' to something discordant. As Dissanayake says:

> Another way of looking at it is to recognize that meaning is aesthetic. Ordinary day-to-day life is formless, incoherent. When shaped and embellished or transformed as in ritual or play or art it takes on a greater or more significant reality so that when we find something to have coherence it seems to be 'aesthetic'. When we feel something to be aesthetic we recognize that it is coherent. (1980, p.404)

In Susan's *Saying Goodbye to the Sea* portrait (see Figure 6.17), metaphor and symbolism are utilised to mirror the disturbed feelings Susan felt as a child.

### Statement of Intention: *Saying Goodbye to the Sea*

Susan said: 'Paint me as a child stood saying goodbye to the sea, I would stand there and pretend to be Boudicca. My father was always happier when we were on holiday by the sea, and I always feared returning home, where my father's rages were uncontrolled.' Susan chose the Pre-Raphaelites, Joseph Wright and the painting *Morning* by the Newlyn School as stylistic references for the portrait.

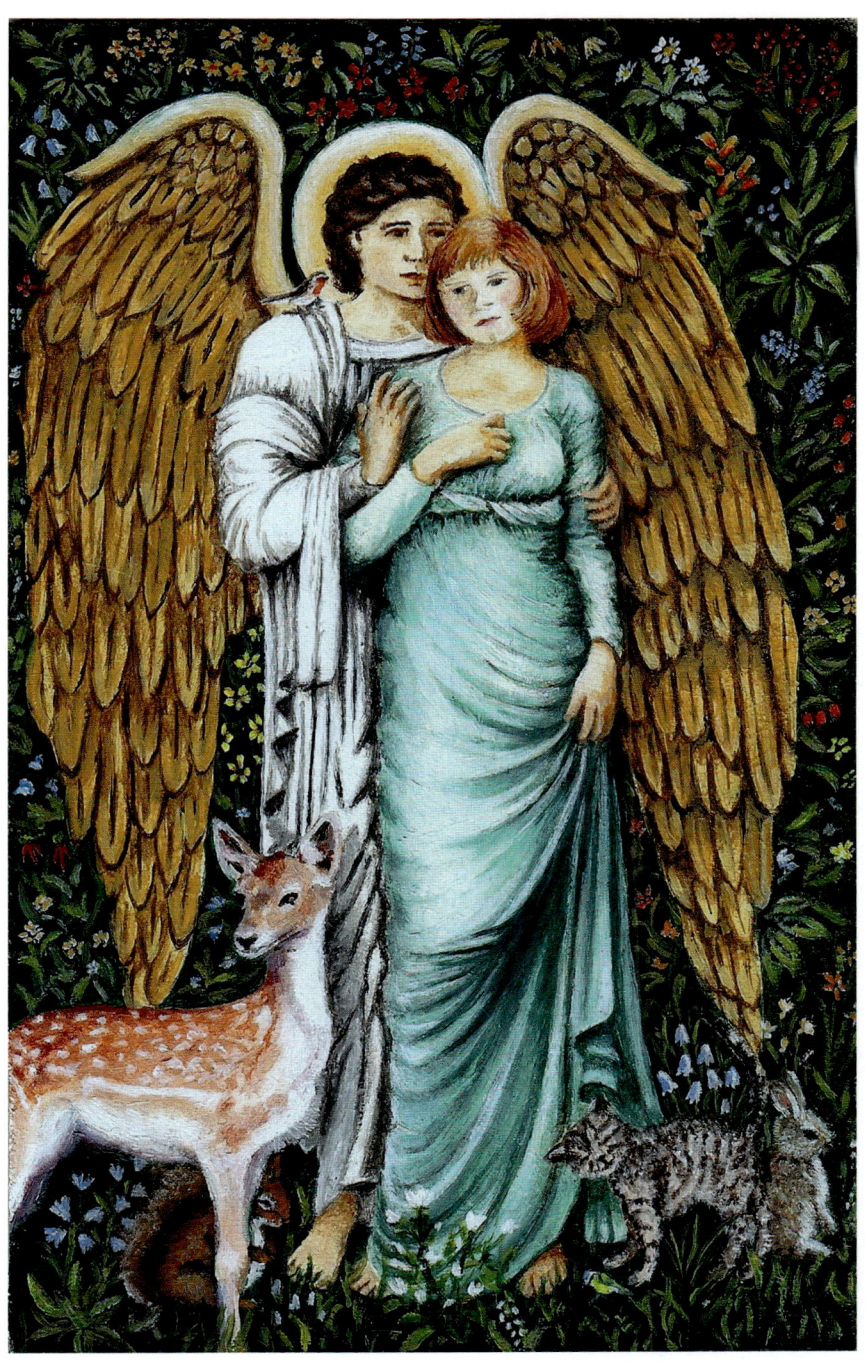

Coloured Plate i *Held by an Angel* by Susan Carr (co-designed by Hilary), 2011.

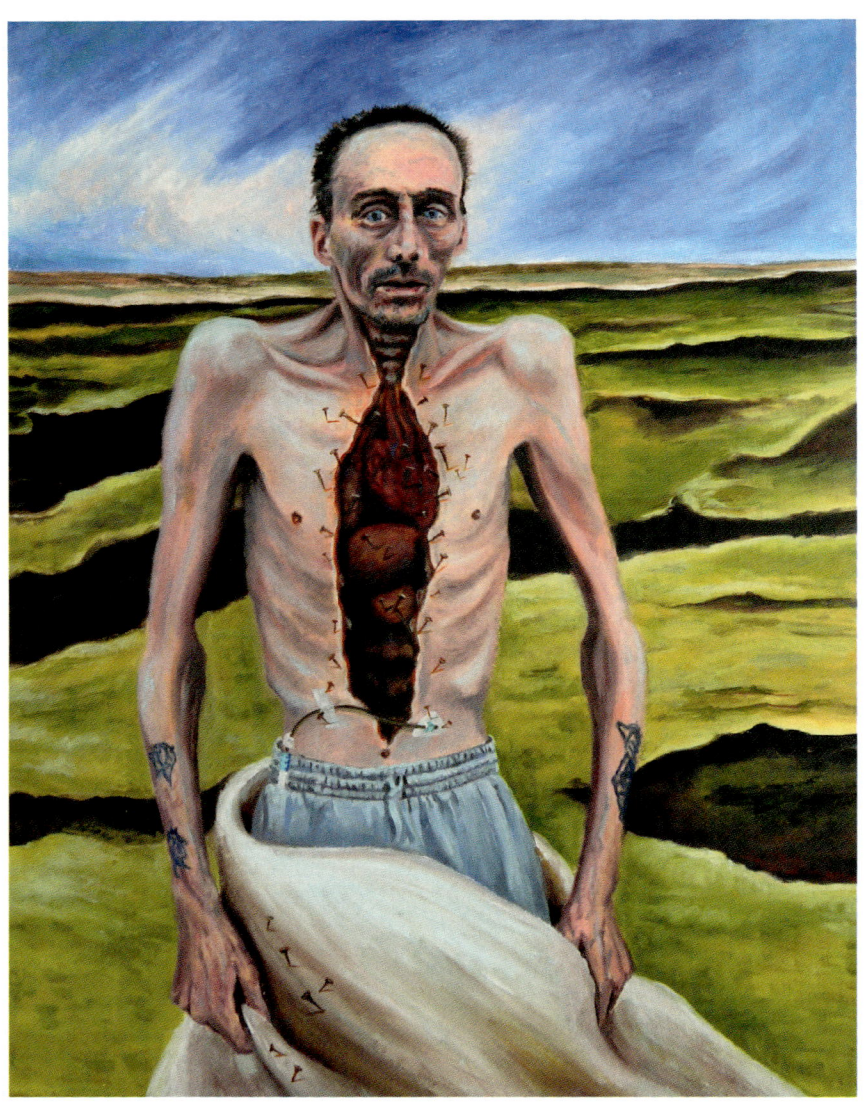

Coloured Plate ii *Broken Lungs* by Susan Carr (co-designed by Paul), 2013.

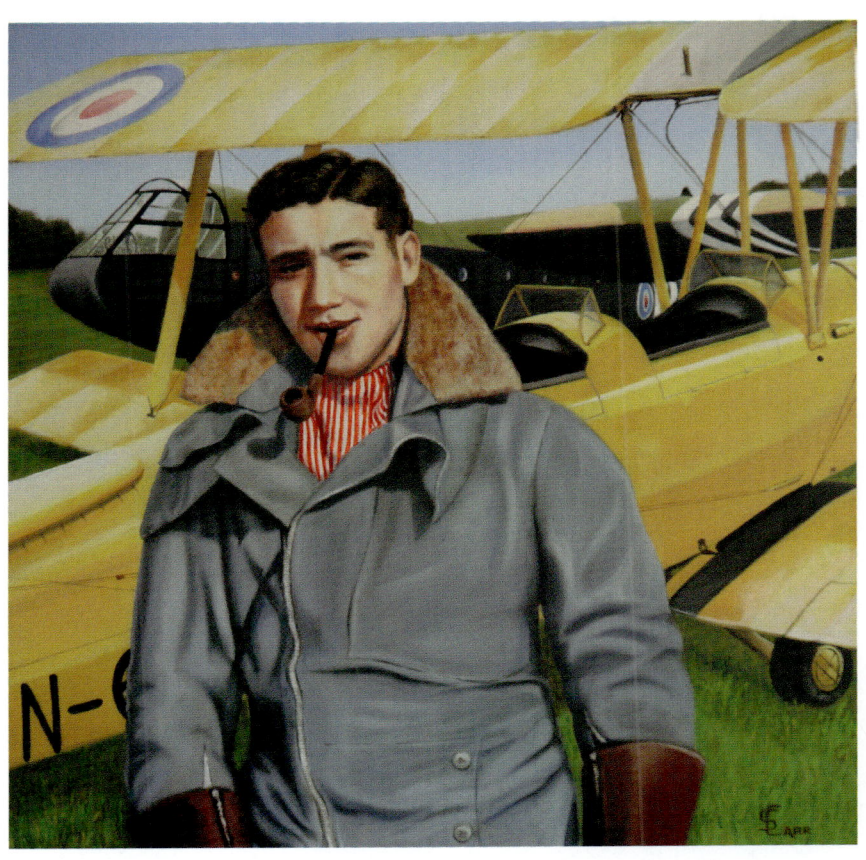

Coloured Plate iii *Flying Ace* by Susan Carr (co-designed by Bill), 2011.

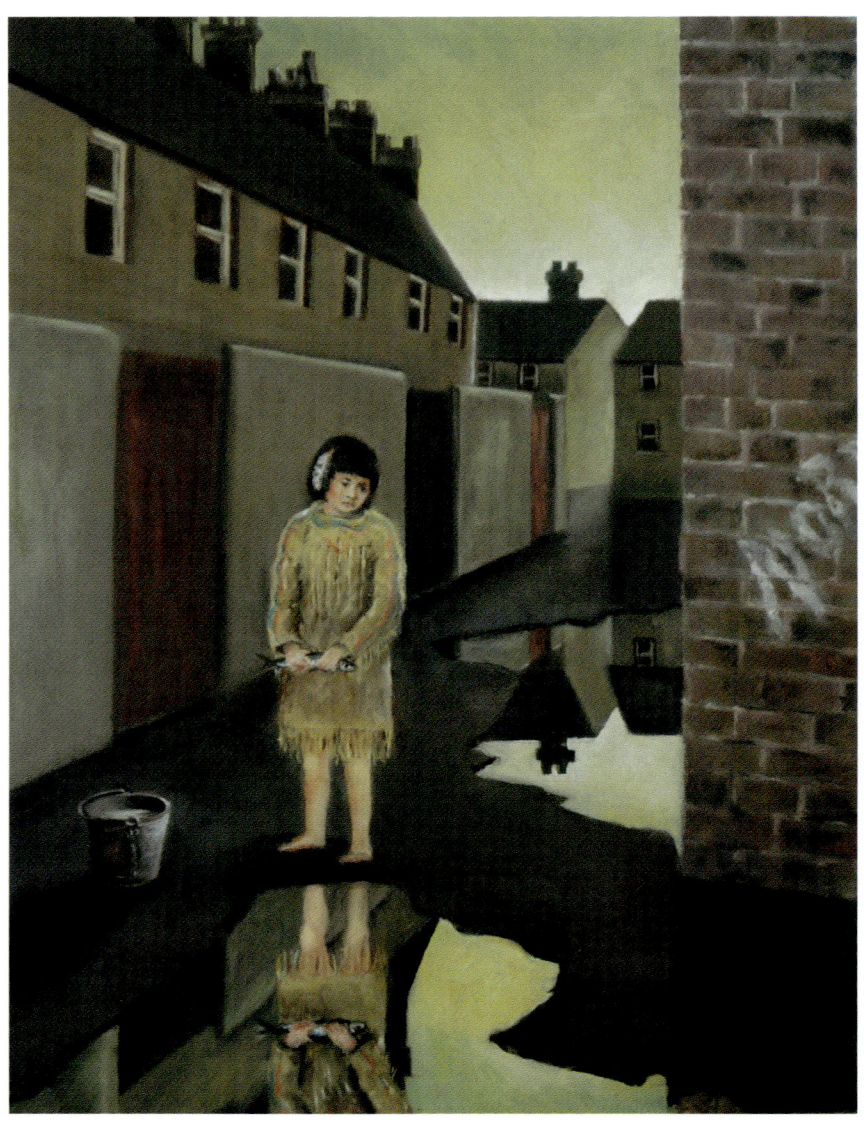

Coloured Plate iv *Fish Out of Water* by Susan Carr (co-designed by Norma), 2012.

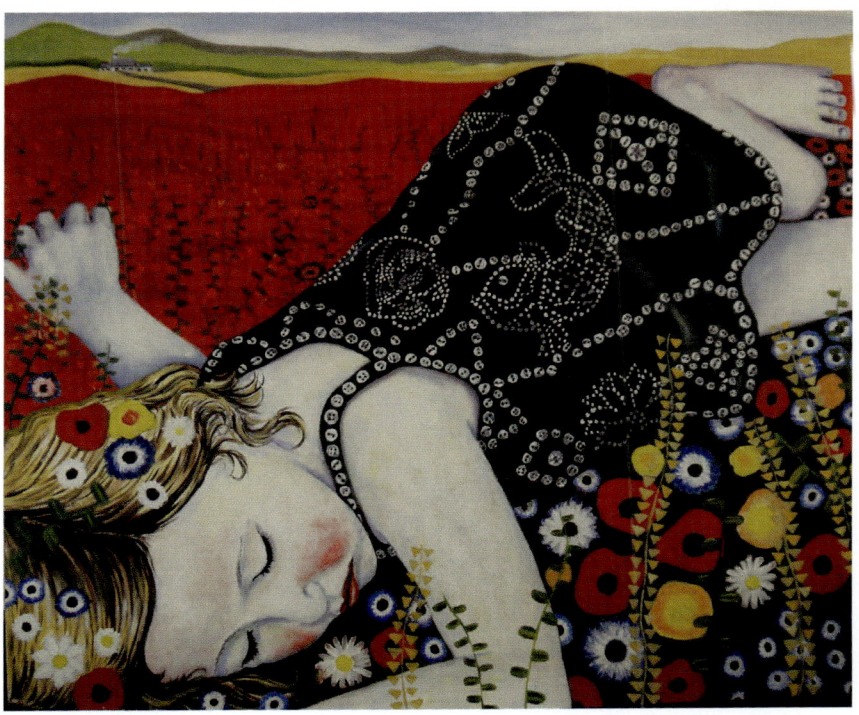

Coloured Plate v *The Poppy Field* by Susan Carr (co-designed by Rose), 2011.

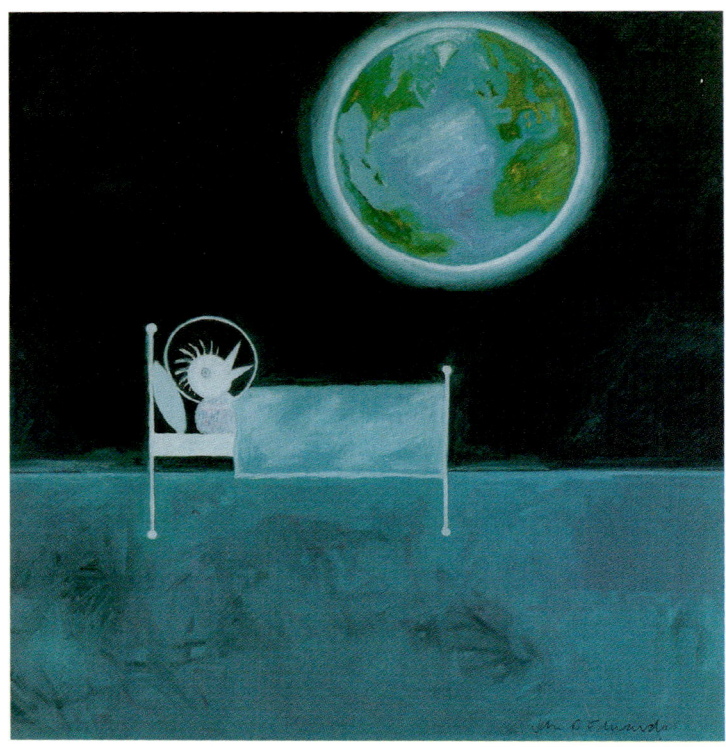

Coloured Plate vi *Out of This World* by John D. Edwards © 1999.

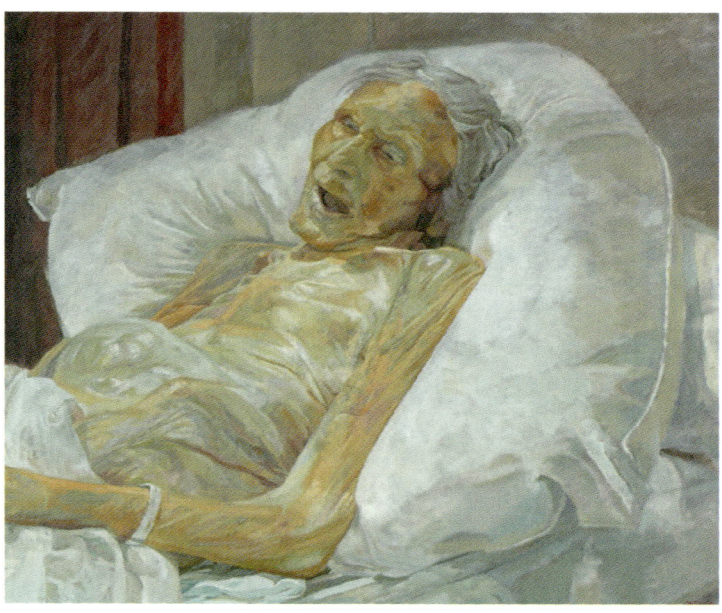

Coloured Plate vii *Last Portrait of Mother* by Daphne Todd © 2009.

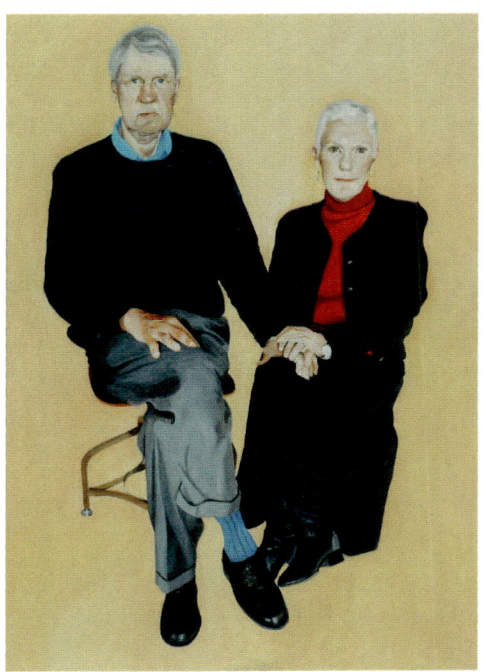

Coloured Plate viii *Robin and Mardi* by Mark Gilbert © 2007 (*Portraits of Care* Project).

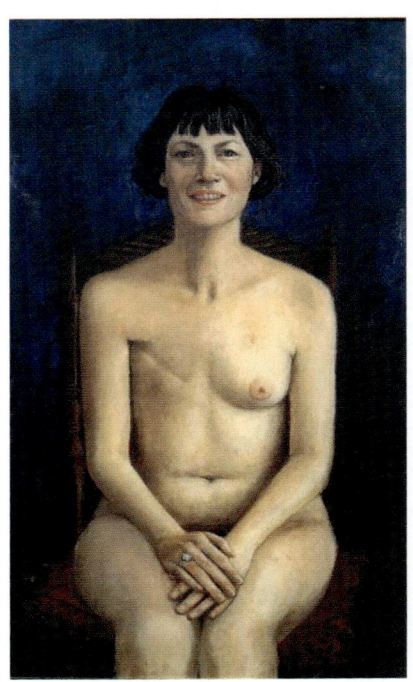

Coloured Plate ix *Evelyn* by Heath Rosselli © 1997.

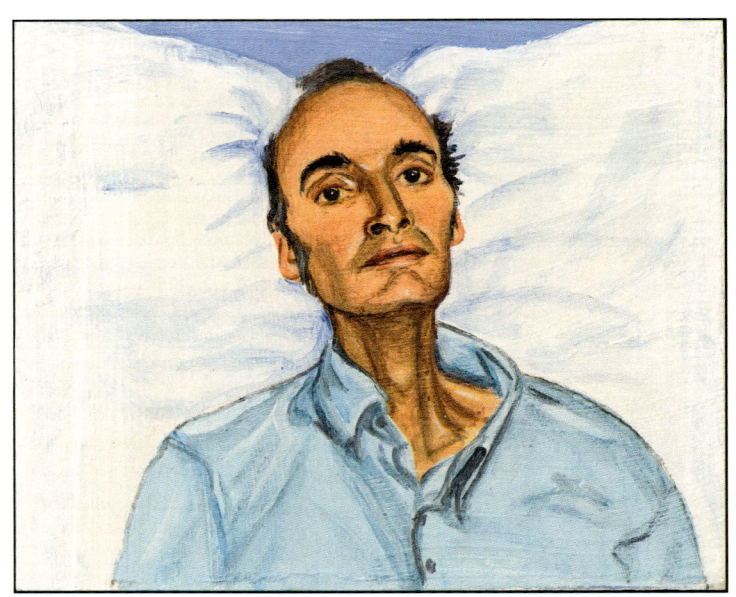

Coloured Plate x *Steve* by Antonia Rolls © 2007.

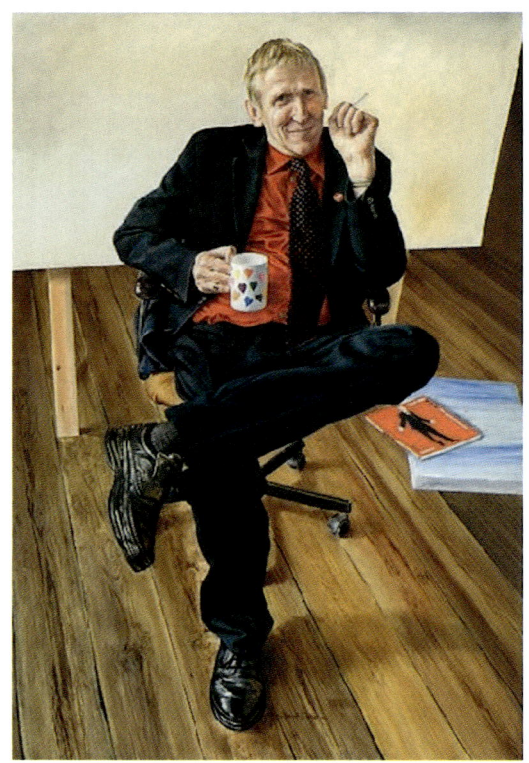

Coloured Plate xi *Dead Man Posing, Portrait of Philip Ledbury* by David Fisher © 2009.

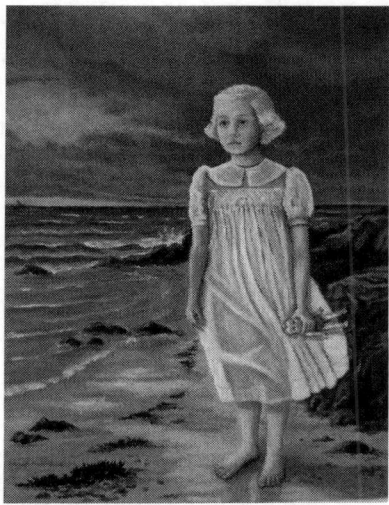

Figure 6.17 *Saying Goodbye to the Sea* by Susan Carr (co-designed by Susan), 2012.

In the visual analysis of this painting I identified these three aspects of Susan's self-identity...

Wild-Boudicca Child

Uncapturable-Mermaid Child

Idealised-Conforming Child

...and created the following essence statements:

**Statement of Emergent Knowing:** *Saying Goodbye to the Sea*
I stand strong and defiant facing the waves, shouldering the storm, safe inside my imagination. I long to stay by the sea, but must retain my idealised self through obedience and hide my true powerful self.

**Statement of Emergent Learning:** *Saying Goodbye to the Sea*
Susan fears returning to her childhood home, where her father's rage is uncontrolled. Staying by the sea would mean that the 'holiday spirit' continues, and the strangle hold on the doll's neck could be released.

By attaching 'beauty' as a metaphor for recovery and self-reclamation to this portrait, Susan is able to *revision* her remembrance of this difficult time, capturing again a sense of 'balance' and holding the dualities of hope and despair, enabling the development of a sense of *aesthetic resonance* and coherence.

> SC: You're changing that remembrance… [indicating *Saying Goodbye to the Sea*]
>
> S: Yes, definitely. I get all good feelings of this, you know. The sadness of saying goodbye to the sea is balanced by being there in the first place, you know, to be there and to be protected, but to be protected in a nice way, have things made for you and all the love that's implied in that.[15]

Rediscovering her lost child-self through the portraits and finding beauty within them was also important for Norma, as she possessed no photographs of herself as a baby or young child, saying that this part of her life was missing, and that any photographs she'd had were either lost or destroyed in a fire. The portraits of herself as a child may then equate to a *repossession* of her past child-self. Seymour (2002) suggests that 'by repossessing the past a person may abandon or rework an earlier life script: the "cleaned slate" may enable the person to reconstitute him or herself in a more purposeful manner' (Seymour 2002, p.239). Certainly, these portraits became significant in their ability to change meaning and add coherence through attaching *aesthetic resonance*. This is indicated in Norma's portrait of herself as a child, entitled *Lost* (Figure 6.18).

> SC: You have seen this one [*Lost* portrait] before, haven't you? …
>
> N: *Oh, it looks beautiful, looks lovely.* […] *Very sad, lost little girl. It's lovely.*[16]

---

15 SC = Susan (Artist-Therapist-Researcher). S = Susan (Patient-Researcher). End of project interview 19/10/2012.
16 SC = Susan (Artist-Therapist-Researcher). N = Norma (Patient-Researcher). End of project interview 26/09/2012.

# MIRRORING AND ATTUNEMENT THROUGH PORTRAITURE

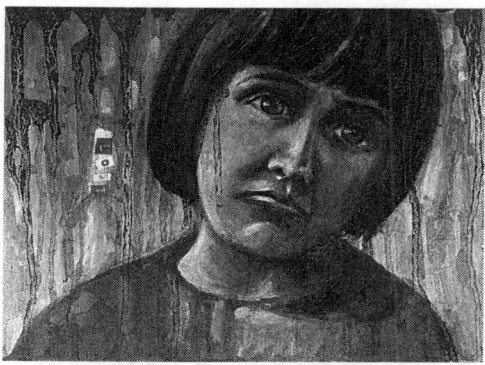

Figure 6.18 *Lost* by Susan Carr (co-designed by Norma), 2012.

Norma's first reaction to seeing the *Lost* portrait of herself as a child was to exclaim how 'beautiful' it is, how it 'looks lovely', that even though it is of a 'very sad, lost little girl' – it is still 'lovely'. This demonstrates how the meaning of the image is subtly changed, not in a way that romanticises illness or loss, as Norma still recognises herself as a 'sad lost little girl', but through validating the experience in a symbolic concrete form, to which *aesthetic resonance* can be added without losing the meaning behind the image.

This therefore added a sense of coherence to these difficult childhood memories, again a way of holding both 'hope and despair', something also evident within Norma's *A Fish Out of Water* portrait (see Figure 6.19).

> **Statement of Intention:** *A Fish Out of Water*
> Norma said, 'Paint me as a child growing up in the back streets of Aberdeen'.

This brief Statement of Intention perhaps reflected Norma's own lack of knowledge about her early years, and I reflected on how to progress with the portrait in Norma's active documentation sketchbook:

> **Notes from Norma's active documentation sketchbook 01/09/2012**
> I know Norma enjoys metaphor and symbolism within Native American artwork that she has shown to me, so I will try to use

this within the portrait. I want to somehow get a sense of Norma's early abandonment and disorientation, whilst also a sense of reconciliation and hope, perhaps of Norma 'finding' herself. Perhaps incorporating a bear into the portrait?

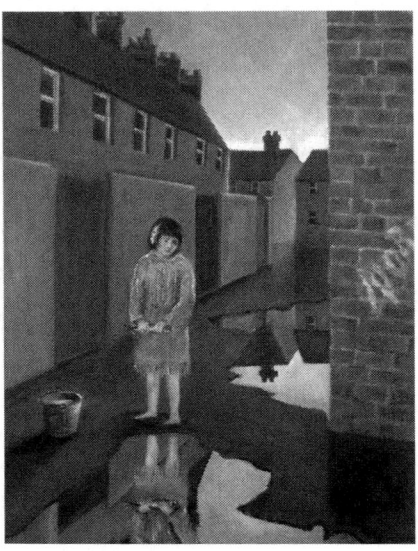

Figure 6.19 *Fish Out of Water* by Susan Carr (co-designed by Norma), 2012 (see also Coloured Plate iv).

Norma said:
I was a tomboy when I was a child
I would go out to play and kick off my shoes and socks
Returning home with black feet –
My Mother said I should be
A member of the black foot tribe –
Now I am…'North Bear'…

Within this portrait, Norma's difficult early life is represented in the yellow/greenish sky and the large puddles symbolising a 'storm', which has passed. The houses and the back alley within which Norma stands are 'empty' and lifeless, the walls are high and the windows are 'blank', the 'gates' have no handles, and no smoke billows from the chimneys, all of which speaks of Norma's early abandonment and lack of a secure attachment. A 'fish out of water' is also a metaphor for an 'unhomelike-being-in-the world' (Svenaeus 2011); however, the fish held by Norma is both 'out of the water', and also (within the puddle reflection) 'in the water'. This 'reflection' in the puddle also becomes the shape of a bear, 'North Bear', Norma's Native American Indian identity.

### Statement of Emergent Knowing: *Fish Out of Water*

Lost in the back streets of Aberdeen, searching for her true identity, a child stands, clinging to life, fighting for breath, transfixed by her own reflection.

### Statement of Emergent Learning: *Fish Out of Water*

Norma demonstrates her strength through stories of survival against the odds and reflects upon what might have been and might still be. Through seeing her reflection in the water, the small lost child finds herself as 'North Bear', a symbol of power and regeneration.

I was aware when painting this portrait that I wanted to add *aesthetic resonance*, not only by making the painting 'beautiful' but by making it *complex*, with multi-layered meanings and riddles, something I knew Norma enjoyed. In order for a sense of surprised recognition and for the symbolism and metaphor to work for Norma, I refrained from telling her what I had planned. Norma therefore really enjoyed the sense of personal discovery when looking at the portrait for the first time, and discovering the 'bear' hidden within the portrait:

N: There he is! [indicating the 'bear' in the puddle].

SC: Yes, there he is indeed, I didn't want to make him immediately obvious.

N: You haven't! That is brilliant.

SC: So, that's the reflection.

N: He's standing there with his paws out, like they do when they're up on their hind legs.

SC: Yes, and it's strange because that fish is *out of the water*, and that fish is *in the water* isn't it because it's in the puddle.

N: *And that's where Norma found North Bear!* [...] That's *beautiful!* It's really nice, so unusual. And it is very much like the backstreets of Aberdeen.[17]

Norma recognises the aesthetic, metaphoric attunement and coherence within the portrait when she says 'that is brilliant...that's beautiful!'

The ability of this portrait to capture Norma's: past and present, inner and outer, early and whole life experiences (characterised by the search for her self-identity) within one portrait, enabled a process of re-discovery, as she says... 'That's where Norma found North Bear!' This portrait therefore becomes for Norma a 'point of reference' within the uncertain landscape of her previous life and the ongoing uncertainty of her illness, something that exemplifies and yet *re-visions* these experiences. Through the addition of *aesthetic resonance* positive memories and connections are able to develop, changing subtly Norma's remembrance of her early life.

Within this section I have outlined a process of *aesthetic resonance*, adding meaning, complexity and coherence within the portraits, enabling patients to recapture a sense of themselves as valuable and beautiful. Susan and Norma were able to redefine childhood experiences and reclaim their child-selves, recognising the difficulties they faced, and enjoying the layered meanings and complexity added to the portrait through the process of attunement.

---

[17] SC = Susan (Artist-Therapist-Researcher). N = Norma (Patient-Researcher). End of project interview 26/09/2012.

— Chapter 7 —

# MAKING SPECIAL, MAKING MEANING

*Homelike-being-in-the-world and Ontological Security*

One of the central themes to emerge from researching portrait therapy was the way in which the painted portrait becomes a medium for making meaning, and that through the meaning-making process patients experience an increased sense of *ontological security* (Giddens 1991, p.38) and *homelike-being-in-the-world* (Svenaus 2011). Within this chapter I show how through the portraits, patients found an increased sense of *belonging*, *remembering* and *continuity*, linking and integrating aspects of *past*, *present* and *future* self-identities. I also describe the experience of portraits as *legacy*, and as an important part of a person's *future* self-identity, thereby equating to a sense of *immortalisation* or *cheating death*.

## Portraits making special, making meaning

Within an increasingly materialist and consumerist society 'the primacy of the body' has become the overriding belief about the 'self', coinciding with a change in belief systems from the dualist/religious belief in 'body and soul' to a reliance on 'scientific' explanations (Evans 2005b, pp.46–47). As Bauman (2004, p.75) says:

> All cultures we know of, at all times, tried, with mixed success, to bridge the gap between the brevity of moral life and the eternity of the universe. ... We are perhaps the first generation to enter life and live it without such a formula.

The dualist distinction between the soul and body gave people the comfort of believing that whilst their bodies may have been attacked by disease, their souls remained intact; however, for materialists 'they themselves become "a diseased body"' (Evans 2005b, p.46), and death becomes the final stripping away of all that constitutes self-identity. Despite this, in my experience of working with patients in palliative care, there is still a strong belief that human beings are 'more' than consciously aware bodies (ibid., p.49), and this is reflected in the eclectic range of religious and spiritual beliefs explored by the patients within their portraits.

The need to support patients' spirituality and meaning-making process has been identified as one of the key aspects of art therapy within palliative care (Balboni *et al.* 2007; Bell 2008; Puchalski *et al.* 2009; Waller and Sibbett 2005, p.xxviii), and portrait therapy, as a spiritual meaning-making practice within art therapy, has a lot to offer in its ability to support individual eclectic beliefs (Farelly-Hansen 2001). In my experience, severe illness often results in a natural drawing towards an eclectic myth making, as a form of self-made spirituality, and portrait therapy has been a way to facilitate this movement, with some of the portraits taking on aspects of religious icons and becoming 'containers' of spiritual experience.

The portraits have also enabled a reduction of patients' existential anxiety (Kierkegaard [1844] 1944), which is described as a form of stress pertaining to our freedom to act and therefore make decisions, and also a fear of the unknown. Existential anxiety can also equate with a fear of *annihilation* (Falk 2005), which is perhaps the most fundamental and primal anxiety human beings face and one that is brought to the fore in life-threatening and chronic illnesses. This underlines the deep human terror of helplessness, which Bauman suggests is contributed to by 'the terror of uncertainty' and 'the horror of the unknown' (Bauman 2004, p.72), which is exacerbated by the failure of science and reason to offer a sense of meaning in life-threatening and chronic illnesses. As Oliver Sacks says following his personal experience of severe illness:

> Science and reason could not talk of nothingness, of hell, of limbo; or of spiritual night. They had no place for absence, darkness, death. Yet these were the overwhelming realities of this time. ... And I turned to the mystics, and the Metaphysical poets too, for they also offered

both formulation and hope – poetic, aesthetic, metaphoric, symbolic, without the blunt plain commitment that 'religion' involved. (Sacks 1984, pp.89–90)

One of the ways *portrait therapy* helps increase a sense of meaning is through ritual and 'making special' (Dissanayake 1988). Through creating portraits, and bringing them into being in the *present*, they can be used in a ritualised way to develop meaning and feelings of homelike being-in-the-world and ontological security. The term 'ritual' is used here to represent the use of social or private behaviours or rites involving 'sacred or secular symbols' (Cohen 2002), which give 'significance to life passages' (Achterberg *et al.* 1994, p.3). Ritual is often at the forefront of 'formulating experience' and 'can permit knowledge of what would otherwise not be known at all' (Douglass 1966, p.64). Both rituals and portraits are 'bracketed' in that they are set apart from the ordinary and the mundane, are invested with meanings often hidden within heavy symbolism and metaphor, and significance that goes beyond the painted surface (Dissanayake 1995, p.20).

During the photo-elicitation stage of the project Norma, Susan and Rose described having searched for and found alternative spiritual beliefs, i.e. Native American Indian, Buddhist and Spiritualist beliefs respectively, and other patients talked about having no experience of personal religious or spiritual beliefs, e.g. Peter and Paul. In the collage entitled *I Don't Want to Just Disappear* (see Figure 7.1) Hilary explored her feelings of ontological *insecurity* indicating that her sense of ontological *security*, characterised by her religious faith, had been shaken by her illness and the recognition of 'being-towards-death' (Heidegger 1962 [1927]).

Despite constant disturbing images of death, both real and fictional, within popular culture, death is considered the last taboo (Kubler-Ross 1975), and there is in our Western culture an 'unspoken agreement' not to speak about our own death (Sibbett 2005a, p.69). However, without the development of a symbolic language, rich with metaphor and ritual, thoughts and feelings surrounding death cannot be integrated (ibid.).

In Chapter 5, I discussed how Hilary and I co-designed the *Held by an Angel* portrait (see Figure 5.4), and how this portrait became a manifestation of her increased ability to use her imagination. However, when reviewing Hilary's portraits, it seemed that *Held by an Angel* had a dual meaning, with the 'angel' offering 'holding' either in life or death. Luzzatto (2005, p.170) says that visual imagery enables the combination of conflicting symbols within the same painting, and that this combination of contradictory dualities is comforting for patients to see, providing a sense of balance.

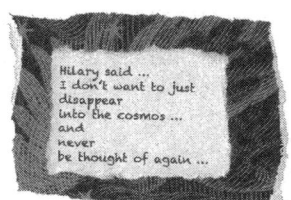
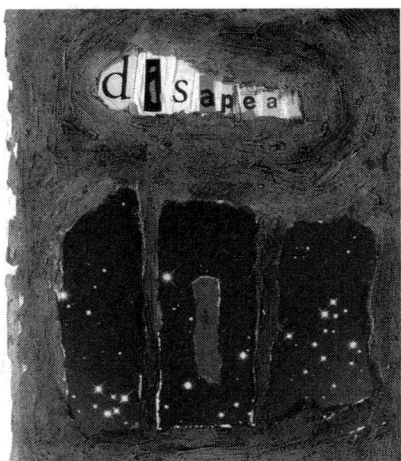

Figure 7.1 *I Don't Want to Just Disappear*, collage by Susan Carr, 2010.

During one of my visits to Hilary, and shortly after completing the portrait *Held by an Angel*, Hilary asked me to give her a photograph of it:

> ### Notes from Hilary's active documentation sketchbook 27/06/2011
> Today Hilary asked me if she could have a photograph of the *Held by an Angel* painting as she wanted to keep it with her at all times, saying if she went into hospital again she would take it with her so she could see it from her bed. I wondered if this image had become a kind of religious icon for Hilary, something invested with powers of protection or healing; physical, emotional and psychological?

The significance of Hilary's *Held by an Angel* portrait becomes manifest therefore in the way it was 'made special' (Dissanayake 1988) and invested with the resonance of a ritualised religious icon, serving as a constant reminder of *being held*, and a testimony to the care of Hilary's 'guardian angel'. The portrait also becomes a testimony of *my care*, and as a meaning-laden object, the portrait resonates with the remembered intersubjective co-designing process, the hours taken by me to paint it, and through this the worthwhileness of Hilary's *self* and *life* is suggested and confirmed, enabling Hilary to feel a sense of ontological security. This is perhaps why Hilary wanted a copy of the portrait to 'keep with her at all times'. (Peter also asked for small copies of his and Mark's portraits to 'keep with him at all times', placing them in his wallet.)

When I discussed Hilary's portraits (Figure 7.2) with my supervisor, he saw them as a reflection of Hilary's *past, present* and *future* self-identities.

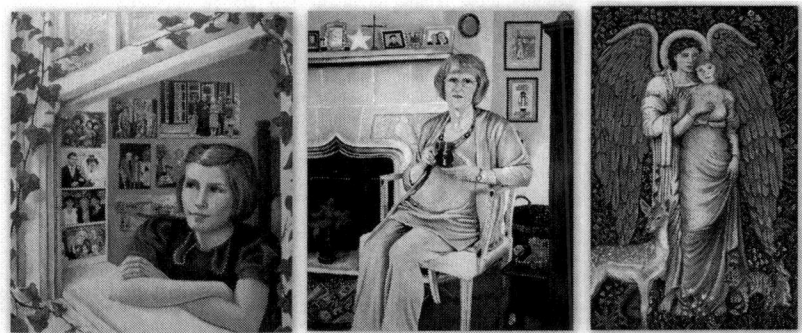

Figure 7.2 Montage of Hilary's three portraits: *The Window, The Heart of the Home*, and *Held by an Angel* by Susan Carr (co-designed by Hilary), 2011.

I reflected on this in Hilary's active documentation sketchbook.

## Notes from Hilary's active documentation sketchbook 01/03/2013

Today I took prints of all the portraits to show Alastair [my university supervisor], and discussed them with him. I was surprised when Alastair said that Hilary's portraits were the only ones which focused on the past, present and future self-identities. Alastair saw the 'past' identity being Hilary as a child in *The Window* portrait; the 'present' identity being *Heart of the Home*; and the 'future identity' being *Held by an Angel*. I had not thought of Hilary's portraits in this way before. In this logic, Alastair thought of the 'Held by an Angel' portrait as portraying Hilary's future 'deceased' identity, whilst I thought of it as Hilary being 'held' spiritually in the *present*?

The portrait as ritualised object, invested with spiritual meanings, is also highlighted within the smudging ceremony carried out by Norma to 'bless' and name the portrait-sculpture *My Baby/My Self* (Figure 5.16).

Norma and I co-designed the portrait-sculpture *My Baby/My Self*, as a way to transform the abandonment that Norma experienced as a baby, as well as to mourn the loss of seven of her own babies. When I was making the muslin 'baby', I was conscious of trying to make the 'baby' as realistic as possible; this included adding rice to the body, head and limbs to give it an authentic feel and weight (see Figure 7.3).

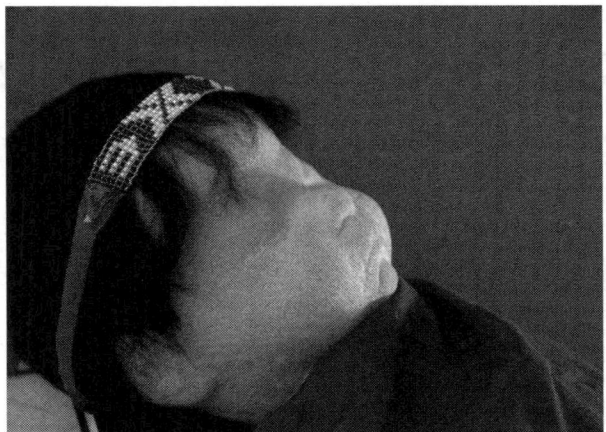

Figure 7.3 'Baby' detail from *My Baby/My Self* by Susan Carr and Norma, 2012.

I remember when I made *Unwelcome Contradictions* (see Figure 5.15) I did not do this, and the 'baby' felt too light and unrealistic when held. However, I did wonder if I had made the 'baby' *too* realistic and before the smudging ceremony I felt I had to warn Norma about how realistic the 'baby' seemed when held. I noticed a distinct change in Norma's demeanour when holding the 'baby' and how easily she assumed the 'caring mother role', gently and reverently holding, rocking and stroking the 'baby'. Norma used a shawl that was special to her to wrap the 'baby' in, adding a sense of continuity and connection and homelikeness, as Norma explains in her end of project interview:

SC: Good, and so next week, hopefully we'll do the smudging ceremony and I'll bring the baby so we'll…

N: Smudge her.

SC: And dress her and…

N: And then put her into the… [cradleboard] … I've got something that I'm going to wrap her in that has come from my great grandmother and it was hand made. So, the baby will be wrapped in that. It will be used this one last time by me, to wrap my seven babies in. Because they were all in it, even my little girl, even though she passed away, I still wrapped her up in it, so there is a part of her in it, because every child that has been wrapped in it has left something into it. *It's made it special.* There's a part of every child in it who was wrapped in it.

SC: Ah, that's lovely.

N: So, that is quite a precious little gift, and it's coming to the exhibition for you. To wrap the little baby in, to wrap my seven babies in.[1]

Although Norma refers to the baby as 'her' (i.e. female) – Norma has lost *male* as well as *female* babies, so perhaps by referring to the baby as 'her' she was focusing on *herself* as an abandoned baby 'now found'. Norma demonstrates her understanding of the process of 'making special' when she talks about her great-grandmother's shawl, and there also seems to be a real sense of 'wrapping herself' as an abandoned baby in the shawl, doing what her mother didn't do when she was born, using the action of 'wrapping' to contain her grief and physically enable feelings of 'closure'. I reflected on the smudging ceremony experience in the active documentation sketchbook.

### Notes from Norma's active documentation sketchbook 19/09/2012

Norma carried out the smudging ceremony in the hospice grounds today. We wrapped the 'baby' and then placed her in the cradleboard, and went out into the garden. It was a lovely clear day. Norma burnt a special bundle of twigs that she had been sent

---

[1] SC = Susan (Artist-Therapist-Researcher). N = Norma (Patient-Researcher). End of project interview 26/09/2012.

from a Shaman in America (a member of her NAI tribe), wafting the smoke over herself, the baby and myself, and naming the baby 'Little Feather'. This was a moving ceremony, and highlighted the importance of being able to 'do' something again for her babies and for herself, even for myself and the baby I lost. I felt humbled by the experience. There was something about being 'mothers' together, who knew how to heal…making something special and meaningful out of something painful.

These sentiments also correlate with the essence statements for *My Baby/My Self*:

### Statement of Emergent Knowing: *My Baby/My Self*

A fragile baby endlessly sleeping, held securely, cared for and wanted, wrapped up with love. Precious riches adorn, laboriously made, for this world or the next?

### Statement of Emergent Learning: *My Baby/My Self*

A baby reunited with a spiritual family, lost babies and the mother identity mourned, as Norma becomes wise woman/elder.

### Statement of Reflexive Resonance: *My Baby/My Self*

The loss of my own baby halfway through a pregnancy meant that I was able to empathise with Norma in her mourning, and enter into the smudging ceremony as one who understands the depths of her despair and the value of art in healing all wounds. Making the baby portrait-sculpture was a therapeutic process both for Norma and myself. Together we became wise, understanding the need for ritual and grace in death and grief.

By creating the baby layette and cradleboard and facilitating the smudging ceremony, Norma was able to give her abandoned baby/self, and her lost babies, the love and care that would have been offered within the Native American Indian spiritual tradition, allowing a sense of closure on painful episodes in her life, and connection to her new spiritual beliefs. Norma was able to physically *do* something for her *self* and her lost babies, something that linked her present Native American Indian identity, with that of her past (Scottish) identity. Norma engaged in a process of 'liminal play' involving ritual objects, enabling change to happen through 'performing symbolic actions' and 'manipulating symbolic objects' (Turner 1982, p.32).

In a contemporaneous portrait of herself (Figure 7.4) Norma asked to be portrayed as the *wise woman/elder* of her Black Foot clan, stood by a lake in the wilds of North America. By placing herself in a landscape she has longed to be in (but due to her illness never has), the portrait is imbibed with all the spiritual significance of Norma being there in reality. It literally took Norma out of her 'liminal space' and placed her where she could feel a sense of homelike-being-in-the-world.

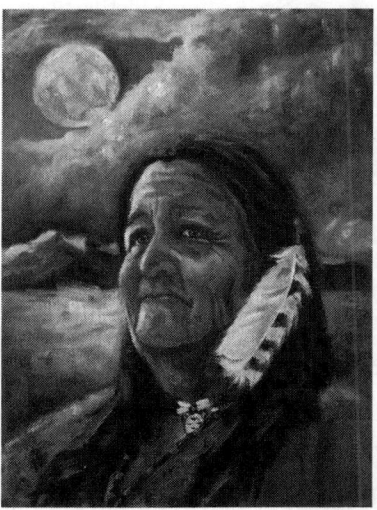

Figure 7.4 *North Bear* by Susan Carr (co-designed by Norma), 2012.

*North Bear* portrays Norma within the land of her adoptive ancestors, in a spiritual space, which acts as confirmation of her Native American Indian identity, one that she can 'show' to others. Norma adds her own significance to the portrait by *seeing* 'bears' within the sea, clouds and moon, something she will enjoy asking others if they can 'see':

N:  I can see part of a bear…can you see where?

SC: [long pause] I don't know really.

N:  It's not a brown bear,

SC: A white bear? You'll have to show me.

N: There's the head of a polar bear.

SC: Oh, is there? Hmmm.

N: If you look really hard, you can see his body just under the water.

SC: Oh, ok. Well, I'm glad there is a bear.

N: But he's not obvious.

SC: He's not obvious, no.

N: And *if you're not looking for a bear, you won't find him*. If you look, you can just see the head about the water. It's a very abstract bear, but you can still see him. If you look at the shadow of the water there, there's a bear and that looks like his leg.

SC: Oh, yes, I can see that now.

N: *And you did it without trying!*

SC: I did yes, that's true. Yes, it just appeared.

N: And there's another bear, I just noticed.

SC: Is there? Where's that then?

N: There's his head.

SC: Oh, yes, it could be...[2]

In this exchange, I felt chastised by Norma for being unable to 'see' the 'bears' she could see, wanting confirmation that the 'bears' had just 'appeared' within the portrait without my consciously putting them there, saying 'and you did it without trying!' There was a sense in Norma that the spiritual (i.e. the 'bears') would find their way into the present through the portraits, and my *intuitive knowing*, without being *told*, was very important to Norma throughout her involvement in this project. I believe this underlined a need in Norma *to be known* on a spiritual level, something that my *attunement* within the portraits depicted in a concrete way, allowing Norma to reflect on and find joy in rediscovering her*self*.

---

2  SC = Susan (Artist-Therapist-Researcher). N = Norma (Patient-Researcher). End of project interview 26/09/2012.

In this section I have described how patients used the portraits and portrait-sculptures in ritualistic and sacralising ways, and how these processes enabled feelings of homelike-being-in-the-world. Hilary and Peter demonstrated the value of the portraits to them through asking for small reproductions to 'keep with them at all times'. Norma used the project to grieve for her abandoned baby-self as well as her own lost babies, bringing her past into the present to be engaged with in the ritualised practices of the Native American Indian smudging ceremony. Norma's final portrait of herself as North Bear, situated within the wilds of North America, depicted a longed-for spiritual experience of *homelike-being-in-the-world*. The portraits therefore enabled the development of ritualistic behaviour, which is tied to the patient's own sense of being and self-worth and the development of new meanings and new ways of *being known*.

## Portraits of belonging and remembering: Linking past, present and future self-identities

All the patients to some extent utilised portrait therapy to connect to something or people they felt a sense of *belonging* to, acting as a bridge to significant others, and a way of connecting to humanity as a whole, or to reaffirm identity 'frames' (Taylor 1989) that patients have belonged to in the past. As Kinnvall (2004, p.742) says, 'As individuals feel vulnerable and experience existential anxiety, it is not uncommon for them to wish to reaffirm a threatened self-identity. Any collective identity that can provide such security is a potential pole of attraction.' This sense of belonging to a collective identity enables feelings of *being part of something larger than themselves*. One of civilisation's earliest self-identity 'frames', and one that is to some extent still prevalent today, is the 'honour ethic' as described by Taylor (1989). This is characterised by the warrior or citizen soldier, who fights for his/her country, as 'to be ready to hazard one's tranquillity, wealth, even life for glory is the mark of a real man' (ibid., p.20). This 'warrior' is therefore deemed to be a person of a higher order than one dedicated to purely economic and peaceful pursuits (ibid.).

The 'warrior' self-identity frame was particularly evident within Bill's portraits. When I began to work with Bill it became very clear that the area of his self-identity he wished to portray through the portraits was that encapsulated by his experiences as a glider pilot in the Second World War. Over the eight months we worked together Bill related his war experience and we co-designed 16 collages and prose poems as response art, and I painted four portraits, all reflecting back these stories of heroism, fear, pain, suffering, brotherhood and loss. In the active documentation sketchbook, I noted the transient thoughts and feelings engendered through listening to, and being with, Bill.

### Notes from Bill's active documentation sketchbook 02/08/2011

Spent time with Bill today talking about his WWII experiences. He told me about how he was shot in the chest and while waiting on a stretcher on the back of a Jeep the enemy opened fire, and he rolled off the back of the Jeep to avoid getting shot again. He said he fell onto his ammo cartridge and broke three of his ribs into the bargain. Bill took my hand and pressed it into the scar in his chest – saying, 'Feel that!' I felt the 'hole' in his ribs where the enemy bullet had struck, and imagined Bill as a young man – lying wounded by the side of the road in Arnhem, in pain and probably full of fear. Afterwards unbuttoning his shirt, he said 'Look, here's the scar where the bullet entered.' Bill said that he thought he was going to die as he lay there wounded – blood filling his lungs – he thought he would drown in his own blood. Through the power of touch and sight I was able to feel Bill's wound and acknowledge his pain and his bravery. I felt Bill showing me this was a direct and visual way to convey the authenticity of his war stories and his suffering. The scar becoming a 'badge' of authenticity?

I wondered about the significance of being present with Bill and witnessing stories of his wartime self-identity, and if this intersubjective relationship might help to mitigate some of the feelings of 'aloneness' he'd felt at the time.

### Notes from Bill's active documentation sketchbook 02/08/2011

As Bill told me of his war experiences he continued to hold on to my hand. And while I sat there, I was aware that even though Bill is now 91 years old, in that moment I was holding the hand of the young wounded Bill, a young man who had a few hours earlier courageously carried an injured soldier through gunfire to safety. This too was the young injured man thrown on a train and sent to a POW camp, alone and afraid, thinking that he would die. It was a very moving experience and I wondered if, by being present with Bill now, by holding his hand as he relived those experiences, that this might help to mitigate the feelings of aloneness he must have felt at the time.

As mentioned in Chapter 5, Bill always added a twist of humour even to the most harrowing of tales. In the collage, *Bill's Gunga Din* (Figure 7.5), Bill talks about one of the German orderlies on the train offering him a moment of compassion and kindness as he lay injured and dehydrated. When relating this story, Bill launched spontaneously into his own wonderful interpretation of the poem 'Gunga Din' by Rudyard Kipling (1892).

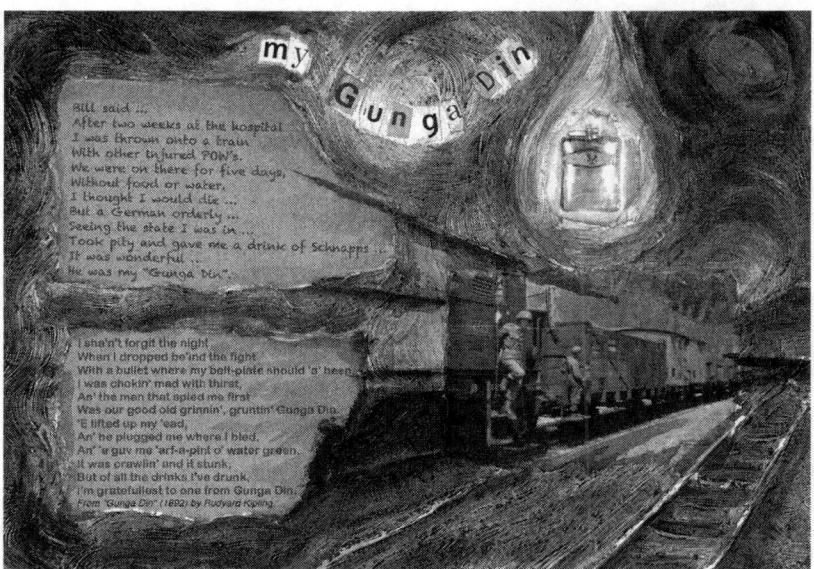

Figure 7.5 *Bill's Gunga Din* by Susan Carr, 2012.

Remembering the sacrifice of his fellow servicemen was a constant theme throughout the collages and prose poems I created for Bill. In Figure 7.6, Bill remembers one young man's personal sacrifice.

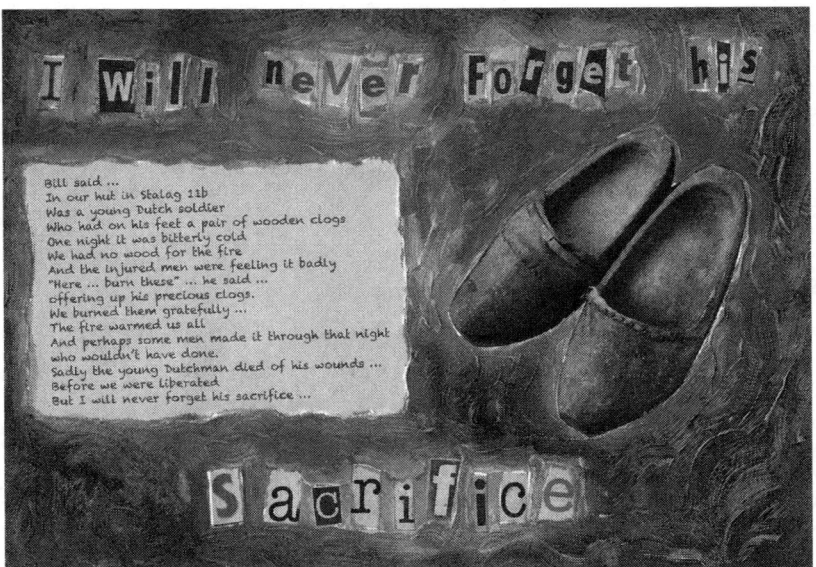

Figure 7.6 *Sacrifice* by Susan Carr, 2012.

I was concerned initially that Bill's preoccupation with his war experiences may have been a way to avoid talking about his present sense of self-identity and a denial of his illness. However, it occurred to me that Bill's present self-identity, which he described as 'the old man', did not even begin to express the self-identity that Bill identified with most strongly, and that ultimately the war experiences, related by Bill, expressed everything he needed to tell me about his self-identity. It told me his values, his concerns, his sense of belonging and brotherhood, it told me what he would and wouldn't do, in short Bill told me 'who' he was, in a way that relating stories of his present self-identity never could. It was the period in Bill's life where his self-identity was *formed* and *broken* and *reformed*, the scars I saw, and felt, were his *badge of membership* (Anzieu 1989) to the veteran brotherhood, an evidence of visible mending, lending an indisputable authenticity to his stories (Anzieu 1989). I wonder therefore if the propensity for older adults to 'talk about the past' is less about a lack of memory of the present, and more to do with maintaining and reaffirming past self-identities, and as such should be considered a vital aspect of psychological and emotional support, and identity work. In Hogan and Warren's (2012) study older women were given the opportunity to depict themselves in ways that challenged the stigmatised view of aging, and some chose images displaying themselves in ways that expressed *youthful exuberance* despite their age, which correlates with Bill's desire to be portrayed as a healthy and vital young man.

When reviewing the three initial portraits I painted for Bill (Figure 7.7), I was concerned that I may have unconsciously *aestheticised* or *romanticised* Bill's war experiences.

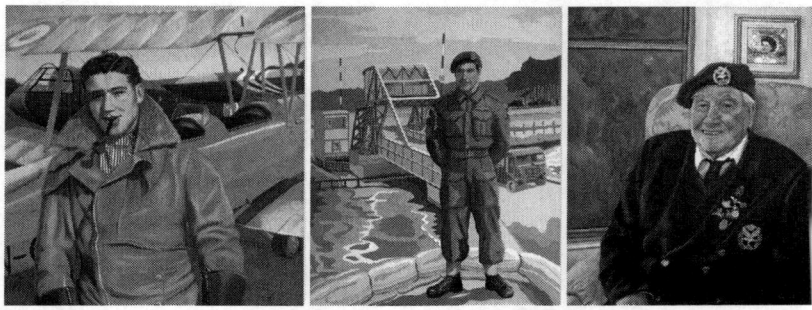

Figure 7.7 Montage of Bill's first three portraits: *The Flying Ace, Pegasus Bridge* and *The Veteran* by Susan Carr (co-designed by Bill), 2011.

### Notes from Bill's active documentation sketchbook 08/12/2011

I was reflecting on Bill's paintings today and wondered if I had unconsciously romanticised or underplayed the horror of his war experiences, in *Flying Ace* and *Pegasus Bridge*. I think that I need to paint a final portrait which goes some way to expressing the horrors of war, not in a 'dangling a dead rat' sense, and perhaps it can even be 'beautiful' but something that recognises Bill's heroism, and the risks he took to serve his country?

At our next portrait session, I discussed with Bill the idea of painting a final portrait, set within a battle scene, based on the collage of Bill's experience of being 'mentioned in despatches' (Figure 7.8).

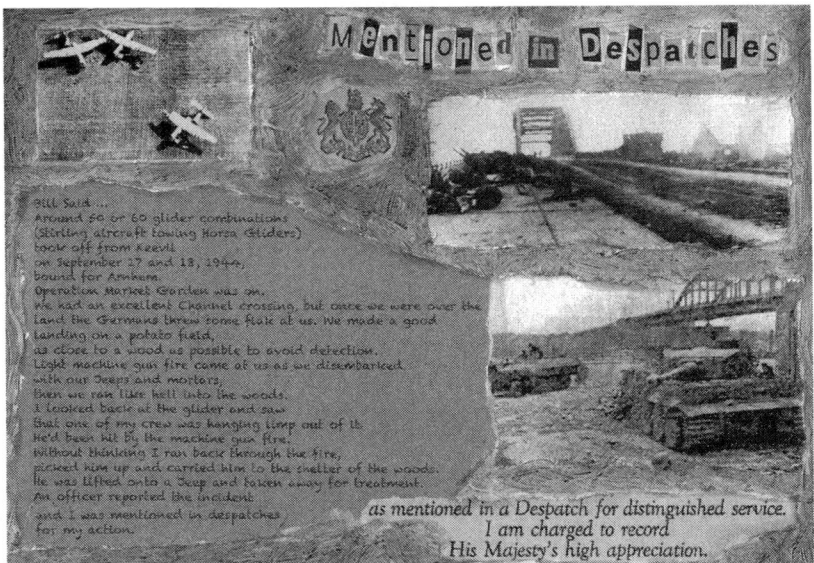

Figure 7.8 *Mentioned in Despatches*, collage by Susan Carr, 2012.

I was conscious of attempting to portray in the resulting portrait *Mentioned in Despatches* (Figure 7.9) the lived experience of action and confusion in a battlefield, and the moment that Bill rescued the injured soldier. I used the paintings of former First World War artist and art therapy pioneer Adrian Hill for reference and inspiration.

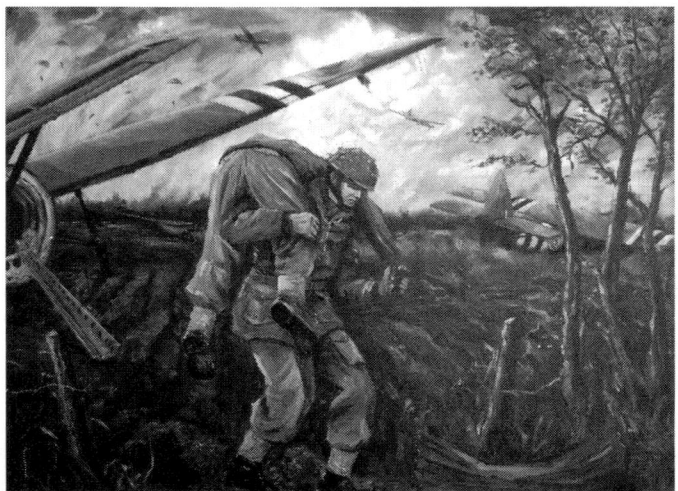

Figure 7.9 *Mentioned in Despatches* by Susan Carr (co-designed by Bill), 2011.

All Bill's portraits seemed to reflect the theme of *belonging* and *remembering* and this is highlighted in Bill's end of project interview:

> SC: So how do you feel about the fact that these portraits will go into an exhibition and be seen by lots of people?
>
> B: Well I shall be pleased because…I tell you what…the Glider Pilot Regiment was the biggest airborne regiment in the War and yet very little is said about it you know, I don't know why…it was a big operation, there were thousands of gliders in it…a big operation. *But I like people to know what it was…I like to be attached to what it was…*[3]

Like Bill, Rose was keen for her portraits to reflect her sense of belonging to something she perceived as 'greater' than herself, and this is explored in her *Bohemian Rhapsody* portrait (Figure 7.10). The prose poem that accompanied this portrait outlined Rose's identification with Freddie Mercury:

> Rose said:
> Paint me like Freddie Mercury
> In Bohemian Rhapsody
> Strong and defiant…
> I'll wear his rings…I have copies you know
> And a rose in my garden named after him,
> Roses are sparky, Like me…
> Like I've had to become
> To survive the uncertainty…
> I used to visit Freddie's house every year
> A kind of pilgrimage
> To read the messages on the wall
> To light a candle…
> Now it's all gone…there is nothing there
> People complained it was too untidy…
> But then life is untidy…
> And I have learned
> Not to complain…but to live…

---

3   SC = Susan (Artist-Therapist-Researcher). B = Bill (Patient-Researcher). End of project interview 24/04/2012.

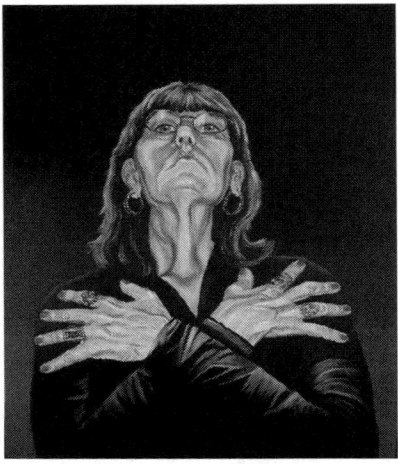

Figure 7.10 *Bohemian Rhapsody* by Susan Carr (co-designed by Rose), 2011.

When I first visited Rose's home it was immediately obvious that she was a fan of Freddie Mercury, as on almost every surface of her lounge there was a picture or reminder of him. Therefore, Rose's request to be painted as Freddie wasn't a great surprise, although her choice of the iconic Bohemian Rhapsody pose was. I arranged with Rose to take some reference photographs for the portrait and Rose dressed for the part, wearing a similar outfit to Freddie's and replica rings for the session. On seeing the photographs I was slightly shocked by the 'corpse like' pose, and Rose also had reservations that she did not reveal at the time, but discussed later in the end of project interview:

SC: Ok…that's great. So, looking at the paintings now, is there anything you would change about them?

R: No… No…

SC: That's good…

R: I was a bit bothered about that to start with [indicating *Bohemian Rhapsody* portrait] when I saw the [reference] photographs.

SC: Bothered about it?

R: Yeah, I thought 'oh dear I don't like that', but the painting has changed it completely, *I like it now.*

SC: I think it has a real strength to it…

R: It's got that...

SC: A real strength...that is in you...

R: ...and determination.

SC: Yes, determination.

R: *That's determined!* [Indicating *Bohemian Rhapsody* portrait][4]

The sense of belonging that Rose felt through aligning herself with her idol, Freddie, was outlined within the essence statements created in the visual analysis process:

> **Statement of Emergent Learning:** *Bohemian Rhapsody*
> In posing as her musical idol Freddie Mercury, Rose is demonstrating her solidarity and identification with him and his suffering, and also her own personal strength, courage and determination to keep on fighting to the end.

Historically the people painted in portraits were of high social status, either the 'great and the good' or the very wealthy, who through their deeds demand our respect, implying that 'their life and integrity is sacred or enjoys immunity, and is not to be attacked' (Taylor 1989, p.25). Through aligning herself with her idol, Rose not only becomes Freddie in that moment, and all he means to her in the way of stardom and celebrity, but also acknowledges the solidarity Rose feels around them both being diagnosed with terminal illnesses and therefore both dwellers of 'liminal' space (Sibbett 2004, 2005a; Turner 1969 [1995]).

The theme of belonging and remembering was also evident in Paul's *English Gothic* portrait (Figure 7.11), where he asked to be portrayed with the three people he had been closest to in his life, these were his grandmother, grandfather and Uncle. Paul's grandfather ran a farm and so it is with this farming community and family that Paul aligns himself, selecting the painting *American Gothic* by Grant Wood (1930) as reference for the portrait, which reflects a sense of homelike-being-

---

4  SC = Susan (Artist-Therapist-Researcher). R= 'Rose' (Patient-Researcher). End of project interview 27/03/2011.

in-the-world. In Paul's active documentation sketchbook, I noted our first discussion around this portrait:

> ### Notes from Paul's active documentation sketchbook 08/10/2012
> Today in our first session I talked to Paul about the project and we discussed how we could incorporate people and things that mean the most to him or reflect his sense of self-identity. Paul said that the three people he had been closest to in life had died, and these were his grandparents and his uncle, who he said was more like a brother to him, being a similar age. Paul became emotional when telling me this, a rare slip of the jovial laid back mask I normally see, and with Paul's show of emotion I also felt moved. I was also acutely aware of a sense of isolation and vulnerability surrounding Paul in his alone-ness, and I wondered if anyone has ever really *known* Paul?

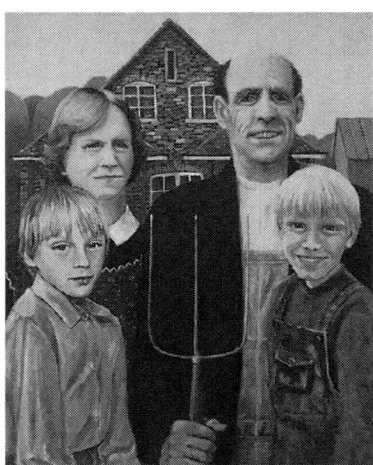

Figure 7.11 *English Gothic* by Susan Carr (co-designed by Paul), 2013.

### Statement of Emergent Knowing: *English Gothic*
> A farming family pose in front of their homestead, steeped in traditional values, growing food for humanity, unafraid of hard work. Calloused hands wield a pitchfork, protecting family bonds...reunited.

### Statement of Emergent Learning: *English Gothic*

Paul identifies with his hardworking farmer grandparents and relations in this painting, remembering the shared experience of working on the farm...worthwhile work, communing with nature and surrounded by family who valued him and his contribution.

Through Paul associating himself with a former autonomous self-identity that contributed positively to society and family, his feelings of self-worth were enhanced and affirmed.

Returning to the past through imagination or symbolic reconstruction, through the portrait, may have been an attempt by Paul to recreate his lost sense of security (Kinnvall 2004, p.744), and increase his sense of belonging. Even if that sense of belonging is part of a *past* identity, through the portraits, it is brought back to the *present*, it is *re-membered*, *re-lived* and *re-integrated*, and thereby invested with a new sense of meaning.

Whilst a sense of belonging is suggested within *English Gothic*, it also symbolises being-towards-death, as, although Paul is portrayed with the three people he was closest to in his life, all except Paul are deceased. Paul literally puts himself in the company of the dead – suggesting that his own death will be a kind of homecoming. When viewed from this perspective this portrait becomes a holder of multiple dualities, of life and death, hope and despair, past and future, belonging and separation, and Paul is able to explore his own forthcoming death, through exploring and coming to terms with the death of those closest to him.

The sense that portraits are able to hold dualities correlates with Susan's experience of co-designing and seeing the portrait-sculpture *The Paper Dress* (Figure 7.12).

### Statement of Intention: *The Paper Dress, Stitching Words Together*

Susan said that as a child her mother had made all her clothes, a favourite had been a little dress with heart shaped pockets. Susan said that she had inherited none of her mother's skills with a needle and was a writer instead. We decided to use photocopies of pages from an academic book Susan had written, and photographs of herself as a child, to make a full-sized paper replica of the child's 'dress with the heart shaped pockets'. This was to acknowledge that Susan's mother 'stitched fabric together' and Susan 'stitched words together', linking them both through *The Paper Dress* with the heart shaped pockets.

The use of needle and thread within this portrait-sculpture evoked images of the 'good enough (m)other', repairing or making, and artist Louise Bourgeois equates the power of the needle to magical reparation and forgiveness (Darwent 2010).

Portraits usually depict subjects who are clothed, whether that be everyday clothes, historical or fancy dress; these all signify temporality, fixing subjects within particular historical eras (Pointon 2013, p.20). Portraits also engage with materiality through the clothes and objects depicted within the portrait, and also through the very fabric of the portrait itself (Pointon 2013, p.128).

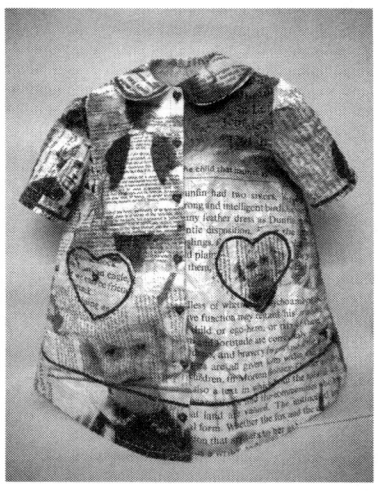

Figure 7.12 *The Paper Dress* by Susan Carr (co-designed by Susan), 2012.

In her end of project interview Susan talks about how a sense of connection was made between herself and her mother through *The Paper Dress* portrait-sculpture:

SC: Yes, that's good. So, in a way that's about telling your life story but looking at it in a different way, because we are looking at how we can make pictures, or lasting images about it. Do you think that changes how you look at it?

S: I think you creating the collages and portraits helped change the way I look at my past because if you asked me for my life story, I wouldn't necessarily have said the things I've said. What we are looking at is an *emotional life story*, which you have to find metaphors to express, which I think is what this does. You know, I would perhaps concentrate on getting the degrees and writing and you know, maybe, meeting the Queen and all that kind of thing, but they are not my emotional life story. *And my emotional life story is much more important to express.* It's nice for someone else to express the emotions that you can't. I mean, this is what thinking about the art enables you to do, *this isn't about me having dresses made, it's a whole part of my relationship with my mother and things like that. I think it's much more important to express.*[5]

*The Paper Dress* portrait-sculpture, therefore, enabled a sense of connection between Susan and her late mother, bringing the past and present together in the one object, allowing Susan to reconcile the difference she felt between herself and her mother with a renewed sense of connection, meaning and *continuity*. Susan also explores the loss of her mother in this portrait-sculpture, continuing the theme of exploring death and mourning through examining the loss of her 'daughter to a beloved mother' identity. The sense of continuity inherent within her portraits is something Susan talks of:

SC: I have done a little more on the [*In the Library*] portrait [...]

S: I think you've got everything there, gosh. *You can see the continuity* there, can't you? [indicating all four of the portraits].[6]

Susan's four portraits are shown in Figure 7.13.

Within this section I have described examples where patients found an increased sense of belonging, re-membering and continuity through the portraits, linking and integrating aspects of past, present and future self-identities. Bill's WWII experiences depicted within the portraits, collages and prose poems revealed everything he needed to tell me about his self-identity, and how it had been formed, broken and reformed,

---

5   SC = Susan (Artist-Therapist-Researcher). S = Susan (Patient-Researcher). End of project interview 10/10/2012.
6   SC = Susan (Artist-Therapist-Researcher). S = Susan (Patient-Researcher). End of project interview 18/10/2012.

despite the gap of nearly 70 years since the war. Rose celebrates her sense of belonging and connection to Freddie Mercury in her portrait *Bohemian Rhapsody*, someone she recognises as a fellow inhabitant of liminal space. Paul finds a sense of homelike-being-in-the-world in his *English Gothic* portrait, depicted with his deceased relatives, at the same time acknowledging an acceptance of being-towards-death. Susan finds a sense of connection with her deceased mother in *The Paper Dress* and a sense of *continuity of being* within her four portraits. As Duesbury (2005, p.207) says, working within palliative care is characterised by not only the 'intimate depth' of the work but also the 'breadth'...'We are working with past, present and future as an entirety.' This is evident within the patients' efforts to make connections between their different temporal self-identities, giving a sense of ongoing continuity of self that is necessary for 'ontological security' (Giddens 1991, p.35) and 'homelike-being-in-the-world' (Svenaeus 2011).

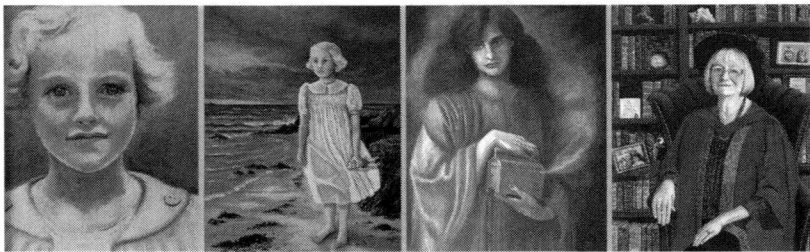

Figure 7.13 Montage of Susan's four portraits: *Little Susan, Saying Goodbye to the Sea, Being Pandora* and *The Library* by Susan Carr (co-designed by PR Susan), 2012.

## Embodied empathy and self-love:
### Being, doing and becoming

Embodied empathy has been described as 'the way the body swells when it enters a wide hall. It sways, even in imagination, when it sees wind blowing in a tree' (Vischer quoted in Elkins 1996, p.137), and an 'embodied intersubjectivity' or 'corporeal commonality' (Finlay 2009, p.6) becomes the 'horizon of experience' through which we can access another's experience (Wertz 2005, p.168).

When writing Rose's case-study and analysing her portraits, I was struck by the physicality inherent within all of them (Figure 6.4). They all capture Rose 'in action' in a moment of *doing* or *becoming*, she is not 'passive' in any of them. Delegates mirrored this physicality when I exhibited *Bohemian Rhapsody* and several other portraits at a London art therapy conference in 2013; I noticed that when people were talking about the portrait, they often made the 'arms across the chest' gesture to describe it.

The link between empathy and imagery has been explained through Rizzolatti *et al.*'s (1996) discovery of 'mirror neurons' which revolutionised the way automatic physical responses to sensory images (seen either directly in life, or in art), are understood, contributing to the knowledge that human beings have a 'body based understanding of the world' (Gallese and Lakoff 2005, p.466). Understanding our bodies from the perspective of mirror neurons suggests that mimicking this 'arms across the chest' gesture signals an empathic engagement with Rose through the portrait, as muscles contract and relax in the exact same way Rose's do in the portrait. They are literally putting themselves in Rose's position. I reflected upon this in the active documentation sketchbook:

### Notes from Rose's active documentation sketchbook 21/05/2013

Thinking of the 'arms across the chest' gesture in *Bohemian Rhapsody*, I wondered if it had any special meaning in sign language, and after some brief research on the internet I discovered it had. It means 'love'! I wonder if Freddie Mercury knew the meaning of his gesture when he made it? Maybe he did because he knew how much he was loved by his huge following of fans, so perhaps he was giving back a little of the love he received in the gesture. Either way, it seems to fit with a sense that Rose is expressing love in this portrait, love and acceptance for herself, as well as her love for Freddie.

This sense of self-love and appreciation is reflected in Rose's 'determination' to make the most of herself:

> R: It's like my t-shirt has got on it 'don't stop me now!' that's a Queen song. I've got a t-shirt with it on.
>
> SC: Yes…

R: *I am determined to make the most of myself.*[7]

Portraits are unique manifestations in that they are objects which represent persons, and as such they can be touched, handled and reflected upon, and as a companion/witness, I am also able to say that I too *love* a portrait or a collage. This is an acceptable way of expressing *love* for a patient, albeit again *third hand*, even so the significance is not lost on the patients. When I said, *I loved* a portrait, patients smiled and nodded and more often than not agreed with me and my implication that, yes, their portrayed sense of self-identity, that we had co-created together, was *lovable*. Patients also talked freely about how much they *loved* the portraits, collages and prose poems. Here Susan talks about the *Rainbow Snake* collage and how it encompasses 'everything' she had talked about, good and bad (see Figure 7.14).

S: Yes, it's so detailed, it's really good! Yes, that's everything there. Hmm, I *love* that one![8]

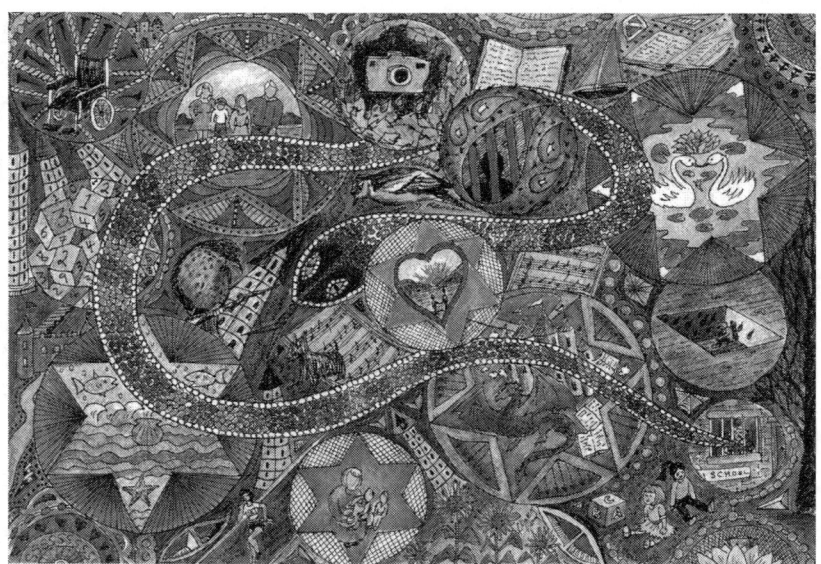

Figure 7.14 *The Rainbow Snake* by Susan Carr, 2012.

---

7 SC = Susan (Artist-Therapist-Researcher). R = Rose (Patient-Researcher). End of project interview 22/03/2011.
8 SC = (Artist-Therapist-Researcher). S = Susan (Patient-Researcher). End of project interview 10/10/2012.

This is the poem Susan wrote entitled 'The Rainbow Snake':

> Silent and sinuous
> The Rainbow Snake carries my life through the Universe.
> Dull coils and bright coils.
> Blue coils, indigo and violet coils – no one hears
> them crying in the silences of space,
> But tears were born in the origins of existence;
> Red coils, orange and yellow coils – no one hears
> them laughing in the silences of space,
> But laughter was born in the origins of existence.
> For me there have been whirling planets of activity,
> Things done, things achieved;
> Briefly visited, but left behind in immeasurable
> distances of time and space.
> For me there have been pulsing stars of joy,
> Babies born, marriage shared;
> A love experienced, that lights the way through
> immeasurable distances of time and space.
> But now a pinprick, a hole in the fabric of
> existence, grows ever nearer, ever bigger.
> Where does it lead?
> Does it bridge a fold in time and lead to
> new existence, glad renewal?
> As the green coils of the Rainbow Snake emerge
> through the spring leaves on a new journey?
> Does it lead to non-existence? Or eternity? Or...?
> The Rainbow Snake cannot stop, cannot pause,
> cannot wait for me to know or choose.
> Just a pinprick, just a hole in the fabric of
> existence, pointing to beyond.
> But what will happen when all existence
> arrives inexorably at that point?
> Will that pinprick, that hole in the fabric of existence, growing
> bold, swallow all that began so infinitely long ago?
> Breathe it out, maybe, into the maelstrom of a new first moment;
> Or reveal itself as portal to another place? Or...?
> The Rainbow Snake whispers nothing of this and moves on.
>
> (Susan, 7 October 2011)

In her end of project interview Susan also talks about loving the portraits:

> SC: This one was about the idea of the mermaid, wasn't it?
>
> S: Yes, I *love* those.
>
> SC: And we've got the other one, as a child.
>
> S: Yes, I *love* that one too.[9]

People often talk about 'loving' *things*, even trivial things; however, I think that admitting love for something that represents *one's self* – particularly in the light of self-identity disruption and the stigma of illness – is a significant step forward. This is a benefit of 'third hand' (Kramer 1971) practice and 'response art' (Fish 2012). Through making images *for* clients, *emotional distance* is created but also, conversely, so is *emotional connection*. I have noticed in my art therapy work that if a client makes an image, they find it very hard to look at it without seeing all the faults within it, and one flaw (which no one else will ever notice) overshadows the meaning of the image for them. However, when I make the image for the patient the situation is reversed, and they are free to 'love' the image, and do not seem to notice the 'flaws' that I, as its creator, see all too easily.

The benefits of developing self-love are wide and far-reaching, as has also been shown with Paul in Chapter 6, through increasing self-care and pride in his appearance and a renewed sense of agency. In her end of project interview Susan also notices similar benefits and talks about taking more care of herself by putting on make-up, etc.

Another theme, which emerged from the analysis, is how the portraits, as *intentionality-made-visible*, reveal a sense of *becoming*, which is an acknowledgement of embodied self-identities in a state of *transition* or *change*. Within one of the themes identified by Aita *et al.* (2010, p.7) in their study *Portraits of Care*, they noted 'a sense of ongoing identity formation especially during transitions in health status' (ibid., pp.7–8). This *identity formation* may correlate with the sense of *becoming* noted within portrait therapy. This is highlighted in Rose's *Poppy Field* portrait (Figure 7.15).

---

[9] SC = Susan (Artist-Therapist-Researcher). S = Susan (Patient-Researcher). End of project interview 18/10/2012.

# MAKING SPECIAL, MAKING MEANING

> Rose said:
> I was Born and bred in London
> and yet...
> Every summer...till I was 10 years old
> Mum and Dad took me to Yorkshire
> And left me at my Aunts...
> For 5 weeks.
> I ran around barefoot, wild and free,
> And lay down in a poppy field
> Where no one could see me...

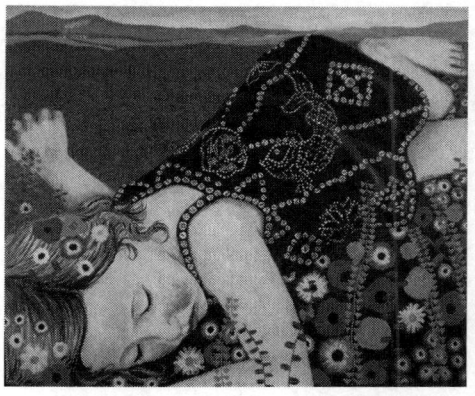

Figure 7.15 *The Poppy Field* by Susan Carr (co-designed by Rose), 2011.

When co-designing *The Poppy Field*, Rose said she would often use a mentalisation of a poppy field, as a 'safe space' to go to in her mind when she is stressed or anxious. By combining this positive mentalisation with Rose's childhood experience of being taken to Yorkshire and left for five weeks with her aunt, the portrait could therefore be recalled by Rose as a 'vivid' *positive* image (Werner-Seidler and Moulds 2011, p.1100), a creative device to use when she is stressed, anxious or depressed. The essence statements for this portrait also show the transition between 'isolated city child' and 'earth-spirit warrior child' and the implied adaptation entailed:

## Statement of Emergent Learning: *The Poppy Field*

There is a sense of continuation of being and spiritual presence in mother nature, which supports and heals Rose. *The Poppy Field* depicts the moment of identity transition and adaption in which 'isolated-city-child' becomes 'earth-spirit-warrior child'.

Within the phenomenological analysis of Rose's portraits, four essences of self-identity were found. These were:

### 'Resilient, see me/hear me Rose'

<u>'Invisible, silenced Rose'</u>

*'Earth-Spirit-Warrior-Child'*

'Isolated-City-Child'

Through *The Poppy Field* portrait, Rose accesses her 'earth-spirit-warrior-child' self-identity once again, and experiences the *transition* between 'isolated-city-child' and 'earth-spirit-warrior-child' demonstrating an autonomous sense of *becoming*. This sense of *transition* and *adaptation* correlates with the development of 'resilient, see me/hear me' Rose, found within the end of project interview voice analysis.

## Listening for Contrapuntal Identity Voices:

**1. Listening for 'Resilient, see me/hear me Rose'.**

2. <u>Listening for 'Invisible, silenced Rose'.</u>

R: [...] <u>Why because you are ill, let it stop you doing things</u>? **You should think I *can* still do it, that's how I look at it.**

SC: Yes...

R: <u>For instance, I can't drink, 'cause I can't go to the pub and have a pint because I would be sick</u> **but it doesn't stop me going and sitting with friends, I can still go and sit there and have a water or something. You've just gotta change it round.**

SC: Yeah, just adapt?

R: **Yeah adapt it.**[10]

---

10 SC = Susan (Artist-Therapist-Researcher). R = Rose (Patient-Researcher). End of project interview 22/03/2011.

When commencing the analysis of *The Poppy Field* and metaphorically 'stepping inside' the painting or *indwelling* (this process is described in Chapter 9, Table 9.1), I realised that I had inadvertently painted Rose laying in an approximation of the 'recovery position', perhaps indicating on my part an unconscious addition of 'hope' to this painting – a hope of 'recovery'.

On reflection I realise that this unconscious use of the recovery position could also indicate a sense of *denial* of Rose's MND diagnosis, and a false sense of holding 'hope' for Rose? However, the ambiguities evident within this painting enable the holding of dualities such as life and death, hope and hopelessness, denial and acceptance, and these dualities are also depicted within the *Paint Me Like a Picasso* portrait (Figure 5.20).

In this section I have described the patients' experience of portraiture as a way to increase the sense of a worthwhile and valuable self/life, and the portraits' capacity, through mirror neurons, to elicit feelings of embodied empathy within its viewers. This gives patients a sense of embodied empathic engagement with their own portrait, but also a recognition that other viewers of the portraits will feel this too. The portraits also become a focus and channel for 'love' with patients and myself able to express 'love' for the portraits without this being misconstrued. This was helped by the portraits being created 'third hand', meaning patients were able to express their 'love' for the portraits without feeling inhibited by anxiety about perceived flaws in the painting, or accusations of *narcissism* (i.e. an unhealthy obsession with one's appearance or self).

## Legacy and temporality: Immortalising the sitter/cheating death

One of the ways that life-threatening and chronic illness disrupt a person's self-identity is through a change in their perception of time and the future (Crossley 2003, p.439). Acknowledging our temporality is perhaps akin to acknowledging our mortality and therefore the passage of time acts as a reminder of the weakness of the human body damaged by illness (Seymour 2002, p.141).

Seymour defines time in relation to illness thus:

> Time is physical and mechanical, experiential and cultural: temporality is the context for our lives. [...] Clear in the knowledge that it is time that will triumph in the end, we spend our lives negotiating the boundaries of our enslavement. Encouraged by small gains, we bargain and negotiate, obscure and reconceptualise our relationship with time, but victory is always tentative; time is inexorable. Time is the fundamental element in the unfolding of our mortal lives and in their impending termination. (Seymour 2002, p.136)

While working with the patients I became aware that one of the unique qualities that portraits offer is: *time* combined with *positive focused attention*, and that this combination results in *vivid positive memories* (Werner-Seidler and Moulds 2011). The equation is simple but effective: *we remember* when someone gives us his or her *undivided attention and time*, and during a portrait sitting or the co-designing process this combination is provided. It could be argued that this combination is also a feature of therapeutic relationships within the many and varied approaches to art therapy; however, there are several unique aspects to the time and attention given in portraiture. The first is that the portrait becomes a tangible *testimony* of this time and attention; it exists *because of* the time and attention given by the artist/therapist in order to paint it. Second, a proportion of the time and attention happened *away* from the patient in the studio, therefore the time and attention *continued* outside of their presence, allowing a sense of *being-held-in-mind* by the art therapist with implications for patients' self-worth. Also, their *being-held-in-mind* is *testified* within the portrait and continues when exhibited in a gallery and displayed in the patient's homes, enabling a sense of a valued *future* self.

I have noticed in my art therapy work in palliative care that patients often describe feeling stuck in a 'void' between their 'past identity' (I was), which feels lost to them, their 'present identity' (I am) which they do not recognise, and their 'future identity' (I will be) that is a feared unknown. As Oliver Sacks has said when writing about the disrupting impact of illness on his self and identity:

> There was a gap – an absolute gap – between then and now; and in that gap, into the void, the former 'I' had vanished. (Sacks 1984, p.63)

Svenaeus (2011, p.339) proposes that, in illness, an 'alienation' develops between a person's temporal experience of past and future:

> Illness ruptures my life, to the point that the past and the future appear in a new light – or perhaps a new darkness – in which they acquire a strange quality of being, simultaneously mine and yet no longer mine. (Svenaeus 2011, p.342)

As the body is both 'a physical object, made of matter, *and* the seat of consciousness', distance or a void can arise between the physical/biological body and the lived/experienced body (Carel 2013, p.351). However, I suggest that the body-as-object can be *reclaimed* in the portrait process, through patients directing how they want their subjective selves to be portrayed. The portrait therefore becomes a 'subject-object' (Carel 2011, p.37), a link between the patient's body as object/material and their body as subject/consciousness. Similarly, past, present and future identities can be contained within the portraits, enabling a revisioning, re-connection and integration of the fragmented self-identity.

In her end of project interview Rose talks about how through portrait therapy 'it's like someone took notice', gaining a sense of self-worth through that attention, with the *transformational* power of portraiture highlighted when she says 'you made it into *something*…':

SC: And how about the telling of your story and someone listening to you, and then interpreting that through the portrait?

R: Yes because, it's like, *someone took notice* and what to me was just an everyday thing, *you've made it into something*, does that make sense? (SC: yes) You made it interesting.[11]

When I first worked with Paul he described his experience of illness as 'constricting' and 'frustrating' and the theme of being 'trapped' or of *being unable to be 'Paul'* was a constant one (see Figure 7.16). Evans (2005a, p.28) says, 'some patients express claustrophobic feelings of being trapped inside their diseased body, and the person who existed before diagnosis crumbles, becoming a new unwelcome identity'. This is highlighted within Paul's collage (Figure 7.16).

---

11 SC = Susan (Artist-Therapist-Researcher). R = Rose (Patient-Researcher). End of project interview 22/03/2011.

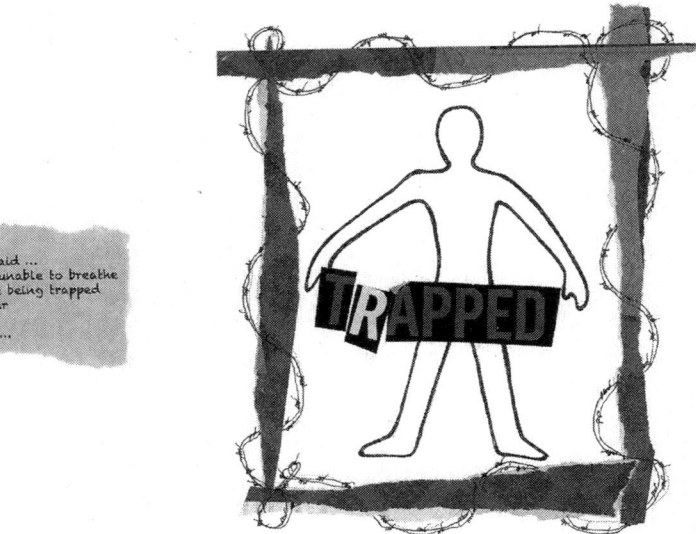

Figure 7.16 *Trapped*, collage by Susan Carr, 2012.

For Paul's third portrait we decided that I would paint him 'from life' at his home. During one portrait session Paul decided to play on his video game while I was painting him. The experience of watching Paul *be* 'Paul' within the virtual world of the game was quite revealing and I gradually became acquainted with 'virtual Paul' (see Figure 7.17). I recorded this in Paul's active documentation sketchbook.

## Notes from Paul's active documentation sketchbook 03/03/2013

Today I painted Paul in his room as he was not feeling well enough to go downstairs. While I was painting him, Paul played on his video game. In the game, Paul became a character who is able to run, jump, climb, fight and effect change on his environment, or to 'be'. This 'Paul' was somebody who (virtual) people took notice of. I felt that Paul was showing me his 'virtual self-identity' or even his pre-illness identity, and perhaps it was also adaptive, in that he could be 'himself' or someone else, even for a short time. I said that in his game he could 'do and be' all those things, and he said that even though it was 'virtual reality' he still got out of breath playing the game. Perhaps he was reminding me that it was only a game, and that he was still 'trapped' in his sick body.

This then formed the basis of Paul's portrait and we called it *Virtual Paul* (Figure 7.17).

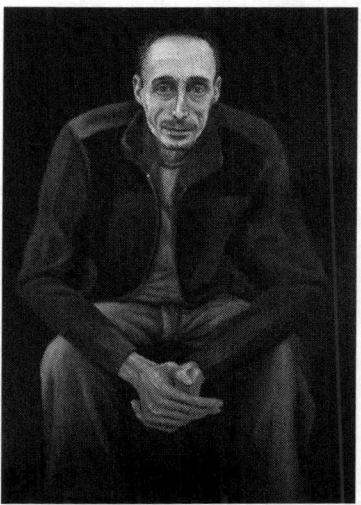

Figure 7.17 *Virtual Paul* by Susan Carr (co-designed by Paul), 2013.

Reflecting on this portrait I find that 'virtual Paul' conversely exists in a liminal space – as do Mark Gilbert's subjects (Figures 3.1 and 3.2), although I was not aware of any thoughts of mimesis at the time. Portraits act as a bridge between the present, past and future, as well as all other imagined 'virtual realities'. Just as Paul is able to be 'at home' in his virtual game, so within the portrait his *capacity to be* changes. Paul injects humour into our discussion about the portrait, reflecting upon the fact that I neglected to paint the chair he was sitting in:

> SC: But I quite like that one [indicating *Virtual Paul* portrait] because it is really stripped back…so there is nothing apart from you in the picture…so it is really focused…
>
> P: I must be quite fit to stay like that! [laughs]
>
> SC: [Laughs][12]

The 'as if' nature of portraits, combined with the mirror neuron effect (Rizzolatti *et al.* 1996), enables us to feel actions in our bodies, meaning

---

12 SC = Susan (Artist-Therapist-Researcher). P = Paul (Patient-Researcher). End of project interview 03/06/2013.

that within the portrait, and *felt empathically* within his body, Paul is, *able to be* 'quite fit'. The Paul caught in the painting's surface is also protected from temporality, curtailing the relentless pace of time, so old age and sickness can no longer affect 'virtual Paul'. As West says:

> ...a portrait also serves magically to freeze time and to extend artificially the life of the represented individual. Portraits can thus appear to be both records of specific events and evocations of something more lasting. The power of portraiture rests largely in this tension between the temporal and the permanent. (West 2004, p.44)

The idea of extending life or immortality within portraiture has historically been tied to Renaissance paintings of religious subjects; however, with the moving away from a belief in organised religion in the West there has been a growing secular focus on 'fame' (Taylor 1989, p.43) and 'celebrity'. Whilst the link with religion is present within Hilary's *Held by an Angel* portrait (see Figure 5.4), for the other patients 'immortality' may focus more on fame and celebrity through the potential exhibition and publication of the portraits. All patients suggested that they were keen for their portraits to go into exhibitions and be seen by others, reiterating the sense of portraits as bridges to *being known*. Radley (2009, p.211) warns that putting works of illness into a gallery setting risks changing its meaning, and takes the artwork further away from those who made it or those for whom it was made (Radley 2009, p.211). However, exhibiting the portraits is one of the key ways that a portrait is able to go and 'do its work' (ibid., p.214). This sense that portraits have a job to do imbibes them with the 'as if' human characteristics of the person portrayed, which becomes part of the patient's *future*, 'immortalised' self-identity.

In her end of project interview Rose talks about how the project has transformed her perception of herself from being a 'nobody' to someone who has 'done something with my life':

SC: But what I am saying is, has it helped you...well you said it has helped you recognise parts of yourself?

R: Yeah...

SC: And maybe given you a stronger sense of self and identity?

R: *Yeah, because now, instead of being a nobody, this is as if I have done something with my life, you know 'cause, that with the poppies, it was just nothing, now it's got meaning, ... I can't describe it...*

SC: No that is fine.[13]

This links to the idea of the portraits as legacy or remembrance, and the idea of legacy has within it an implicit acknowledgement of one's *mortality*. The anticipation of an exhibition of the portraits allows for the development of a belief in a *futureself*, one that does not depend upon being *alive*. Through maintaining the perception of an ongoing 'life', the portraits provide a sustained 'contact' with people in the future (Freeland 2010, p.42), which enables the embodiment and sense of continuation of an irreplaceable uniqueness or 'presence'. Susan talks about how the portraits become part of a patient's *future identity*:

SC: So, how do you feel about these portraits going into an exhibition and being seen by people? [...]

S: Yes, I think there are two good things about that. I think that it offers evidence for the value of this kind of intervention, so hopefully it will help to make it happen for other people. *And secondly, to feel that you're not..., that there's something solid out there that will be you, you know when you aren't there. It's quite nice.*

SC: Other people have thought of that as their future self, you know that we all need that future self to...and I guess your book is like that as well?

S: Definitely, I guess they are similar issues, something that will go on into the future.

SC: Leaving a legacy or something like that?

S: But also, as I say, I hope that the evidence will be persuasive and make people, other people, think about what happens in this kind of therapeutic situation.[14]

Susan reiterates her point later in the interview:

---

13 SC = Susan (Artist-Therapist-Researcher). R= Rose (Patient-Researcher). End of project interview 22/03/2011.
14 SC = Susan (Artist-Therapist-Researcher). S = Susan (Patient-Researcher). End of project interview 18/10/2012.

SC: So, another question, do you feel this kind of project would benefit other people who have a similar illness or similar issues to you?

S: Yes, I think it would help. It helps people in my situation, but I think it would help a broader range of people, I think it would be particularly important to people suffering from depression, to try to create something visual that would lift them...to see the positive aspects of themselves, so yes, I would say people with psychological illnesses and people psychologically affected by physical illnesses, so both sides of the coin. *And a particular thing in the hospice situation is where people know that their own death is not a long way away, so that to help people to feel that they have this kind of projection into the future, that they're not just going into the hospice and dying and the world moves on and forgets that they ever existed, it does give people some kind of existence beyond that point*, so that's another reason for it in the hospice context I would think. However, I certainly would see that it could also have a lot of validity in people with other issues, like severe depression.[15]

The idea of legacy and the alchemy of portraiture meant that for Peter the portraits embodied the person depicted even after that person's death. Peter talks about the 'as if' nature of the portrait *There's Something About Mark, RIP* (see Figure 5.10) and how this seems to have brought Mark 'back' to him and his family:

SC: So how do you feel about these portraits going into an exhibition? [...]

P: That is an added benefit, but *the important thing is seeing the result*. I think when my sons and my wife see that [indicating *There's Something About Mark, RIP* portrait] it will bring tears to their eyes.

SC: Good ones?

P: Oh yes...happy memories...*it is as if he is there with us*, it's so wonderful.[16]

---

15 SC = Susan (Artist-Therapist-Researcher). S = Susan (Patient-Researcher). End of project interview 18/10/2012.
16 SC = Susan (Artist-Therapist-Researcher). P = Peter (Patient-Researcher). End of project interview 27/02/2012.

Within this chapter I have described the patients' experiences of the portraits as legacy, and as an important part of their future self-identity, thereby equating to a sense of immortalisation or cheating death. Portraits capture time within the painting process and this is combined with the art therapist's positive focused attention, resulting in feelings of being-held-in-mind, the formation of positive memories and an increased sense of self-esteem. The 'as if' nature of portraits and Peter's belief that through the portrait Mark 'is there with us' does not equate to a denial of Mark's death, because although we look at a portrait and view 'a person' we do not expect them *to move or speak to us*. We are able to hold the concept of '*as if* reality' and 'physical reality' in our minds at the same time. This 'as if' quality means that the portrait exists for Peter, in both realities, and as such equates to an adaptive acceptance of connection and separation from Mark within the portrait. Also, through *loving* the portraits, collages and prose poems *of* and *about* themselves, patients are reawakening a sense of self-love and empathy, which impacts positively on their self-esteem and home-like-being-in-the-world.

— PART III —

# PORTRAIT THERAPY PROTOCOL AND EVALUATION METHODS

## Chapter 8

# A THERAPIST'S MANUAL

*The Three Phases of Portrait Therapy*

This chapter will provide a detailed description of the protocol for portrait therapy, describing the tools and activities used within its three distinct phases, and advice for therapists to help them use this intervention safely within their practices. The protocol is divided into three distinct phases.

### Phase one: Emotional distancing, elicitation tasks, and the active documentation sketchbooks

As with any other art therapy intervention it is important to advise the patient about confidentiality and its limits before you begin working together. If you are visiting a patient in their own home it is important to follow your organisation's lone working and health and safety policies, and discuss your planned visit with other members of the team who know the patient and their circumstances. It is also important to ensure that you are covered by your own or your employer's professional indemnity insurance for home visits.

Where possible the venue for the portrait sessions should be negotiated with the patient involved, as some may prefer a home visit and some may prefer to hold the sessions at a neutral venue, where an art therapy/counselling room can be booked. If the sessions are to take place at the patient's home it is important to ask the patient if they have a room you can work in where you will be undisturbed. It is important to be strict about keeping the boundaries to this space; however, it is difficult to control in someone else's house and interruptions are almost certain to happen, but the benefits of meeting at the patient's home outweigh the difficulties. For patients living with life-threatening and chronic illnesses, meeting at their home means that they do not have to expend the energy to get to the hospice, or other venue, and it also gives their carer an hour or so of respite. Also, a person's home tells you so much about them, and usually the walls are full of photographs and other memorabilia that it is important to see and discuss. The patients whose case-studies I discuss in this book were also given the option of having a chaperone (a volunteer from the hospice), to sit in on the portrait sessions, but none of the patients took up this offer, perhaps demonstrating that they all felt at ease with myself and the process. However, this may be something you would consider offering.

The first few portrait sessions are all about building a collaborative therapeutic relationship within which the patient feels comfortable talking about their self-identity. Elicitation tasks (i.e. tasks that help gather knowledge from human subjects) can be used together with the patients to help this process; these are described as follows.

### *Button self-identity elicitation task*

The button task is a quick and easy to use creative elicitation task, and an easy way to identify the impact of illness on a person's sense of self-identity. The materials are inexpensive and easy to obtain; buttons are familiar, non-threatening objects and therefore help to reduce the patients' stress and anxiety. Buttons are also easy to handle and most patients can engage easily with this task. If a patient has problems using their hands, they can direct the art therapist to pick out the buttons for them and direct where to place them on the board.

The aim of this task is to enable patients to talk about and remember aspects of their *pre*-illness self-identity and their understanding of the impact of illness on their *post*-illness self-identity. The button task also enables *tacit* knowledge to be made manifest, i.e. knowledge that is difficult to describe through written or verbal communication. The button task also enables a sense of *emotional distancing* to take place, by using an *abstract* approach to talk about difficult issues.

### Materials required

- A box containing 100+ mixed buttons, including: old, broken, shiny, pretty, glittery, military, and plain buttons. I also found it helpful to purchase representational buttons such as: a poppy, a tea pot, a mermaid, etc. These were all used by the patients, as were broken, discoloured and worn buttons.

- A baize or plain material covered piece of medium density MDF board, roughly 31 × 31 cm.
- A camera and a voice recorder (or a smartphone with these facilities).

**Protocol**

Explain to the patient what the task is and why you are asking them to take part in it.

Ask permission to record the session, and if granted set up the voice recorder (this is to avoid having to write down what the patient says during the session). The patient is then asked to choose any buttons that represent aspects of their *pre*-illness self-identity and place these on the baize board in any way they like, to form a 'button sculpt'. It is important to say that there is no wrong or right way of doing this and that it is best to just choose buttons on instinct rather than taking a long time to think about it. The patient is then asked to describe the buttons and explain why they chose them. The overall design or shape of the button sculpt may also be significant and can be discussed. With the patient's permission, a photograph can be taken of the button sculpt for reference; the patient is then asked to return the buttons to the box. The process is then repeated, asking the patient to choose buttons that represent their *post*-diagnosis self-identity.

## *LEGO® self-identity elicitation task*

The use of LEGO® as a creative way to communicate was developed by David Gauntlett (2002) as something called 'LEGO® Serious Play'. I therefore developed the LEGO® task as an additional elicitation task that can be used with patients who possess fine motor skills, and who require further help identifying aspects of their *pre*-illness and *post*-illness self-identities. LEGO® is a familiar, non-threatening and yet expressive material. I used this task selectively with patients because of the need for fine motor skills; however, it may be possible for the patient to direct the art therapist to build the sculptures for them.

### Materials required

- A box of mixed LEGO® (or other similar) building bricks, including people and vehicle parts and bases.
- A camera and voice recorder (or a smartphone with these facilities).

### Protocol

Explain the task to the patient and ask permission to record the session. Invite the patient to make a sculpture that represents aspects of their *pre*-diagnosis/illness self-identity, and then explain the elements that make up the sculpture and what it means to them. The patient is then invited to make a second sculpture which represents aspects of their *post*-diagnosis/illness self-identity. The two sculptures can then be compared and talked about by the patient, and with their permission a photograph can be taken to record the sculptures. The patient is then invited to return the LEGO® to the box.

## *Photo-elicitation task*

Ethnographer Sarah Pink (2009) says that photo-elicitation:

> ...relies on the idea of the photograph becoming a visual text through which the subjectivities of research and research participant intersect. It can evoke memories, knowledge and more in the research participant which might otherwise have been inaccessible... (ibid., p.93)

Photo-elicitation is another technique that helps trigger patients' memories about their past selves. The meanings and emotions shared through photo-elicitation may differ or supplement those gained from verbal inquiry. This is because images are processed by areas of the brain that are evolutionarily older than those areas that process verbal information (Harper 2002). Collier (1957) found that photo-elicitation techniques helped 'prod latent memory' which in turn allowed the release of 'emotional statements about the informant's life'.

### Materials required

- Photographs of the patient, selected by the patient.
- Camera and voice recorder (or a smart phone with these facilities).
- Access to a photocopier/printer.

## Protocol

This task should take place during the first or second portrait session, so it is important to plan ahead with regards to asking patients to bring in photographs of themselves at different ages, at turning points and of significant moments in their lives, e.g. baby, school, graduation and wedding photographs.

The patient is then asked to talk about the photographs they have brought in and their significance. These photographs may then be used as reference for portraits of the patient at a later date, so it is important to ask the patient's permission to take photocopies of their photographs and to record what the patient says about the photographs.

I found photo-elicitation very useful as the photographs acted as a focus for the conversation, and allowed patients to control this through their self-selection of the images to show and talk about. This is an important process and one which is difficult to replicate if patients have no photographs or very few to show. This then requires a more imaginative engagement with the patients' stories of self-identity in order to arrive at an acceptable mental and physical image with which to work.

Although elicitation methods such as photo-elicitation are often associated with increasing participants' emotional connection (Collier 1957 and 1967; Harper 2002), within this study the button and LEGO® tasks seemed to enable an *emotional distancing* to occur for the patients. This was first noticed in the early stages of developing the protocol, when working with patients at the hospice who volunteered to pilot these two elicitation techniques. Several of the patients self-reported an emotional *distancing* effect when using these tasks and this has been borne out within the study. This effect may be partly due to the creative processes within both the button and LEGO® tasks and correlates with Awan's (2007, pp.240–1) findings, as she says that creative tasks, engaged with for a set duration, give individuals time to reflect and formulate their thoughts and feelings, and therefore mediate their response, rather than having to produce an instant perhaps more emotive response.

This finding seems to be consistent with the way the patients used the tasks, with the button and LEGO® tasks evoking memories but less emotion than e.g. the photo-elicitation. These initial tasks were generally undertaken early in the intervention and may have helped patients to talk about their self-identity issues without being overwhelmed by emotional affect. However, this was a small study, so further research into the use of button and LEGO® tasks as emotional distancing techniques would be beneficial.

## *Active documentation sketchbook (ADS) (De Freitas 2002)*

It is important to use an active documentation sketchbook (ADS) (De Freitas 2002), to keep visual and written notes about the portrait therapy process. This sketchbook is used to record and collect images, stories, ideas and reflections pertinent to the creative 'third hand' process, as this helps to make the artistic methodological process explicit and transparent.

### Materials required

- An A4 ringed sketchbook or note pad.
- Mixed media art materials.
- Reference material from patients.

### Protocol

The active documentation sketchbook (ADS) (De Freitas 2002) is used by the therapist as a *reflective* and *reflexive* tool to record their own intuitive and *resonant* thoughts and images about the creative process. This process of note taking and recording enables the identification of themes, meanings and connections in the patients' stories of self-identity. Where this resonates with the therapist's own story these areas of resonance can be acknowledged and 'bracketed out' by creating *statements of reflexive resonance* for each portrait.

The ADS can be used to document any ongoing changes and modifications that are agreed between you and the patient, and becomes a place to review the evolution of the portrait, identify progress or blocks, and to record those phases or layers of the work that will become invisible as the work progresses. I would suggest that creating an ADS is especially important for 'third hand' interventions such as portrait therapy, and vital if it is being used as part of a research project, as information from the ADS is used within the analysis and case-studies as a *bracketed, reflexive* and *reflective* account that contribute to the discussion of the themes and essences found within the data.

The overall aim of the ADS is to make the artistic methodological process explicit, in order to outline a rigorous and respected 'artistic method', specifically appropriate to arts-based research, that is equal in status to a 'scientific method' (Grey and Malins 2004, p.22). This sketchbook should also be something you can share and discuss with your patient.

In summary, phase one of portrait therapy involves using creative emotional distancing tasks, utilising familiar, non-anxiety provoking materials (buttons, LEGO® and photographic), in order to help patients remember their stories of self-identity. This phase on average lasts 1–3 weeks at the beginning of the project, although the tasks could also be used at any stage to help the patient remember aspects of their self-identity, and the ADS is used within this phase to facilitate the making and recording of artistic, reflexive and self-reflective processes and observations.

## Phase two: Reflecting back stories of self-identity: Collage and prose poems as *response* art

The second phase of portrait therapy focuses on creating collages and prose poems as 'response art' (Fish 2012; Miller 2007), containing 'mirroring and attunement' (Wright 2009), reflecting back stories of self-identity related by patients within phase one. Collage as a form of *response art* is an important aspect of portrait therapy as it employs metaphoric and symbolic connotations, rather than literal expressions of an idea. This allows new associations and connections to be made, that might otherwise have remained unconscious (Brockelman 2001; Butler-Kisber 2008; Davis 2008; Vaughan 2005; Williams 2002). Contrary to the 'permanence' of oil paint in the portraits, the collages have a sense of *impermanence* and are most often used by patients to explore difficult feelings, fearful memories and existential questions.

The aim of creating collages and prose poems is that both of these artistic forms reduce the patient's self-identity stories to their essences or essential characteristics and meanings (Furman *et al.* 2007). Response art equates to artwork created by the therapist away from the patient, usually during the week between portrait therapy sessions. This work does need to be thought about carefully, but it need not take too long to create. Getting the essence of the story down on paper is the important part, as is the action of 'holding the patient in mind'. By 'holding in mind' I mean the act of thinking and acting on behalf of another person when they are absent. I found this to be a very healing and important aspect of portrait therapy and something that the patients appreciated very much.

Once created, the collage and prose poem (usually only one per week) is then discussed with the patient and any changes are made to accommodate the patient's ideas or adjustments. This may continue for several sessions, where more stories of self-identity are shared by the patient. How to choose which stories to reflect back to the patient through the collage/prose poems was a problem I pondered for some time; however, it soon became clear that the stories I chose were those I could 'resonate with', or relate to, meaning I chose those stories to which I had an *intuitive resonant response*. Choosing stories you resonate with will add 'authenticity' to the collages and prose poems you create for the patient. These will then become part of the reference material from which ideas for the portraits develop.

I see the prose poems not as a way to re-present the same data, but as a way to 'evoke different meanings' and issues (Leavy 2009, p.64) offering a new 'porthole onto an experience' (ibid., p.68). Prose poems are written without the constraints of 'verse'; however, poetic qualities such as heightened imagery, metaphor and emotional effects are preserved.

Poetry allows us to listen over and under and around the words, to focus and hear that which is said and unsaid, poetry 'defies singular definitions and explanations' and reflects the 'slipperiness' of self-identity (Faulkner 2006, p.99).

## Materials required

- Pens and paper.
- Magazines.
- Mixed media art materials.
- Reference material from the patients.
- Stories of self-identity, either noted within the ADS or as voice recordings.

## Protocol

Choose which self-identity story or experience you are going to reflect back to the patient based on what resonates with you, then make a list of words or themes that spring to mind. Using these words, create a prose poem that reflects back the story to the patient, adding in your own *attunement* or *aesthetic resonance*. This may equate to adding metaphor, symbolism or beauty, depending upon what you feel the patient needs to see. The patient will then have the opportunity to 'own' the image and accept it, or 'reject' it and ask for modifications to be made. This is all part of the self-identity *revisioning* process and should be encouraged. During the PhD project one patient offered their own poem to accompany a collage (i.e. Susan's poem *The Rainbow Snake*), and often poems were created intersubjectively between the patient and myself within the portrait sessions.

In my initial design for this intervention I envisioned the collage and prose poem phase of the project to end when the portrait painting begun; however it was not as clear cut as that and I often felt the need to create further collages and prose poems right up until the final sessions with patients. This highlights the need for continued flexibility within the design, also a propensity in the patients to continually *remember* their self-identity, and make connections with past, present and future selves.

## Phase three: Co-designing and painting the portraits, creating a statement of intention, the portrait reference album and appropriation art

An important aspect of the co-designing process was to identify *a statement of intention* for each portrait, based on a series of negotiations. Sometimes patients had concrete ideas from the beginning about how they wanted to be portrayed or the stories of self-identity depicted. However, some patients needed some help with this, usually by revisiting the collages and prose poems and looking through the portrait reference album (PRA), identifying images they felt 'drawn to'. The use, within one's own artwork, of aspects of historical or 'famous' artworks is known as appropriation art, which can be described as intentionally copying/borrowing, and/or altering objects or images/artwork that already exists (Gemmell 2012). I used appropriation within portrait therapy as a way to engage patients in the art process, through their recognition of famous portraits, or through the patient's unconscious 'drawing towards' certain images, without knowing initially why. Appropriating images has meant that the original works were sometimes used as symbols or metaphors by the patients. Appropriation was popularised by artists such as Marcel Duchamp (e.g. *Mona Lisa L.H.O.O.Q.*, 1919) and Andy Warhol (e.g. *Campbell's Soup Cans*, 1962). Contemporary artists such as Yasumasa Morimura (e.g. *An Inner Dialogue with Frida Kahlo*, 2001) use known images to create a pastiche, which, unlike forgery, does not attempt to deceive viewers that the art created is by the original artist; however, appropriation does depend upon a viewer's ability to *recognise* the original painting and all its cultural and symbolic significance (Gemmell 2012).

## *Creating a statement of intention*
### Materials required

- Paper and pens.
- Active documentation sketchbook.

### Protocol

A 'statement of intention' (Hogan 2013, p.17) within portrait therapy is the negotiated concise description of a portrait, and equates to the patient saying, *'Paint me this way!'* This is then used as the 'brief' for the therapist to use when painting the portrait for the patient. It is therefore very important to make sure this is correct, and that both parties are in agreement. I suggest making some quick thumbnail sketches to show the patient how you envision the portrait will look.

This statement enables the therapist to refer back to the patient's brief and remain focused on their intention for the portrait, and avoid an inadvertent focus on their own artistic style or ideas. However, some interpretation of the statement of intention is inevitable and necessary in order to offer attunement. Working with the patient to write the statement of intention involves negotiations around meaning, symbolism, metaphor, temporality, realism, abstraction, composition and medium. It may help to make a list of these when negotiating with the patient, to remind you what is required.

## Portrait reference album

If the patient is having difficulty thinking of ideas for their portrait, perhaps because of a limited knowledge of portraiture, it is useful to have/create a portrait reference album (PRA) for the patient to refer to. This works as an 'access portal' or 'way in' to portraiture. The PRA is simply a postcard-sized photo album, filled with postcards of portraits created by historical and contemporary famous and unknown artists, that I have collected over the years. It is also possible to purchase books containing these (see e.g. Bell 2000). However I think it is important to select images of 'portraits' that stretch the boundaries of what is considered a portrait; for me this included selecting a mixture of representational and non-representational portrait-sculptures (for a full list of the portraits I included in the PRA please see Appendix 1). It is also important to consider one's own skills as a portrait artist, and avoid adding postcards of works or styles by artists that you would struggle to replicate, e.g. if you add a portrait by Rembrandt the chances are that a patient will say, 'Paint me like that!'

### Materials required

- A photo album that takes postcard-sized photographs.
- Approximately 100 photographs or postcards of historical and contemporary portraits by famous and unknown portrait artists. (This may include representational and non-representational portraits, as well as 3D portrait-sculptures, if the therapist is confident they are able to replicate these styles.)

The PRA should be used selectively, so only if the patient requires help to access the world of art and portraiture, and to spark imaginative ideas including decisions relating to: style, medium or composition. When presented with the album the patient is asked to select portraits or portrait-sculptures that they feel *drawn to*. The patient is also encouraged to think in metaphorical and symbolic ways about how to represent intuitive, tacit, embodied and experiential knowledge within the portraits. A discussion then ensues about how the selected portrait is to be used, e.g. just the style, or as an appropriation? This method was used within Paul's *Broken Lungs* portrait (Figure 5.5).

In summary, phase two involves a series of negotiations with the patients to form *statements of intention* for each portrait, sometimes using the PRA as a way to access the world of portraiture, utilising metaphor and symbolism to depict aspects of self-identity. This phase often overlaps with phases one and three, depending upon how many portraits are being created for a patient, so sometimes further collages and prose poems will be created after the first portrait is completed.

## *Painting the portraits*

Portraits are relational in that they are created by one person for another, and embody the self-identity of the person depicted. Directing how they wish to appear in the portraits enables patients to think about who they are and how they want to be remembered, and the portrait becomes a tangible, physical object, imbibed with the therapist's 'mirroring and attunement'. It is however important to remember that within portraiture there is the potential for a 'contest of wills' between artists and their subjects, over the way a person is portrayed, as an artist may wish to present their own vision or perceptions based on personal insight, which may mean the subject's 'air' or subjectivity is lost (Freeland 2010, p.115). The collaborative co-designing phase of portrait therapy is therefore important in mitigating this, with each patient viewed as the 'expert' on their self-identity and given the choice to be painted in a way that reflects different aspects of their self-identity, i.e.: in the present, prior to their illness, or in their early life. I refer to portrait 'sessions' rather than 'sittings' as 'sittings' imply 'passivity' on the part of the patient – whereas the aim was for empowerment and engagement in the collaborative co-designing process.

## Materials required

- A compact travel easel.
- Painting surfaces, e.g. canvas, paper, wood panel.
- Art materials including pallet and brushes.
- Other artistic mediums as agreed between the patient and the therapist.
- Camera for taking high-quality reference images of the patient.

## Protocol

For portraits painted from life, a pose and location should be agreed upon by the patient and therapist. The patient should be made as comfortable as possible and told that they are free to move and talk and take a break whenever required. Take photographs as reference material to use when continuing the portrait away from the patient. The photographs will also help when setting up the following week, to make sure the same pose is used, and to check the composition works.

For studio created portraits (i.e. working away from the patient using photographs) once the statement of intention and the overall design of the portrait is decided upon, the therapist should create some initial thumbnail sketches to show the patient. These can then be modified if required. Subsequent photographs of the portrait's development can be shown to the patient at regular intervals. (Occasionally an initial idea for a portrait was decided upon and the patient saw the portrait for the first time in its finished state, particularly if the portrait only took a short time to complete. Within this scenario, the therapist must remain open to subsequent modifications if required by the patient.)

The amount of time I spend working on collages, prose poems and portraits away from the patient varies, and depended on the design choices of the patient; however, I have found that time devoted to this was important for the therapeutic process, and also for my own cathartic processes to mitigate feelings of embodied counter-transference (Booth *et al.* 2010). Some portraits took several weeks to complete, whilst others took less than an hour; this depended upon the size, medium and style requested by the participant (e.g. a small cubist or impressionist style portrait could be achieved in an hour or two, whereas larger highly detailed work took several weeks to complete). In hindsight, I would restrict the number of portraits or portrait-sculptures produced for each patient to three as a general rule, and restrict the size of the paintings/sculptures produced; however, it is also important to be flexible and patient-led on this. There is always a danger within palliative care to feel an existential need *to do more for patients*, caused by an institutional fear of *annihilation* inherent within palliative care (Duesbury 2005, p.202); certainly this is something which I have experienced within this project, and highlights the importance of having a clear ending (Edwards 1997) focused on the completion of the portraits, in order to help mitigate this.

## *Semi-structured end of project interviews (EPIs)*

As this was a research project I used semi-structured end of project interviews (EPIs) as a research method to gain insight into the patients' lived experience of portrait therapy. Even if you are not carrying out a research project I suggest you spend time talking to the patient about their experience of portrait therapy and perhaps ask if they would take part in an end of project interview, which can be used in a case-study. (See Appendix 2 for the list of questions I used for the EPI.) Before and during the EPIs patients had the opportunity to view their own original completed portraits, collages and prose poems, in order to reflect upon them and use them as reference for their answers.

**Materials required**

- List of questions.
- Audio recorder.
- The patient's portraits, collages and prose poems.
- The ADS.

**Protocol**

The EPI should take place in a comfortable, confidential space, where the portraits, collages and prose poems can be made accessible to the patient. The interview is semi-structured, with a core set of flexible and open-ended questions. Sometimes you may wish to add specific questions to the list that relate only to the patient being interviewed. (If this interview is part of a research project it is important to record the EPI on a voice recorder and transcribe this verbatim. The process I used to analyse this data is described in detail within Chapter 9.) It is important to spend time with each patient after the analysis and case-study stage, to discuss the interpretations, meanings and findings so that these can be modified if necessary. This gives patients a further opportunity to reflect upon their experience, and to discuss final interpretations and meanings to ensure that it is a true reflection of their lived experience.

— Chapter 9 —

# MAKING CONNECTIONS

*Evaluating Portrait Therapy*

Within this chapter I give a detailed description of the qualitative Arts-based Life/world Phenomenological Analysis (ALPHA) that I used to analyse portrait therapy. I will describe the tools and activities I drew upon and their ability to evaluate the diverse range of elements resulting from the intervention, e.g. portraits, collages, prose poems, voice recordings and the written word. I also offer advice and guidance for therapists regarding its use in evaluation and research.

My aim in developing ALPHA was for a simple and flexible analysis framework within which to research something as complicated and dynamic as self-identity, with the creative process providing additional 'variability and depth' (McNiff 2008, p.32). As I sought to understand the patients' *lived experience*, I decided that a phenomenological approach to data collection and analysis, within a broader case-study framework (Yin 2009), would be most appropriate.

ALPHA is a qualitative research method based in a *post*-positivist approach (i.e. recognising that all views of reality are essentially subjective); however, prejudice still exists within health and medical research towards a *positivist* measurement of cause and effect. This is characterised by calls for evidence-based practice (EBP), based on randomised controlled trials (RCTs), and a dominance in the National Health Service for therapies such as Cognitive Behavioural Therapy (CBT), with its emphasis on explicit systematic procedures and the measuring of effectiveness through tick box questionnaires. I refer to RCTs particularly as there have been recent calls in the art therapy literature for more RCT-based research in palliative care (Wood *et al.* 2011, p.144), as well as a historical debate on their usefulness to art therapy research (Edwards 1999; Parry 1997). Art therapists and psychotherapists have countered this with support for case-studies as ways to produce 'our own kind of knowledge' which can then be 'tested,' to produce 'our own kind of evidence' (Gilroy 1996, p.55; Denzin 2009). After all...

> The importance of establishing efficacy must not smother innovation; in the search for more effective ways of helping people, there has to be a phase of clinical theory development and closely observed case-studies before controlled outcome evaluation. The latter cannot precede the former and the former must be fostered and encouraged. (Parry 1997, p.12)

One of the key ways to achieve Parry's 'clinical theory development' is to use qualitative research methods, and these have expanded exponentially in recent years, with a wide range of methods now being employed within social science research (Denzin and Lincoln 2005), and the use of the arts in research becoming an ever-expanding field (Barrett and Bolt 2007; Cole and Knowles 2008; Jongeward 2009; Knowles and Cole 2008; Leavy 2009; Pink 2012; Sullivan 2010). Moon (2014, pp.3–4) describes the foundation for theory building in art therapy as a process that is essentially 'interpersonal, interdisciplinary, and contextual' (ibid., p.2), a way to 'make sense of something ... a process of using experiences, observations, experimentation, and intuition to construct ideas about how something works' (ibid.), and is the 'collective responsibility' of art therapists working in the field (ibid., p.10).

For this project 'clinical theory development' included: questioning the taken-for-granted normalised assumptions regarding: 'who' makes the artwork in art therapy, the universal requirement for confidentiality irrespective of context, the interpretation of images based on the client's unconscious drives and processes, and the patient–expert divide. These epistemological commitments have formed the very basis of art therapy practice since early in its inception, and as Moon (2014, p.5) says, art therapists who operate 'unquestioningly and uncritically' would perhaps be 'mystified' by making such challenges.

## Multiple case-study design

Case-studies can be described as in-depth investigations of a group, event, person or community, with data gathered from a variety of sources. Yin (2009, p.23) describes a case-study as an 'empirical inquiry' which 'investigates a contemporary phenomenon within its real-life context; when the boundaries between phenomenon and context are not clearly evident; and in which multiple sources of evidence are used'.

Following the analysis phase I used the emergent themes and voices of self-identity to write case-studies for each patient, drawing in the different data elements for an overall view and discussion. The decision to use a case-study design was influenced by the need for a qualitative research method that could incorporate the multiple data collection and dual data analysis methods within this study (Yin 2012, p.10). Finlay (2011, p.175) suggests that case-studies are 'most appropriate' for a relation-centred approach to phenomenological research, particularly when conducted by psychotherapists who are already familiar with reflexive and relational approaches to working' (ibid.).

Art therapist David Edwards (1999, p.6) identifies the case-study as a method of enquiry which addresses key aspects of clinical work in art therapy. Specifically it: focuses on 'the "individuality" of the client and the way they communicate through actions, words and images', it embraces the 'richness, diversity, messiness and complexity' of clients' lived experience and the art making process. It doesn't require that we turn 'subjects (i.e. people) into objects', and it allows us to write about research in a way that is 'recognisably human'. Case-studies are also inexpensive compared to large scale studies, and encourage the inclusion of the voices, personalities and creativity of the clients and therapist/researcher (Edwards 1999, p.6).

An important consideration was the way each of the individual cases could stand alone as an explication of the patient's lived experience, whilst cross-case analysis enabled the drawing of convergent understandings or 'triangulation' (Yin 2012, p.13). Some critics suggest that due to the small number of cases researched, it is not possible to generalise the findings or establish reliability; however, the relevance of one or more person's experience to others in a similar situation is a key way that case-studies gain validity (Hogan 1997, p.237). Also within phenomenological studies the aim is for detailed accounts of participants' lived experience and for researchers to make *tentative generalisations* from the cross-case analysis (Smith *et al.* 2009); however, as Warnock says, 'delving deeper into the particular also takes us closer to the universal' (Warnock 1987, cited in Smith 2004, p.42). The focus of the cross-case analysis is therefore concerned with explicating the patients' unique experiences and how these relate to the patient group as a whole, and the implications of this for wider contexts.

## Methods for visual analysis

I begin by explaining the methods of phenomenological analysis that I adapted to create ALPHA. In selecting and adapting methods for analysis I was aware that I was constructing a 'theoretical and ontological' filter through which to analyse the patients' portraits of identity (Mauthner and Doucet 1998, p.23). Whilst I accept that this choice will affect the results achieved, the process itself aims to be transparent, enabling other researchers to trace the procedures followed as well as follow my reflexive decision making process (ibid.). It is often in the analysis stage of research that the power differentials over patients are most highlighted (Mauthner and Doucet 1998, p.23), and whilst it is impossible to avoid some degree of researcher-interpretation within the analysis and conclusions, I hope to have mitigated this by working with the patients to negotiate interpretations and meanings within the case-studies.

### *Arts-based Life/World Phenomenological Analysis (ALPHA)*

There are many debates about what constitutes 'appropriate' phenomenological research (Finlay 2009, p.13) and no 'clear-cut recipes explaining how to engage in phenomenological analysis' (Finlay 2011, p.228); therefore Finlay suggests developing an approach that 'works for you' (ibid.).

ALPHA incorporates both *phenomenological reduction* (Husserl 1977 [1929], 1970 [1954]) and *phenomenological hermeneutic interpretation* (Heidegger 1962 [1927]; Gadamer 1975), in order to bring together the *life* experience (the return to the things themselves through reduction to essences) and the *world* (the re-introduction of cultural and historic meanings and understandings) of lived experience. It therefore recognises that *life* or experience does not happen in a vacuum, it is always situated in the *world*, and therefore understandings and meanings are co-created relationally through both *primary pre-reflective knowing* and *secondary reflective learning*, in order to make sense of experience. This acknowledges the critics of Husserlian phenomenology who have claimed that phenomenological reduction ignores the cultural and historical being-in-the-world and its meaning.

This combination of phenomenological approaches equates to a 'stepping into' the portraits, to experience them 'as if' you are within the landscape of the image, experiencing it anew; and then stepping out, and stepping back from the portrait, in order to experience its significance within the sociocultural life world of the patient. I then used these two experiences to create essence statements of *knowing* and *learning* respectively.

I have used six steps for the ALPHA reduction to essences which is outlined in Table 9.1.

Table 9.1 Six steps for the Arts-based Life/World Phenomenological Analysis (ALPHA)

| ALPHA: reduction to essences | Protocol | Rationale |
| --- | --- | --- |
| 1. Make a *Statement of Reflexive Resonance* for the portrait. | This process brackets out, but acknowledges any personal resonances, or what the image means for the artist-therapist-researcher. | This is a reflection on the phenomena from a personally reflexive and reflective position. This serves to bracket out one's personal interpretation of the phenomena. |
| 2. Step into the image. Experience being in the image as if it is the first time you have been there, employing intuition, wonder and curiosity. | Write down any sensory, intuitive and resonant words and phrases that come to mind (Lett 1998, p.332). Bracket out any prior knowledge or assumptions already mentioned in the *statement of reflexive resonance*. | Husserl's (1970 [1954]) *transcendental* phenomenology involves bracketing out prior knowledge and assumptions to enable a 'return to the things themselves' and a pure description of the essence of a phenomena, to elucidate the phenomena, to find out what can be known. This process uses *pre-reflective* experiencing (Spinelli 1995, p.24) as a way to immerse one's self in the phenomena, and achieve an 'amplified awareness' (Lett 1998, p.340) or 'indwelling' (Moustakas 1990, p.24). |

*cont.*

| ALPHA: reduction to essences | Protocol | Rationale |
|---|---|---|
| 3. Step back from the image, create distance and focus on the bigger picture including cultural or symbolic references. | Write down any words or phrases that come to mind. | This description gathers cultural and symbolic meanings to elucidate the sense patients are making of the phenomena. This process uses reflective experiencing, dwelling on the data to discover meaning and sense. |
| 4. Sorting and titling self-identities (Lett 1998, p.332). | Group the words generated by steps 1 and 2 into lists of similar words to make self-identity categories for the patient. Title the lists as voices of self-identity. | This is a process of gathering, sorting and reflecting upon the data, to create lists of words based on their sensed connectedness and shared meaning. |
| 5. Extracting the essences (Lett 1998, p.332). | Create an essence statement/description of experience for each list/theme/self-identity, based on the words within it. | This is a process of identifying the essential features or themes of the phenomena. |
| 6. Synthesis of essences. | Write two final essence statements: *Statement of Emergent Knowing:* This statement focuses on the essences derived from stepping into the image and experiencing it anew. *Statement of Emergent Learning:* This statement combines and brackets back in the cultural and symbolic references identified in step 2. | Heidegger's (1962 [1927]) *hermeneutic* phenomenology goes beyond the description of essences to discover the *meaning* of an experience by including *interpretation*. This is a way of combining the data to discover something further about the phenomena itself, through the synthesis of essences. |

This method of analysis leads to identifying personal themes and aspects of self-identity, as well as essence statements of emergent knowing and learning. This process acknowledges that as human beings we experience the world and each other through diverse multi-sensory and intersubjective ways.

In the Visual Analysis Matrix (Table 9.2) I give an example of how I used this process, generating a list of words and essence statements in order to evaluate Rose's *Poppy Field* portrait. The resulting essence statements are drawn from lists of words derived from 'stepping into the portrait' and experiencing it anew, and then a new list generated from 'stepping back' from the portrait and considering the cultural and symbolic significance of the portrait, or how it 'fits' within the world. These lists of words are then used to create the identity titles for each list and an essence statement for each list. These statements are then used to create statements of emergent knowing and learning.

Table 9.2 Example of how to 'extract the essences' from the portraits

| Zoom in | Zoom out | Sorting and titling | Extracting the essences | Synthesis of essences |
|---|---|---|---|---|
| Step into the image, experience being in the image, as if for the first time, employing intuition, wonder and curiosity, write down sensory and resonant words and phrases. | Step back from the image, create distance, focus on the bigger picture, write down a list of words, e.g. cultural or symbolic references. | Group the words generated by steps 1 and 2 into lists of similar words to make self-identity categories. Title the lists as voices of patients' self-identity. | Create an essence statement/ description of experience for each list/ theme, based on the words within it. | Write two final essence statements combining those found in step 4: *Statement of Emergent Knowing* and *Statement of Emergent Learning* |

*cont.*

| Zoom in | Zoom out | Sorting and titling | Extracting the essences | Synthesis of essences |
|---|---|---|---|---|
| Poppies, farm Landscape Poppy field Flowers Smoke, Earth Little black dress Pearly Queen Flowers in her hair, pink cheeks Shadows of clouds No shoes Pearly queen buttons Fish and flower Rose, daisy, corn Hills, sky, peace Idealised Bright colours Striking Jewel-like High contrast Diagonal divide Flower detail reflected in dress Blood red Battlefield? Spirit child Earth child Warrior child City child Smell the corn, earth, smoke, flowers, fresh air Feel the warmth of the earth, and sun, a soft breeze Prickles of the corn on skin Waiting to be found? Hear the birds and insects Silence and space | Klimt, symbolist Idealised? Symbolic, dreams Realist mythical Oil painting Body as landscape Undulating Body reflecting hills Child diagonal across canvas lying in field Cropped child Summer time Poppy field Little girl hiding? Alone, asleep Tendrils Earth and sky Black dress Hide and seek Uncomfortable Lost, lonely, isolated? Body twisted Invisible Pale white/blue bare arms and legs, vulnerable Right hand grasps flowers Recovery position? Cropped child Diagonal division Abandoned Waiting 5 years old? Hide and seek? Eyes shut so invisible? Can you see me? Will I be found? | **Embracing Mother Earth Earth Child Spirit Child Warrior Child** Smoke Flowers Landscape Poppies Shadows of clouds No shoes Tendrils Space, silence Birdsong, fresh air, peace Bright colours. Pink cheeks **Hide and Seek** Waiting to be found? Will I be found? Am I lost? Abandoned Lonely Alone, asleep Hiding? Body twisted Eye shut so invisible Counting to 100? City child Uncomfortable Invisible Pale white/ blue skin, bare arms and legs Isolated Abandoned Waiting Vulnerable Misplaced | I lie in a divided space Diagonally across hemispheres In the recovery position Poppies surround me. Earth-spirit child can hide herself in order to hide others. She can live in her imagination, and create her own reality. I lie in wait counting to 100? Will I be found, or will I lie here forever, forgotten, abandoned, searching, hiding, I continue to count... City girl in her little black dress Cannot be seen and cannot see you Displaced between worlds | *Statement of Emergent Knowing:* As Earth-spirit-warrior child I can hide myself in order to hide others. I can live in my imagination, and create my own reality. In my silence unseen and alone, and yet Embracing Mother Earth – I find myself. *Statement of Emergent Learning:* There is a sense of continuation of being and spiritual presence in Mother Earth/ Nature, which supports and heals Rose. The Poppy Field depicts the moment of identity transition and adaption in which 'isolated-city-child' becomes 'earth-spirit-warrior child'. |

## Voice-centred interpersonal analysis

For the analysis of verbal data gathered within the end of project interviews I used an adaptation of *voice-centred relational analysis*, developed by Brown and Gilligan and their colleagues in the USA (see Brown and Gilligan 1991, 1992, 1993; Brown *et al.* 1988; Gilligan 1982) during their feminist research into the lives of women and girls in the fields of developmental psychology and education (Mauthner and Doucet 1998, p.8). The method is rooted in relational theory and hermeneutics (Brown and Gilligan 1992) and aims to explore, within individuals' verbal accounts, the relationship they have with the people around them and with themselves, and also the social and cultural contexts of where they live (Mauthner and Doucet 1998, p.9).

Portraits are silent and yet they 'speak' a universal language; it therefore seems logical to look for 'voices' of self-identity as well as themes when analysing the portraits using ALPHA. This leads to identifying several different self-identity voices personal to each patient, which can then be listened for and identified within the *voice-centred relational analysis* (Balan 2005; Gilligan *et al.* 2003; Mauthner and Doucet 1998). I chose to adopt more than one approach to the analysis for this study, as I felt that focusing on just one method might have biased the interpretation to 'fit' the chosen model, and that by using two, a more rigorous analysis could be achieved.

I used the protocol of Gilligan *et al.*'s (2003) voice-centred relational analysis method (as outlined by Balan 2005), as a method I could easily adapt to find multiple self-identities with the portraits. Gilligan *et al.*'s (2003) method consists of four main steps that involved multiple 'listenings' to voice recordings of participants. These were:

1. To listen for the plot.

2. Listening for and underlining 'I-Me' statements to make an 'I Poem'.

3. Listening for and underlining contrapuntal (multiple) voices.

4. Composing an analysis.

I therefore adjusted and simplified this analysis for portrait therapy as follows:

1. Listening for and highlighting contrapuntal (multiple) voices of identity, as identified within the portraits analysis.

2. Listening for and highlighting the emergent themes.
3. Composing an analysis in the form of the case-studies.

The 'multiple listenings' for voices of identity served to check the validity of, and enhance the phenomenological analysis of the portraits. Listening for the emergent themes enabled a cross-case analysis of the themes to take place. A series of 'listenings' assumes that self-identity voices are 'contrapuntal' rather than 'monotonic', meaning that different voices can be heard entwined or alongside each other (Gilligan *et al.* 2003, p.150). It is important to *listen* for voices of self-identity – rather than *read* them, because *listening* requires a different sensory modality, with intention and meaning contained within: tone of voice, inflection, pauses and emphasis. This process enables a further period of 'indwelling' (Moustakas 1990, p.24) or 'dwelling with the data' (Finlay 2011, p.228), recognising that analysis is an ongoing process.

### Protocol: Identifying patients' *voices of self-identity*

Once the self-identity voices have been identified from the analysis of the portraits, transcribe and print out the patient's end of project interview, and then, whilst listening to the audio recording of this, use different coloured highlighter pens to highlight where you hear the individual self-identity voices, as previously identified from the analysis of the portraits. Note where the different voices take precedence over other voices, or other dominant voices. Notice the way these voices interact and which are dominant or subversive. This enables the patients' voices of self-identity to be searched for within the text and is a way of double checking that the voices of self-identity emerging from the visual analysis can also be found in the patients' speech, thereby increasing rigor and validity.

### Protocol: Identifying master themes

Look for correlations between each of the patients' lived experiences and identify master themes identifiable in each case-study. Move relevant sections of each patient's end of project interview transcripts into lists of texts relating to each of the master themes.

These can then be used to describe where the patients' experiences converge and therefore how this can be generalised.

I have chosen this method as it attempts to keep the patients' voices intact, and enables a direct link between the verbal and visual data, as well as insight into how the different 'voices of self-identity' interact, dominate or intercede within the end of project interviews.

Once the themes have been identified, sections of the patients' EPIs can be placed under headings for each theme identified; this can then be used within the case-study as evidence. An example of this process is shown in Table 9.3.

Table 9.3 Example of identifying themes found in the analysis in the EPI data

| Increasing patients' 'creative capacity' to adapt to illness | Portraits making meaning, increasing a sense of homelike-being-in-the-world and ontological security | Mirroring and attunement, intersubjective and symbolic ways of knowing and being and relating |
|---|---|---|
| 'It made me realise I could still explore different things' (Rose EPI). | 'Yeah, because now, instead of being a "nobody" this is as if I have done something in my life' (Rose EPI). | 'You told me the story of my life...' (Peter EPI). |
| 'What it has done is help me accept the loss of Mark' (Peter EPI). | 'I felt worthless and useless when we first started this project. But by having to relive my life, by telling the story, I've realised that I've actually become stronger through the illness. The iller I've got, the stronger I've got. And that no, I'm not useless – I've got a purpose in life, and I'm fulfilling it' (Norma EPI). | 'Your input more or less got me to a "T"...' (Paul EPI). |

## *Reliability and validity in phenomenological research*

Issues around reliability and validity are considered differently in phenomenological studies, where 'essential meaning, the sense of the empirical rather than facts' is highlighted (Quail and Peavy 1994, p.47). Giorgi (1989) suggests that trustworthiness within phenomenological research can be established through the researcher presenting a convincing and thorough investigation, and establishing worthwhile results when measured against the original aims of the study. It is also important to demonstrate 'methodological congruence (rigorous and appropriate procedures) and experiential concerns that provide insight in terms of plausibility and illumination about a specific phenomenon' (Pereira 2012, p.19).

To ensure a robust analysis I suggest using Finlay's four 'Rs' of 'good' phenomenological research, i.e. research must be 'rigorous, resonant, reflexive and relevant' (Finlay 2011, p.180).

Within this chapter I have described and discussed the methods used to generate the data for analysis within the final two phases of the project. In phase one the emphasis was on the use of button, LEGO® and photo-elicitation tasks, to help patients describe their lived experience of self-identity and the impact of life-threatening and chronic illnesses, and the development of the active documentation sketchbook as a creative, reflexive and reflective space to document the processes involved. Phase two focused on the use of collages and prose poems as *response art*, reflecting the patients' stories back to them in a visual and poetic form, and the subsequent negotiation of *statements of intention* for the portraits.

Phase three included a discussion of the reasoning behind the use of portraiture as a third hand art therapy intervention, and the protocol used for painting the portraits, which may have included painting from life, or using reference photographs and the *appropriation* of works by other artists through the portrait reference album. I have highlighted potential problems with this method and how I have attempted to resolve or minimise these. Phase three ended with the semi-structured end of project interviews. I have shown that patients were given the opportunity to adjust or amend their end of project interview transcripts if they so wished.

Phase four included the visual analysis of the data generated by this project; I have outlined the reasoning behind the selection of *reflexive-relational* (Finlay 2011) and *experiential* (Lett 1998) phenomenological analysis methods to adapt for the visual data, and the perceived advantages for this project. I described the combination of transcendental and hermeneutic phenomenological approaches to the analysis, which facilitated the description, and interpretation of the lived experience of the patients, as well as the bracketing out of my preconceptions and reflexive resonance. I also described how this study correlates with Finlay's (2011) four 'Rs' of 'good' phenomenological research.

Phase five consisted of the adaption of *voice-centred relational analysis* (Balan 2005; Gilligan *et al.* 2003; Mauthner and Doucet 1998), which enabled patients' voices of identity to be identified and used within the case-studies. I have adapted this method to *listen for* (and highlight within the transcripts) the different voices of identity as identified in the *arts-based life-world phenomenological analysis* through a process of multiple 'listenings'. I also described my rationale for a multiple case-study design and how this fits with a phenomenological study. These case-studies were then checked by patients for their final adjustment and approval, ensuring that the descriptions and negotiated interpretations accurately reflected their lived experience of the intervention.

— Chapter 10 —

# AFTERWORD

*Drawing Conclusions*

When I began developing this intervention it was with the belief that portraiture had the potential to act as an attuning 'mirror' for the patients to see themselves in more clearly, a way to *revision* and *remember* their sense of self-identity. However, this doesn't adequately reflect the *power* of art, and as Trotsky says: 'Art…is not a mirror, but a hammer: it does not reflect, it shapes' (Trotsky 2005, p.120, first published in 1924). Trotsky's quote suggests therefore that portraiture is more effective than simply *reflecting* self-identities implies, there is *power* in portraiture, and it does *shape* people, and the ability of portraiture to transform paint and canvas into a powerful and meaningful representation of a person is arguably the emotive power that enabled patients to *re-shape* their disrupted self-identities.

The initial elicitation phase of the project was a process of unravelling and revealing the many layers of self-identity evident within the patients' stories. These stories were generally episodic and fragmented, they did not necessarily begin their life story at the 'beginning' and end at the 'present', they sprang out of the button and LEGO®tasks and photographs of events that were *turning points* in their lives. One of the most important aspects of this process was to find and recognise these turning points, and these were depicted within the portraits as moments of *becoming* (e.g. as in Rose's *Poppy Field* portrait (Figure 7.15) and Norma's *Fish Out of Water* portrait (Figure 6.19). This helped patients to *re-member* their creative child-selves and the adaptive strengths they possessed.

## Results from the end of project interviews

Within their end of project interviews all the patients claimed that their involvement in the project had been a positive one, using words to describe their experience such as: *extremely interesting, imaginative, fascinating, very good, informative, rewarding* and *emotional*. All (seven out of seven) patients indicated that through the project they had discovered new or forgotten parts of their self-identity. Patients also indicated that the project had helped them feel *heard*, and that it had given them an overall *stronger* sense of self-identity. When asked how their families had reacted to the portraits and collages, all said very positive things, and of the 37 portraits completed only two portraits were disliked by their families, and these were embodiments of patients' pain and suffering. All said that they thought the project would help other people diagnosed with a similar illness to them, with four out of seven adding that it would also benefit people with other issues, such as depression. When asked how they felt about the paintings going into an exhibition all responded positively, using words such as: *wonderful, I shall be pleased, I like that idea, very proud, an honour*. Patients were asked if they felt in any way exploited by the project and all said 'no', with three out of seven adding that it had been the reverse of exploitative.

Although this study did not specifically aim to find generalisations within the patients' accounts with the particular focus being on individual self-identity, common themes were identified. I do however acknowledge that a different art therapist undertaking portrait therapy with the same group of patients may have produced different but no less valid results, due to the personalised 'attuning' aspect of this particular intervention.

## Themes from the analysis

In the following sections I discuss the significance of the findings as clustered under the three master themes found in the analysis, as well as identifying key aspects of clinical theory development, and implications for future research. I then offer a final reflection on my own personal experience of providing portrait therapy for patients.

## Master theme 1: Increasing patients' creative capacity to adapt to illness

Within the analysis, I found evidence to support the view that portrait therapy increases a person's *creative capacity to adapt to illness*. I see this as a process of *empowerment*, adaption and *growth*, offering the potential for ongoing adjustment to self-identity as the patient's life-threatening and chronic illness progresses.

I described how Hilary found an increased capacity for *imaginative thinking*, finding relief and comfort in a portrait, showing herself finally and eternally *Held by an Angel*. I identified *humour* as an *adaptive* process facilitated and developed within portrait therapy, helping patients to manage their experience of liminality and unhomelike-being-in-the-world. Humour also enabled patients to ask the metaphorical question '*Do you get it?*' and therefore '*Do you get me?*', highlighting the importance of humour as a function of *being known*. Hilary and Peter demonstrated the value of the portraits by asking for copies to 'keep with them at all times'. Norma used the project to 'find' and grieve for her abandoned baby-self, as well as her own lost babies, bringing her past into the present, to be engaged with in the ritualised practices of the Native American Indian smudging ceremony.

*Mourning losses* was a key adaptive process facilitated by this intervention, and patients used the portraits as *externalising objects*, capable of *containing* and *holding* hidden pain and suffering, enabling both *emotional connection* and *distancing* to take place, and new meanings to be developed. Through engagement in creative and adaptive *rituals*, Norma and Peter described how the portraits enabled experiences of *closure* regarding important bereavements and losses within their lives. The findings also suggest an increase in the patients' feelings of control and autonomy, and the rediscovery of adaptive strategies used in their pre-illness lives, resulting in increased adaption through self-care and agency.

## Master theme 2: Portraits making meaning: Increasing the lived experience of homelike-being-in-the-world *and* ontological security

As discussed in Chapter 1, a sense of 'home-like-being-in-the-world' (Svenaeus 2011) is often lost when people are plunged into 'liminal space' (Sibbett 2005a, pp.12–37; Turner 1969 [1995]) or the 'world of illness' (Radley 2009) following the diagnosis of a life-threatening and chronic illness. The visual and verbal data has shown that the patients used the portraits and portrait-sculptures in ritualistic and sacralising ways, enabling feelings of *ontological security* and *homelike-being-in-the-world*, characterised by a sense of belonging. All the patients to some extent utilised this project to connect to something or someone they felt a sense of *belonging* to and as such the portraits acted as bridges to significant others and to humanity as a whole. Paul found a sense of homelike-being-in-the-world in his *At Home* portrait, which also enabled him to develop an increase in agency and self-care. All the patients said they gained an increased sense of a *worthwhile* and *valuable self/life*, with their portraits becoming a focus and channel for 'love', enabling patients and myself to express 'love' for the portraits without this being misconstrued.

This process of *re-membering* and *belonging* engendered feelings of *continuity* within the patients, linking and integrating aspects of their *past, present* and *future* self-identities. Susan found a sense of connection with her late mother in *The Paper Dress* portrait-sculpture and a sense of continuity of being within her four portraits. Despite the gap of nearly 70 years, Bill's WWII experiences, depicted within the portraits, collages and prose poems, revealed *everything he needed to tell me* about his self-identity and how it had been *formed, broken* and *re-formed*. Rose celebrated her sense of belonging and connection to Freddie Mercury in her portrait *Bohemian Rhapsody*, someone she recognises as a fellow inhabitant of *liminal* space.

The evidence suggests that portrait therapy enabled patients to develop their personal search for spiritual meaning through a process of 'making special' (Dissanayake 1988) and this correlates with Aita et al.'s (2010) study where exhibition viewers noted that the portraits portrayed evidence of a search for meaning. The patients also expressed an experience of portraits as *legacy* and as an important part of their *future* self-identity, thereby equating to a sense of *immortalisation* or *cheating death*. The portraits captured *time* within the layers of paint applied and this, combined with the therapist's *positive focused attention*, resulted in feelings of *being-held-in-mind* and the formation of *positive memories*.

This evidence therefore supports the view that portrait therapy enables an increase in: meaning making, ontological security, and the lived experience of *homelike-being-in-the-world*, all of which may contribute to a stronger, more coherent sense of self-identity.

## Master theme 3: Mirroring and attunement through portraiture; intersubjective and symbolic ways of knowing, being and relating

The data provided by the analysis suggests that portraits created by 'third hand' methods are effective visual channels for *mirroring* and *attunement*. Through this process patients became aware of previously *unknown* and *untold* aspects of self-identity, sharing stories of self-identity they had *never told anyone else before*, which correlates with findings from the Saving Faces portraiture project (Hutchison, Gilbert and Farrand 2000).

The portraits enabled mirroring and attunement that was both an *intra*subjective validation of self-identity for the patients through viewing portraits and collages that *they needed to see themselves*, as well as an *inter*subjective validation provided by portraits they needed *others* to see. This is based on the view that portraits as subject-objects can be seen as active *participants* in the world, able to bear witness to the patients' physical presence and subjectivity, and as such able to influence and change the views of people and society. Through the mirroring and attunement within his *At Home* portrait, Paul found a renewed sense of *agency* and liberation from his fear of leaving the house, enabling him to revisit, for a final time, a place which he 'loved' and where he was *known*. Through viewing *The Two Normas* portrait Norma was able to *see the difference* between two important aspects of her self-identity and realise for the first time how they support each other.

Mirroring and attunement included a process of *aesthetic resonance*, which equated to my intuitive additions of 'beauty', symbolic meaning and complexity, resulting in an overall sense of *coherence* within the portraits. This process enabled patients to recapture a sense of their own significance and themselves as *valuable* and *worthwhile*. Susan and Norma were able to redefine childhood experiences and reclaim their child-selves, enjoying the layered meanings and complexity added to the portraits. The development of an *intersubjective symbolic capability* with the patients was crucial to this process, enabling patients to unravel layers of meaning within the portraits. The portraits mirrored the patients as 'whole people', which correlates with Aita *et al.'s* findings (2010, p.5).

The analysis demonstrated that portraits have the ability to 'hold' and 'contain' dualities such as *hope* and *despair*, mitigating feelings of *cognitive dissonance* (Festinger 1962). In *Being Pandora* (see Figure 6.16), good and evil, power and helplessness are explored and Susan is left holding *hope* within the 'box'. In *Broken Lungs* (Figure 5.5), Paul explores the dualities of *inside* and *outside* realities, and literally 'opens up' and 'lets us in' to his inner world of pain and suffering.

Aita *et al.'s* study noted that exhibition attendees recognised the presence of 'hope' and yet also the centrality of 'mortality' within the portraits (2010, p.5), suggesting a correlation with the findings of this project regarding the holding of dualities.

Mirroring and attunement through portraiture allows a different way of seeing and *knowing* a person, through the sustained positive focused attention and empathic listening required to accurately re-present the patients' vision of themselves.

## Portrait therapy and clinical theory development

My aims in relation to theory building within art therapy and palliative care relate specifically to the development of portrait therapy, extending and combining the art therapy models of 'mirroring and attunement' (Wright 2009), the art therapist's 'third hand' (Kramer 1971), and Carel's philosophical theories on 'health within illness' (Carel 2008). For the purposes of portrait therapy, I extended the boundaries of Wright's theory to include portraits painted *for* others, as a way to enable patients to achieve a stronger, more coherent sense of self-identity. The evidence from this study suggests that the portrait does become, for the patient, a surrogate for the 'good enough (m)other' of infancy, holding, attuning, reflecting and validating their sense of self-identity.

The discovery of Edith Kramer's 'third hand' theory (1971) gave me, as the artist/therapist, 'permission' to develop an intervention that focused on the 'art object' as the healing form, rather than focusing on the 'art making process'. This reversal enabled the analysis to be focused almost entirely on the healing qualities of the art objects, i.e. the significant resonant forms within the portraits. Ultimately Kramer believed the aim of art therapy was to create aesthetically coherent artworks, and the evidence suggests that this was enabled through portrait therapy, despite the lack of patient engagement in the physical art-making process.

This study necessitated questioning the taken-for-granted normalised assumptions within art therapy regarding:

- Who makes the artwork in art therapy?
- The universal requirement for confidentiality irrespective of context?
- The *dys*-engagement with aesthetics as a healing force?

These questions and their implications are discussed in the following sections.

### *Who makes the artwork in art therapy?*

The expectation common to most art therapy models, that patients will create the artwork within art therapy and talk about this within the sessions, has its 'limitations' (Maclagan 2011, p.8), particularly in palliative care where patients are often too unwell, fatigued, disabled, or for any other reason unwilling or unable to make art. This means that many patients who might benefit from art therapy self-exclude, and for those who attend and make no art, the session becomes reliant on 'talking therapy', which while beneficial in its own way is not the point of *art* therapy and does not harness the power of creative processes to transform meanings and experience.

The data from this project suggests that in palliative care, the making of art by an art therapist *for* patients, including portraits, collages and prose poems, is a useful and healing way of working. However, when art therapists make images *for* patients/clients, they make themselves vulnerable and risk making mistakes, but the findings suggest that portrait therapy *benefits* from being a *third hand* encounter and that this is part of its efficacy. Self-portraits created by patients would have excluded the important aspects of *mirroring and attunement, empathic focused attention, aesthetic resonance* and *being held in mind*, and was quickly ruled out by the patient focus group when designing the study.

## *The universal requirement for confidentiality irrespective of context*

This project has shown that in certain circumstances, particularly when validating self-identity, confidentiality may be inappropriate or even counterproductive. All the patients in this study indicated that they wanted their portraits to be shown in publications and exhibitions and yet art therapists are often reticent about asking patients permission to display their artwork.

Anonymising the portraits would have defeated the object of the intervention and yet in the National Health Service Confidentiality Policy (April 2013) it states in point 4.1.3 that, 'Person-identifiable information, wherever possible, must be anonymised by removing as many identifiers as possible whilst not unduly compromising the utility of the data.' To anonymise a portrait would have meant blanking out patients faces, meaning they could never bear witness to the presence or self-identity of the patients.

Whilst confidentiality has been put in place for good reasons to safeguard and protect patients' privacy, its blanket use seems to suggest that patients are *unable to make their own decisions* around confidentiality. This assumption seems to infringe the Mental Capacity Act (2005), which states in section 1.3 that, 'A person is not to be treated as unable to make a decision unless all practicable steps to help him to do so have been taken without success' and in section 1.2 that, 'A person must be assumed to have capacity unless it is established that he lacks capacity.' My contention is that decisions are often made by art therapists *for* patients, without recognising the patients' rights to choose for themselves.

It is important to remember that a blanket confidentiality policy also serves to keep those who are ill separate and hidden, and to silence their voices. Radley (2009) suggests that the 'acceptability' of representations of illness, are often 'a useful measure of where matters concerning illness (and the sick as a group) stand in the scale of public concern' (ibid., p.17). Ultimately, it is important to be aware that patients have a right to be seen and heard, to reciprocate, and most importantly to be supported in their right to decide for themselves.

## *The* dys-*engagement with aesthetics as a healing force*

Whilst I do not argue against a focus on pain and suffering within the many approaches to art therapy, the results from this study correlate with McNiff's (2004, p.60) suggestion that ignoring the power of aesthetics to transform ugliness and pain may impose limits on the potential of art created within art therapy to heal in diverse ways. I agree with Knill's (1995) proposal for an 'aesthetic response' within art therapy and the integration of the cathartic with the aesthetic (Knill *et al.* 2005), something which is evident within the *aesthetic resonance* added to the portraits and equates to holding dualities such as 'beauty' and 'suffering' within the one image.

The attachment of empathically attuned *aesthetic resonance* to patient's images of self-identity is a key element of portrait therapy, and a powerful healing force. As Wilkinson and Chilton (2013, p.8) say, 'Capitalizing on such "signature strengths" as creativity, playfulness, appreciation of beauty, and other elements of positive art therapy might inspire transformation of our practices and communities, not only to cope with stressors but also to attend to, appreciate, and attain the best in life.'

## Portrait therapy with other client groups: Implications for further research

Within the end of project interviews, I asked patients if they thought that the intervention would help other people living with similar illnesses. All the patients expressed the view that it would be helpful, with some adding that it may also help people with other issues such as depression.

I believe that portrait therapy would be beneficial for many different client groups, especially those who experience trauma (of any kind) as a disruption to their sense of self-identity. These may include (but are not restricted to) people living with addiction, bereavement and loss; physical disability or disfigurement; depression and anxiety; combat stress, post traumatic stress syndrome, etc.

Additional research evaluating the effectiveness of portrait therapy with people who experience *trauma* as a disruption to their self-identity would build upon the results from this and Aita *et al.*'s study, adding to knowledge in this area – as would the research of portrait therapy as a third hand art therapy intervention for children, teenagers and people from other ethnic groups facing life-threatening and chronic illnesses.

The findings within this study correlate with Aita *et al.*'s where they reiterate 'the importance of recognising the identity of the person even when both the patient and those around (him) are overshadowed by the medical condition' (2010, p.10). This has important implications for the training of healthcare professionals in ways that affirm and support the fragile self-identities of their patients, something I believe is central to *holistic* care and the empowerment of the individual.

Recognising the shortcomings of our culture, and our health service, is an important function of culturally aware art therapists, and if we do not question or critique cultural constructs, then we collude with that culture (Moon 2014), with the stigmatisation of illness and the denial of death, and fail to recognise the needs of individuals facing life-threatening and chronic illnesses. The findings have highlighted the need for increased awareness by healthcare professionals regarding the power they possess, through their actions, words or interventions, to either validate or demean the self-identities of their patients/clients. Recognising and reaffirming positive past, present and future self-identities, particularly for older adults, should be considered a vital aspect of their psychological and emotional support. This challenges the widespread prescription of antidepressants for people who are living with identities disrupted by illness or who are essentially lonely or *unknown* (Hansen *et al.* 2007).

The portraits within this project are socially responsive artworks (Hocoy 2007) in that they highlight a need and point out the current lack of time and opportunity, for self-identity validation and mirroring and attunement within relationships between healthcare providers and patients. I suggest that 'third hand' interventions such as portrait therapy have the potential to offer real benefits to patients, at a time when they feel the medical profession has 'given up on them', an intervention with the potential to offer amelioration of suffering and increased quality of life.

This project builds on Carel's (2008) thesis and adds to knowledge in the field of medical humanities, in that it offers further evidence to support the idea that people living with life-threatening and chronic illnesses experience illness primarily as a disruption to the lived body, but also as a disruption to their sense of self-identity. Further research into self-identity disruption as part of the lived experience of illness would add to knowledge in this field.

## Implications for art therapy training

This project has implications for the training of art therapy students, and I suggest theoretical and experiential training for first year students could include 'third hand' and 'mirroring and attuning' techniques, e.g. creating collage and prose poems as 'response art' initially for other students and subsequently for their clients within palliative care placement settings. Students could also practise the button and LEGO® emotional distancing techniques with other students in experiential training sessions, before using them with their clients at their placements. This project also highlights the importance of art therapy students' creative art practice with a particular emphasis on continued professional development in the area of portraiture. Life drawing/portrait sessions could become part of the curriculum, as well as developing their creative art practice to include an awareness of aesthetic resonance. Art therapy students in their final year could use the portrait therapy protocol as experiential work with other students, and art therapy students with placements within *palliative care* could then use the portrait therapy protocol to work (under supervision) with patients. Whilst portrait therapy may be beneficial to other client groups who experience trauma as a disruption to their self-identity, further research is needed before training can be suggested for this.

### *Reflecting on experience: Portraits as unique ways of knowing the self and being known*

The findings from this study suggest that portrait therapy is an embodied way of knowing the self and of paying *empathic focused attention*, offering a unique way of accounting for the body and the physical presence of a person. Instead of 'losing' anything through the adoption of 'third hand' art therapy techniques, empathic attunement and aesthetic resonance is gained. The body becomes newly visible in a way that is not possible in narrative, acknowledging its importance as humanity's only way of experiencing the world and being experienced. The portraits reflect, through the eyes and hands of the artist/therapist messages of: companioning, witness, presence and the holding in mind of the person portrayed.

From the evidence generated by this study I contend that the feeling of *knowing the self* is intrinsically linked to *being known*, therefore patients have a need to *be known* in order to *know themselves*. This relational view of self-knowledge highlights the requirement to 'understand identity not as a fixed, natural state of being, but as a process of *becoming*' (Kinnvall 2004, pp.747–8 [my emphasis]) and the portraits act like *bridges* or conduits, where *knowing* is offered *through being known*, both by the artist/therapist and by others, through the viewing of the portraits. This may indicate that the negative impact of isolation and loneliness upon the body and the immune system (Jaremka *et al.* 2012) is linked to being *un*known by others, but also the self.

The evidence suggests that there is a fundamental need or urgency to know the self or *be known* when one is faced with impending death and that the portraits enable this by *being the bridges between* and therefore providing the *difference* between:

> Seeing and *being seen*
>
> Recognising and *being recognised*
>
> Knowing and *being known.*

As bridges, linking these opposing concepts, portraits become *a unique way of knowing the self,* therefore the above equation can be developed into:

> Seeing *through* being seen
>
> Recognising *through* being recognised and
>
> Knowing *through* being known.

As Carel (2004, p.230) says:

> Meaning is not generated by the speaker, rather it is located intersubjectively, somewhere between the reception of the listener and the intention of the speaker. If there is no one to receive my speech I become mute. I cannot speak or make sense at all, not even to myself.

Radley (2009, p.90) believed that the act of making testimony was the key to healing, saying:

For people who have undergone extreme suffering, testifying in this way – by means of speech, text or paint – is not a distillation of knowledge but knowing oneself again only through making testimony.

However, the results suggest that it is knowing the self *through being known*, which is key. This is subtly different in that it requires a *reflected* testimony, an *attuned knowing* by another person, that of the '(m)other' or artist/therapist. This has important implications for healthcare professionals who do not 'know' their patients – for the widespread prescription of antidepressants for patients at end of life (Grau 2006) who experience life-threatening and chronic illnesses as a disruption to their self-identity. This project has highlighted the need for those living with life-threatening and chronic illnesses to express who they are/were within an empathic relationship, and particularly older adults who may express a *different* self-identity to the one they are currently 'living'. Being known for 'who' they are, not 'what' society perceives them to be, with all the stigma and judgement implied in that. The findings suggest that being plunged into the liminal space of life-threatening and chronic illnesses requires a *creative* solution, or a creative, collaborative and flexible kind of *knowing*, to ameliorate *suffering*.

Portraits as empathic attunement therefore have the power to 'call us into relationship' (Gablik 1991, p.114) and to establish feelings of connection and understanding between ourselves and others. All of which adds support to the concept of portraiture as a therapeutic intervention, enabling self-identity coherence and increased quality of life.

As an intervention for vulnerable people there are important reasons why *portrait therapy* should be an *art therapy* intervention carried out by a trained art therapist (with skills in portraiture and 'third hand' interventions) rather than a portrait artist. As this study, the Saving Faces (Farrand 2000) project and Portraits of Care study (Aita *et al.* 2010) have shown, there seems to be an interesting *portrait effect* in that having a portrait painted often enables people to open up to the artist and tell them stories of self-identity they have *told no one else before*. It is important therefore, when working with vulnerable people, to know how to witness, contain and perhaps transform this knowledge. Second, as Kramer pointed out, third hand techniques require the therapist to suppress their own 'pictorial ideas or preferences' (Kramer 1986, p.71). As well as working on a creative level, art therapists are trained to understand the 'interpersonal dynamics' (Wood 2005, p.84) that exist between the art therapist and patient, the need to develop a therapeutic relationship with secure boundaries, and are required to undergo regular clinical supervision to ensure their own and the patients' safety. Artists may not have access to this kind of learning or support, and may not understand the ethical issues regarding confidentiality and its limits.

If as art therapists we are to produce *our own kind of evidence* (Gilroy 1996, p.55), we ourselves need to be involved in the finding of it and the explaining of it, and third hand interventions offer just such an opportunity. This will not be gained simply by observing the behaviour of others, but by stepping out of the shadows and making border crossings into unknown landscapes (McNiff 1992). This involves *giving time* and working collaboratively with our clients, *to enable them to tell us what they need, what works and why*.

Importantly the findings from this study support the claim made by Kramer (1971, p.40) that creating portraits of clients has the ability to 'reassure them and strengthen their feelings of identity' (ibid.). It also corroborates the claims made by Moon (2002, p.214), that creating portraits of clients is one of the most direct ways that art therapists can 'witness' their clients, to promote feelings of being acknowledged rather than judged, and to 'take time to notice and at some level, to care' (Moon 2002, p.215).

## A final reflection

Accompanying Rose, Hilary, Peter, Bill, Susan, Norma and Paul on their journey of self-discovery and reflection has been a humbling and extraordinary privilege, and yet with each completion I felt a sense of guilt, that I was free to continue with my life, whereas they were left to continue alone in their liminal world of illness. However, our time together left a trail of collaboration and creativity evident in the portraits, collages and prose poems, acting as a lasting reminder of this journey, and as points of reference for the patients in the uncertain landscape that lies ahead.

As I near the end of this book I reflect upon my own triadic self-identities involved in this project and the addition of a fourth – my writer/author identity. I have come to realise that my *artist* and *writer* self-identities are like 'jealous lovers', clamouring for my attention – when I am at my computer writing, I am aware of my artist identity sulking and scowling in the background, and I know that when I return to her she will resist my advances, and sabotage all my initial artistic attempts. However, my writer, artist, therapist and researcher identities have all joined together in helping me find my 'voice', and through this, to know myself better. If this process has taught me anything it is that *if I do not know myself, I cannot know my patients*; similarly if I do not make art to feed my soul, then I become empty and I have nothing to offer them. By stepping out of the shadows and painting portraits *for* patients, my own artistic identity becomes visible and I have to own my part in *creating experience* and *creating meaning with* my patients. Therefore, the success of portrait therapy depends on my willingness to be *available*, to become *vulnerable*, and to remain *flexible*, in their service.

Sadly, in the past months five of the patients I worked with on this project have died. Working in palliative care there is an anticipation that patients will die, and yet each death came as a shock and left me questioning whether I had done *enough* to help them. Thinking about this I was reminded again of Winnicott's 'good enough (m)other' and also the sense that death always leaves unfinished business. Each loss inevitably affects who I am, through the loss of a relational sense of self-identity, unique to each patient and myself.

I have attended each patient's funeral and created a final creative acknowledgement of our collaborative relationship (see Figure 10.1), both ritualistic practices that enable the creating of a *farewell gesture* important for closure. As Wood (2005) says, 'The process of building up and letting go of relationships is intrinsic to working in cancer care, and in the end, we must be satisfied with this...' (ibid., p.97).

Within the portraits something tangible remains of the subjectivity of the person portrayed, providing evidence of their personal significance and the sacredness of human life. Through this project and enabling patients to find their voices, I also found my own voice, as I started to speak and show this work to the world. As such, developing portrait therapy has also been about my own identity, about reconciling the *artist, therapist* and *researcher* within me into a coherent whole.

AFTERWORD

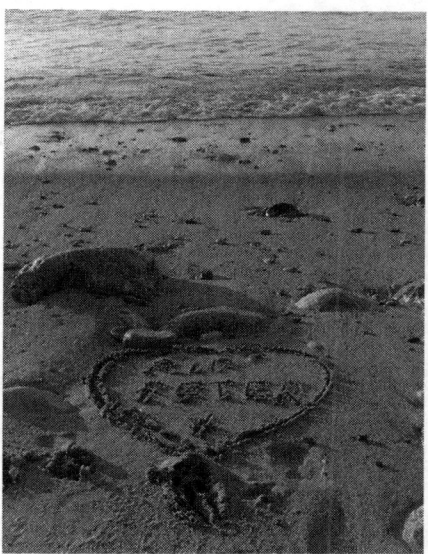

Figure 10.1 *RIP Peter*.

Now the portraits must 'go and do their work'. As Pinkola Estes once said, 'Art is not just for oneself, not just a marker of one's own understanding. It is also a map for those who follow after us' (1992, p.13).

— Appendix 1 —

# PORTRAIT REFERENCE ALBUM

*(90 portraits/sculptures dating from 1661 to 2010)*

| Title | Artist and date |
|---|---|
| *Young Woman Holding a Black Cat* | Gwen John, 1920–5 |
| *Constellation* | Mika Kato, 2004 |
| *Rest* | Edwin Harris, 1855–1906 |
| *Cupid Delivering Psyche* | Edward Burne-Jones, 1871 |
| *Fibre Portrait* | Jill Parry, 2009 |
| *Arctic Hare Skullcap* | Katherine Coe, 2009 |
| *Distill* | Sarah Clement, 2010 |
| *Twins Border* | Sarah Clement, 2010 |
| *Pillar of Salt (Lot's Wife)* | Sam Webber, 2008 |
| *The Return Home* | Roselina Hung, 2007 |
| *Self-Portrait (The Past Five Years)* | Roselina Hung, 2006 |
| *Mom & Dad 1* | Roselina Hung, 2008 |
| *The Order of Release* | Sir John Everett Millais, 1853 |
| *Mariana* | Sir John Everett Millais, 1851 |
| *The Blind Girl* | Sir John Everett Millais, 1856 |
| *Young Girl* | Sir John Everett Millais, 1852 |
| *Self-Portrait* | David Caldwell, 2009 |
| *John* | Benjamin Cohen, 2008 |
| *Brian* | Benjamin Cohen, 2008 |
| *Liam* | Elizabeth Payton, 1996 |
| *Zandvoort Fisher Girl* | Elizabeth Adela Forbes, 1912 |
| *Glauke: Pensive* | Edwin Longsden Long, 1883 |
| *April Love* | Arthur Hughes, 1856 |
| *Self Portrait* | Rembrandt, 1661 |
| *Self-Portrait (1914)* | Sir Stanley Spencer, 1914 |
| *Portrait Presume de son geolier* | Jacques-Louis David, c1820 |
| *Self-Portrait* | Eugene Delacroix, c1818 |

## PORTRAIT REFERENCE ALBUM

| | |
|---|---|
| *The English Boy* | Ford Madox Brown, 1860 |
| *Girl Before the Mirror* | Pablo Picasso, 1932 |
| *The Weeping Woman* | Pablo Picasso, 1937 |
| *Emilie Flöge* | Gustav Klimt, 1902 |
| *Three Ages of Women* | Gustav Klimt, 1905 |
| *Endangered Species IV* | Paul W Ruiz, 2008 |
| *Saltimbanque II* | Paul W Ruiz, 2008 |
| *Child Portrait* | Gee Vaucher, 2010 |
| *Self Portrait Sketch* | Paul S Brown, 2005 |
| *Girl Reading* | Charles Edward Perugini, 1878 |
| *Carnation, Lily, Lily, Rose* | John Singer Sargent, 1886 |
| *Jacques Barenthon* | John Singer Sargent, 1883 |
| *Ena and Betty Wertheimer* | John Singer Sargent, 1901 |
| *William Butler Yates* (drawing) | John Singer Sargent, 1908 |
| *Andromeda: Grand Hôtel de l'Observatoire* | Joseph Cornell, 1954 |
| *Circe Invidiosa* | John W. Waterhouse, 1892 |
| *Garton Orme at the Spinet* | Jonathan Richardson the elder, 1707 |
| | |
| *Broken Column* | Frida Kahlo, 1944 |
| *Tree of Hope Keep Strong* | Frida Kahlo, 1946 |
| *The Two Fridas* | Frida Kahlo, 1939 |
| *My Body is No Longer a Temple* | Hollis Sigler, 1995 |
| *Out of this World* | John D. Edwards, 2008 |
| *Carry Me This Way* | Michele Angelo Petrone, 1996 |
| *Portrait on Violin* | P. J. Crook, 2010 |
| *Drip Portrait* | Indigo (contemporary street art) |
| *Dame Judi Dench* | Alessandro Raho, 2004 |
| *Mike's Brother (Sir Paul McCartney)* | Sam Walsh, 1964 |
| *Nighthawks* | Edward Hopper, 1942 |
| *American Gothic* | Grant Wood, 1930 |
| *The Drifter* | Jack Vettriano, 1994 |
| *Mo Mowlam* | John Keane, 2001 |
| *Alfred Tennyson* | Samuel Laurence and Sir Edward Coley Burne-Jones, 1840 |
| | |
| *Sir Ian McKellen* | Clive Smith, 2002 |
| *Self-Portrait* | Lucian Freud, 1963 |
| *Lady Emma Hamilton as Calypso* | George Romney, 1792 |
| *Self-Portrait* | Sir Joshua Reynolds, 1780 |
| *Woman's Head* (collage) | Meriel Potts, 2011 |
| *A Wood Nymph* | Robert Poetzelberger, 1886 |
| *Isabel 1 & 2* | Loretta Lux, 2009 |

| | |
|---|---|
| *The Drummer* | Loretta Lux, 2004 |
| *Self-Portrait* | Vincent van Gogh, 1889 |
| *A Mermaid* | John W Waterhouse, 1900 |
| *Girl in the Window* | Peter Matthews, 2009 |
| *Black Suit Red Wine* | Fabian Perez, 2012 |
| *Pandora's Box* | Dante Gabriel Rossetti, 1869 |
| *Self Portrait (with hardware)* | Zac Freeman, 2010 |
| *Assemblage 1* | John Whipple, 2009 |
| *A School Girl* | Sir George Clausen, 1891 |
| *A Village Maiden* | Sir George Clausen, 1892 |
| *The Stone Pickers* | Sir George Clausen, 1887 |
| *Phonebook Paper Dress* | Jolis Paons, 2009 |
| *Peace (Paper Couture)* | Lia Griffith, 2010 |
| *Esmé Robbe* | George Henry Boughton, 1897 |
| *Never Morning Wore to Evening* | Walter Langley, 1894 |
| *Cherish* | Susan Cutts, 2011 |
| *Footsteps Past and Present* | Susan Cutts, 2008 |
| *Lullaby* | Susan Cutts, 2004 |
| *Irren-Anstalt Band-Hain* | Adolf Wölfli, 1910 |
| *Blood Man* | Howard Terpning, 1988 |
| *Child of the Earth* | Virgil Stephens, 2008 |
| *On the Beach* | Arthur Rackham, 1910 |
| *Amelia* | Sascalia, 2009 |
| *Tuba K.* | Mark Gilbert, 2000 |
| *Dead Man Posing (Philip Ledbury)* | David Fisher, 2009 |

## Appendix 2

# SEMI-STRUCTURED END OF PROJECT INTERVIEW QUESTIONS

1. How have you found the experience of being painted and having paintings made of you?
2. How did you find the collaborative process?
3. Did you find out new things about yourself? Can you give any examples?
4. Did it help you find different parts of yourself and self-identity that you had perhaps lost or didn't know existed? Can you give any examples?
5. Would you have liked to have been involved with the actual making/painting of the portrait? Why do you think this is?
6. How do you feel about the fact that these portraits will go into an exhibition and be seen by lots of people? Is that an important aspect of the project for you?
7. Is it important to you that your contribution to this project might help other people in a similar situation to you? Why do you think this is?
8. How did you find my visits to your home?
9. How did you find telling your story to me and my interpretation of that into a painting?
10. Did that help you feel heard? Can you explain why?
11. How do you feel about my interpretations of your statement of intention within your portraits?

12. Has this project helped give you a stronger sense of yourself and your identity? Can you give me examples of why this might be?

13. Has this project helped you make meaning of your life? Or find a new meaning? Can you give any examples?

14. Do you have any ideas how portrait therapy could be improved?

15. Do you feel that portrait therapy would benefit other people who have a similar illness or issues to you?

16. If you have shown them to your family, how have they reacted to the portraits and collages?

17. Has this project made you feel exploited in any way?

18. Would you like your real first name or a pseudonym attached to your painting when it is exhibited or printed?

19. Are you happy for your diagnosis to be mentioned in literature accompanying your portraits?

20. Do you have any questions or comments of your own?

# REFERENCES

Achterberg, J. (1985) *Imagery in Healing: Shamanism and Modern Medicine.* Boston: Shambhala.

Achterberg, J., Dossey, B. and Kolkmeier, L. (1994) *Rituals of Healing: Using Imagery for Health and Wellness.* New York: Bantam.

Adams, A. (2009) 'Face to Face: Looking at and Portraying Disfigurement.' Audio recording of the panel discussion which took place at the Mall Galleries on Tuesday 19 May.

Adamson, E. (1984) *Art as Healing.* London: Coventure.

Addington-Hall, J. (2002) 'Research sensitivities to palliative care patients.' *European Journal of Cancer Care 11*, 3, 220–224.

Aita, V., Lydiatt, W. and Gilbert, M. (2010) 'Portraits of care: medical research through portraiture.' *Journal of Medical Ethics and Medical Humanities 36*, 1, 5–13.

Akhtar, S. and Samuel, S. (1996) 'The concept of identity: developmental origins, phenomenology, clinical relevance, and measurement.' *Harvard Review of Psychiatry 3*, 5, 254–267.

Alea, N. and Bluck, S. (2003) 'Why are you telling me that? A conceptual model of the social function of autobiographical memory.' *Memory 11*, 2, 165–179.

Allen, P. (1992) 'Artist-in-residence: an alternative to "clinification" for art therapists.' *Art Therapy: Journal of the American Art Therapy Association 9*, 1, 22–29.

Allen, P. (2001a) 'Art therapists who are artists.' *American Journal of Art Therapy 39*, 4, 12–20.

Allen, P. (2001b) 'The Open Studio Process as a Way to Practice Art Therapy.' In, J. Rubin (ed.) *Approaches to Art Therapy: Theory and Technique* (Second Edition) (pp.178–188). New York and London: Brunner-Routledge.

Anzieu, D. (1989) *The Skin Ego* [*trans.* Chris Turner]. New Haven, CT and London: Yale University Press.

Arnheim, R. (1986) *New Essays on the Psychology of Art.* Berkeley, Los Angeles, London: University of California Press.

Arnheim, R. (1990) 'The artist as healer.' *The Arts in Psychotherapy 17*, 14.

Awan, F. (2007) 'Young People, Identity and the Media: A Study of Conceptions of Self-Identity Among Youth in Southern England.' PhD Thesis, Bournemouth University. Accessed on 11/03/2017 at https://goo.gl/jUsism.

Balan, N. (2005) 'Multiple voices and methods: listening to women who are in workplace transition.' *International Journal of Qualitative Methods 4*, 4, 63–86.

Balboni, T., Vanderwerker, L., Block, S., Paulk, E. *et al.* (2007) 'Religiousness and spiritual support among advanced cancer patients and associations with end-of-life treatment preferences and quality of life.' *Journal of Clinical Oncology 25*, 5, 555–560.

Barnett, M. (2001) 'Interviewing terminally ill people: is it fair to take their time?' *Palliative Medicine 15*, 2, 157–158.

Barrett, E. and Bolt, B. (2007) *Practice as Research Approaches to Creative Arts Enquiry.* London and New York: I.B. Tauris.

Barthes, R. (1985) *Camera Lucida: Reflections on Photography* [trans. R. Howard]. New York: Farrar, Straus and Giroux.

Bauman, Z. (2004) *Identity: Conversations with Benedetto Vecchi.* Cambridge and Malden: Polity Press.

Becker, E. (1997) *The Denial of Death.* New York: Free Press.

Bell, J. (2000) '(Intro.)' *500 Self Portraits.* London: Phaidon.

Bell, S. (2002) 'Photo images: Jo Spence's narratives of living with illness.' *Health: An Interdisciplinary Journal for the Social Study of Health, Illness and Medicine 6*, 1, 5–30.

Bell, S. (2008) 'Drawing on the End of Life: Art Therapy, Spirituality and Palliative Care.' University of Sheffield Doctoral Thesis.

Benner, P. (2003) 'Finding the Good Behind the Right: A Dialogue Between Nursing and Bioethics.' In F. Miller, J. Fletcher and J. Humber (eds) *The Nature and Prospect of Bioethics, Interdisciplinary Perspectives* (pp.312–319). Totowa, NJ: Humana Press.

Benner, P. and Wrubel, J. (1989) *The Primacy of Caring: Stress and Coping in Health and Illness.* California, Massachusetts, Ontario, Sydney, San Juan, Madrid, Tokyo, Singapore: Amsterdam Addison-Wesley Publishing Company.

Betensky, M. (1995) *What Do You See? Phenomenology of Therapeutic Art Expression.* London: Jessica Kingsley Publishers.

Bion, W. (1962) *Learning from Experience.* London: William Heinemann.

Bion, W. (1967) *Second Thoughts.* London: William Heinemann.

Blows, E., Bird, L., Seymour, J. and Cox, K. (2012) 'Liminality as a framework for understanding the experience of cancer survivorship: a literature review.' *Journal of Advanced Nursing 68*, 2155–2164.

Bolen, J. (1996) *Close to the Bone: Life-Threatening illness and the Search for Meaning.* New York: Touchstone.

Bolton, G. (2004) 'The healer's art.' *Progress in Palliative Care, 12*, 3, pp.138–141.

Booth, A., Trimble, T. and Egan, J. (2010) 'Body-centred counter- transference in a sample of Irish clinical psychologists.' *The Irish Psychologist 36*, 12, 284–289.

Brilliant, R. (1991) *Portraiture.* London: Reaktion Books.

Brockelman, T. (2001) *The Frame and the Mirror: On Collage and the Postmodern.* Evanston, IL: Northwestern University Press.

Brough, J. (2001) 'Temporality and Illness: A Phenomenological Perspective.' In S. Toombs (ed.) *Handbook of Phenomenology and Medicine* (pp.29–46). Dordrecht, The Netherlands and Norwell MA: Kluwer Academic Publishers.

Brown, C. (2008a) 'Very toxic – handle with care: Some aspects of the maternal function in art therapy.' *International Journal of Art Therapy 13*, 1, 13–24.

Brown, C. (2008b) 'The importance of making art for the creative arts therapist: an artistic inquiry.' *The Arts in Psychotherapy 35*, 201–208.

Brown, J. (2010) '"Devotional" Painting of Artist's Dead Mother Shortlisted for Award.' *The Independent*, 28 April 2010. Accessed on 10/03/2017 at https://goo.gl/KWabvH.

Brown, L., Argyris, D., Attanucci, J., Bardige, B. *et al.* (1988) *A Guide to Reading Narratives of Conflict and Choice for Self and Relational Voice.* Cambridge, MA: Harvard Graduate School of Education.

# REFERENCES

Brown, L. and Gilligan, C. (1991) 'Listening for Voice in Narratives of Relationship.' In Mark Tappan and Martin Packer (eds) *Narrative and Storytelling: Implications for Understanding Moral Development* (New Directions for Child and Adolescent Development) (pp.43–62). San Francisco: Jossey-Bass.

Brown, L. and Gilligan, C. (1992) *Meeting at the Crossroads: Women's Psychology and Girls' Development.* Cambridge, MA: Harvard University Press.

Brown, L. and Gilligan, C. (1993) 'Meeting at the crossroads: women's psychology and girls' development.' *Feminism and Psychology 3,* 11–35.

Broyard, A. (1992) *Intoxicated by my Illness and Other Writings on Life and Death.* New York: Fawcett Columbine.

Bruce, V. and Young, A. (1986) 'Understanding face recognition.' *The British Journal of Psychology 77,* 305–327.

Buber, M. (2004 [1937]) *I and Thou* (Second Edition). London: Continuum.

Buckner, R. and Carroll, D. (2006) 'Self-projection and the brain.' *TRENDS in Cognitive Sciences 11,* 2, 49–57.

Burt, H. (ed.) (2012) *Art Therapy and Post Modernism: Creative Healing through a Prism.* London and Philadelphia: Jessica Kingsley Publishers.

Butler, J. (2004a) *Undoing Gender.* New York: Routledge.

Butler, J. (2004b) *Precarious Life: The Powers of Mourning and Violence.* London and New York: Verso.

Butler-Kisber, L. (2008) 'Collage as Inquiry.' In G. Knowles and A. Cole (eds) *Handbook of the Arts in Qualitative Research* (pp.265–276). Thousand Oaks: Sage.

Cahn, E. (2000) 'Proposal for a studio-based art therapy education.' *Art Therapy: Journal of the American Art Therapy Association 17,* 3, 177–182.

Canals, R. (2011) 'Studying Images through Images: A Visual Ethnography of the Cult of Maria Lionza in Venezuela.' In S. Spencer (ed.) *Visual Research Methods in the Social Sciences: Awakening Visions* (pp.235–238). Abingdon and New York: Routledge.

Cancienne, M. and Snowber, C. (2009) 'Writing Rhythm: Movement as Method'. In P. Leavy (ed.) *Method Meets Art: Arts-Based Research Practice* (pp.198–214). London, New York: The Guilford Press.

Carel, H. (2004) 'Philosophy as Listening, the Lessons of Psychoanalysis.' In H. Carel. and D. Gamez. (eds) *What Philosophy IS* (pp.235–238). London and New York: Continuum.

Carel, H. (2007) 'Can I be ill and happy?' *Philosophia 35,* 95–110.

Carel, H. (2008) *Illness: The Cry of the Flesh.* Stocksfield UK: Acumen Publishing Ltd.

Carel, H. (2011) 'Phenomenology and its application in medicine.' *Theoretical Medicine and Bioethics 32,* 33–46.

Carel, H. (2012) 'Phenomenology as a resource for patients.' *Journal of Medicine and Philosophy 37,* 96–113.

Carel, H. (2013) 'Illness, phenomenology, and philosophical method.' *Theoretical Medicine and Bioethics 34,* 345–357.

Carel, H. (2014) *Phenomenology of Illness.* Oxford: Oxford University Press.

Carel, H., Kidd, I. and Pettigrew, R. (2016) 'Illness as transformative experience.' *The Lancet 388,* 1152–1153.

Carr, S. (2011) 'Reflecting identities: using portraiture with people suffering from life-threatening illnesses.' *British Medical Journal Supportive Palliative Care 1,* 2, 236.

Carr, S. (2014) *'Revisioning Self-Identity:* the role of portraits, neuroscience and the art therapist's "third hand".' *International Journal of Art Therapy 19,* 2, 54–70.

Carr, S. and Hancock, S. (2017) 'Healing the inner child through portrait therapy illness, identity and childhood trauma.' *International Journal of Art Therapy 22,* 1, 8–21.

Cauvel, J. (1999) 'The transformative power of art: Li Zehou's aesthetic theory.' *Philosophy East & West 49*, 2, 150–173.

Chambers, E. (2009) 'Surgical Portraiture and the Hospital Environment as Site and Subject' (pp.1–14). Paper presentation at Crossings: Art, Medicine, Visual Culture conference, Manchester, Association of Art Historians.

Charmaz, K. (1983) 'Loss of self: a fundamental form of suffering in the chronically ill.' *Sociology of Health and Illness 5*, 2, 168–195.

Charmaz, K. (1995) 'The body, identity, and self: adapting to impairment.' *Sociological Quarterly 36*, 4, 657–680.

Charmaz, K. and Rosenfeld, D. (2006) 'Reflections of the Body, Images of Self: Visibility and Invisibility in Chronic Illness and Disability.' In D. Waskal and P. Vannini (eds) *Body/Embodiment: Symbolic Interaction and the Sociology of the Body* (pp.35–50). Aldershot UK, Burlington USA: Ashgate Publishing Ltd.

Clark, A. (2010) 'Ethical issues in image-based research.' *Arts & Health 2*, 1, 81–93.

Clark, A. (2012) 'Visual Ethics in a Contemporary Landscape.' In S. Pink (ed.) *Advances in Visual Methodology* (pp.17–36). London, California, New Delhi and Singapore: Sage Publications.

Clarkson, P. (2003) *The Therapeutic Relationship*. London & Philadelphia: Whurr.

Clayton, J., Butow, P., Arnold, R. and Tattersall, M. (2005) 'Fostering coping and nurturing hope when discussing the future with terminally ill cancer patients and their caregivers.' *Cancer 103*, 9, 1965–1975.

Clayton, J., Hancock, K., Parker, S., Butow, P. *et al.* (2008) 'Sustaining hope when communicating with terminally ill patients and their families: a systematic review.' *Psycho-Oncology 17*, 7, 641–659.

Cohen, M. (2002) 'Death Ritual: Anthropological Perspectives.' In P. Pecorino (ed.) *Perspectives on Death and Dying*. Online Textbook. Accessed on 08/03/2017 at https://goo.gl/RLjXlw.

Cole, A. and Knowles, G. (2008) 'Arts-informed research.' In G. Knowles and A. Cole (eds) *Handbook of the Arts in Qualitative Research*. Los Angeles: Sage.

Collier, J. Jnr. (1957) 'Photography in anthropology: a report on two experiments.' *American Anthropologist 59*, 843–859.

Collier, J. Jnr. (1967) *Visual Anthropology: Photography as a Research Method*. New York: Holt, Rinehart & Winston.

Connell, C. (1992) 'Art Therapy as part of the palliative care programme.' *Palliative Medicine 6*, 18–25.

Connell, C. (1998) *Something Understood: Art Therapy in Cancer Care*. London: Wrexham Pubs.

Cooper, A. (2016) 'A good death?' *Journal of Social Work Practice 30*, 2, 121–127.

Corbin, J. and Strauss, A. (1987) 'Accompaniments of Chronic Illness: Changes in Body, Self, Biography and Biographical Time.' In J. Roth and P. Conrad (eds) *Research in the Sociology of Health and Care* (pp.249–281), Greenwich CT: JAI Press.

Corbin, J. (2003) 'The Body in Health and Illness.' *Qualitative Health Research 13*, 2, 256–267.

Costello-Du Bois, J. (1989) 'Drawing out the unique beauty: portraits.' *Art Therapy: Journal of the American Art Therapy Association 6*, 2, 67–70.

Craig, G. (2009) 'Intersubjectivity, phenomenology and multiple disabilities.' *International Journal of Art Therapy 14*, 2, 64–73.

Crewe, N. (1980) 'Quality of life: the ultimate goal in rehabilitation.' *Minnesota Medicine 63*, 586–589.

# REFERENCES

Crossley, M. (2003) '"Let me explain": narrative emplotment and one patient's experience of oral cancer.' *Social Science and Medicine 56*, 439–448.

Darwent, C. (2010) 'Louise Bourgeois: Inventive and Influential Sculptor Whose Difficult Childhood Informed Her Life's Work.' *The Independent*, 2 June, 2010.

Davis, D. (2008) 'Memoir, Fantasy, Media Analysis: A Collage-Informed Body of Experience.' Paper presented at the Annual Meeting of the American Educational Research Association, New York.

Dean, R., Kinsman, A. and Gregory, D. (2004) 'Humor and laughter in palliative care: an ethnographic investigation.' *Palliative and Supportive Care 2*, 139–148.

De Freitas, N. (2002) 'Towards a definition of studio documentation: working tool and transparent record.' *Working Papers in Art and Design 2*, Hertfordshire University. Accessed on 08/03/2017 at https://goo.gl/m8vC0l.

Denzin, N. (2009) 'The elephant in the living room: or extending the conversation about the politics of evidence.' *Qualitative Research 9*, 139.

Denzin, N. and Lincoln, Y. (2005) *The Sage Handbook of Qualitative Research* (Third Edition). Los Angeles, London, New Delhi, Singapore and Washington, DC: Sage Publishing.

Dissanayake, E. (1980) 'Art as a human behaviour: toward an ethological view of art.' *Journal of Aesthetics and Art Criticism 38*, 4, 397–406.

Dissanayake, E. (1988) *What is Art For?* Seattle: University of Washington Press.

Dissanayake, E. (1995 [1992]) *Homo Aestheticus: Where Art Came From and Why*. Washington: The University of Washington Press.

Douglass, M. (1966) *Purity and Danger: An Analysis of Concepts of Pollution and Taboo*. New York: Frederick A. Praeger.

Duesbury, T. (2005) 'Art Therapy in the Hospice: Rewards and Frustrations.' In D. Waller and C. Sibbert (eds) *Art Therapy and Cancer Care* (pp.199–209). London: Open University Press.

Edwards, D. (1997) 'Endings.' *The International Journal of Art Therapy 2*, 2, 49–56.

Edwards, D. (1999) 'The role of the case study in art therapy research.' *The International Journal of Art Therapy 4*, 1, 2–9.

Edwards, J, D. (2007) *How Cancer Saved My Life*. London: Bolam Rose.

Eisner, E. (2005) *Reimagining Schools: The Selected Works of Elliot W*. London and New York: Routledge.

Eisner, E. (2008) 'Art and Knowledge.' In G. Knowles and A. Coles (eds) *Handbook of the Arts in Qualitative Research* (pp.3–12). Los Angeles, London, New Delhi, Singapore and Washington, DC: Sage Publishing.

Elkins, J. (1996) *The Object Stares Back: On the Nature of Seeing*. New York: Simon & Schuster.

Elliott, A. (2008) *Concepts of the Self*. Cambridge and Malden: Polity Press.

Elliott, A. (ed.) (2011) *Routledge Handbook of Identity Studies*. London and New York: Routledge.

Etherington, K. (2004a) *Becoming a Reflexive Researcher: Using Our Selves in Research*. London and Philadelphia: Jessica Kingsley Publishers.

Etherington, K. (2004b) 'Research methods: reflexivities-roots, meanings, dilemmas.' *Counselling and Psychotherapy Research: Linking Research With Practice 4*, 2, 46–47.

Etherington, K. (2004c) 'Heuristic research as a vehicle for personal and professional development.' *Counselling and Psychotherapy Research: Linking Research With Practice 4*, 2, 48–63.

Etherington, K. (2008) *Trauma, Drug Misuse and Transforming Identities: A Life Story Approach*. London and Philadelphia: Jessica Kingsley Publishers.

Evans, K. (2005a) 'On Death and Dying.' In D. Waller and C. Sibbett (eds) *Facing Death: Art Therapy and Cancer Care* (p.1–11). Maidenhead, UK: Open University Press.

Evans, K. (2005b) 'Body Image and The Construction of Identity.' In D. Waller and C. Sibbett (eds) *Art Therapy and Cancer Care* (pp.38–49). London, Maidenhead, UK: Open University Press.

Exley, C. and Letherby, G. (2001) 'Managing a disrupted life course: issue of identity and emotion work.' *Health 5*, 1, 112–132.

Falk, B. (2005) 'Fear of Annihilation: Defensive Strategies used within Art Therapy Groups and Organizations for Cancer Patients.' In D. Waller and C. Sibbett (eds) *Art Therapy and Cancer Care* (pp.172–184). London, Maidenhead, UK: Open University Press.

Falvo, D. (1999) *Medical and Psychosocial Aspects of Chronic Illness and Disability* (Second Edition). Aspen: Gaithersburg, MD.

Farelly-Hansen, M. (ed.) (2001) *Spirituality and Art Therapy: Living the Connection*. London and Philadelphia: Jessica Kingsley Publishers.

Faulkner, S. (2006) 'Reconstruction: LGBTQ and Jewish.' *International and Intercultural Communication Annual 29*, 95–120.

Fenton, J. (2008) 'Finding one's way home: reflections on art therapy in palliative care.' *Art Therapy: Journal of the American Art Therapy Association 25*, 3, 137–140.

Festinger, L. (1962) 'Cognitive dissonance.' *Scientific American 207*, 4, 93–107.

Field, N. (1989) 'Listening with the body: an exploration in the countertransference.' *British Journal of Psychotherapy 5*, 4, 512–522.

Fine, M. and Glendinning, C. (2005) 'Dependence, independence or inter-dependence? Revisiting the concepts of "care" and "dependency".' *Ageing & Society 25*, 601–621.

Finlay, L. (2009) 'Ambiguous encounters: a relational approach to phenomenological research.' *Indo-Pacific Journal of Phenomenology 9*, 1, 1–17.

Finlay, L. (2011) *Phenomenology for Therapists: Researching the Lived World*. Malden, Oxford, Chichester: Wiley-Blackwell.

Finley, S. and Knowles, G. (1995) 'Researcher as artist/artist as researcher.' *Qualitative Inquiry 1*, 1, 110–142.

Fish, B. (1989) 'Addressing Countertransference Through Image Making.' In H. Wadeson, J. Durkin and D. Perach (eds) *Advances in Art Therapy* (pp.376–389). New York: John Wiley & Sons.

Fish, B. (2012) 'Response art: the art of the art therapist.' *Art Therapy: Journal of the American Art Therapy Association 29*, 3, 138–143.

Frank, A. (1997) *The Wounded Storyteller: Body, Illness and Ethics*. Chicago: University of Chicago Press.

Frank, A. (2000) 'Illness and autobiographical work: dialogue as narrative destabilization.' *Qualitative Sociology 23*, 1, 135–156.

Franklin, M. (1990) 'The esthetic attitude and empathy: a point of convergence.' *The American Journal of Art Therapy 29*, 2, 42–47.

Franklin, M. (2010) 'Affect regulation, mirror neurons, and the third hand: formulating mindful empathic art interventions.' *Art Therapy: Journal of the American Art Therapy Association 27*, 4, 160–167.

Fraser, G. and Gordon, L. (1994) 'A genealogy of dependency: tracing a keyword of the U.S. welfare state.' *Signs 19*, 2, 309–336.

Freeland, C. (2007) 'Portraits in painting and photography.' *Philosophical Studies 135*, 95–109.

Freeland, C. (2010) *Portraits and Persons*. Oxford, New York: Oxford University Press.

Fuller, P. (1980) *Art and Psychoanalysis*. London: Writers and Readers Cooperative.

# REFERENCES

Furman, R., Langer, C., Davis, C., Gallardo, H. *et al.* (2007) 'Expressive research and reflective poetry as qualitative inquiry: a study of adolescent identity.' *Qualitative Research* 7, 3, 301–315.

Gablik, S. (1991) *The Reenchantment of Art.* London: Thames and Hudson Ltd.

Gadamer, H. (1975) *Truth and Method.* New York: Seabury Press.

Gallese, V. and Lakoff, G. (2005) 'The brain's concepts: the role of the sensory-motor system in reason and language.' *Cognitive Neuropsychology* 22, 3, 455–479.

Gauntlett, D. (2002) *Media, Gender and Identity: An Introduction.* Abingdon and New York: Routledge.

Gauntlett, D. (2007) *Creative Explorations: New Approaches to Identities and Audiences.* Abingdon and New York: Routledge.

Gauntlett, D. and Holzwarth, P. (2006) 'Creative and visual methods for exploring identities: a conversation between David Gauntlett and Peter Holzwarth.' *Visual Studies* 21, 1, 82–91.

Gemmell, G. (2012) 'Appropriation art (or how to steal like an artist).' *Artspace,* 28 November.

Giddens, A. (1984) *The Constitution of Society: Outline of the Theory of Structuration.* Berkeley and Los Angeles: University of California Press.

Giddens, A. (1991) *Modernity and Self-Identity: Self and Society in the Late Modern Age.* Cambridge: Polity.

Gilligan, C. (1982) *In a Different Voice: Psychological Theory and Women's Development.* Cambridge, MA: Harvard University Press.

Gilligan, C., Spencer, R., Weinberg, M.K. and Bertsch, T. (2003) 'On the Listening Guide: A Voice-Centered Relational Method.' In P. Camic, J. Rhodes and L. Yardley (eds) *Qualitative Research in Psychology: Expanding Perspectives in Methodology and Design* (pp.157–172). Washington, DC: American Psychological Association.

Gilroy, A. (1996) 'Our own kind of evidence.' *The International Journal of Art Therapy* 1, 2, 52–60.

Gilroy, A. (2006) *Art Therapy, Research and Evidence-Based Practice.* London: Sage.

Giorgi, A. (1989) 'Some theoretical and practical issues regarding the psychological phenomenological method.' *The Saybrook Review* 7, 2, 71–85.

Goffman, E. (1959) *The Presentation of Self in Everyday Life.* Hamondsworth, New York, Victoria, Ontario, Auckland: Penguin Books.

Goffman, E. (1963) *Stigma. Notes on a Spoiled Identity.* Englewood Cliffs, NJ: Prentice-Hall.

Gormley, A. (2002) 'BBC Forum Questions and Answers.' In BBC, *Opening of Tate Modern,* 2002. Accessed on 11/03/2017 at https://goo.gl/pFxyLK.

Grau, C. (2006) 'Eternal sunshine of the spotless mind and the morality of memory.' *Journal of Aesthetics and Art Criticism* 64, 1, 119–133.

Grey, C. and Malins, J. (2004) *Visualising Research: A Guide to the Research Process in Art and Design.* Aldershot and Burlington: Ashgate Publishing.

Grice, E. (2009a) 'Portrait With a New Lease of Life.' *The Telegraph,* 2009.

Grice, E. (2009b) 'The Painting That Went and Did Its Work.' *The Telegraph,* 28 January, 2009. Accessed on 09/03/2017 at https://goo.gl/mDrGDo.

Hansen, D., Rosholm, J., Gichangi, A. and Vach, W. (2007) 'Increased use of antidepressants at the end of life: population-based study among people aged 65 years and above.' *Age and Ageing* 36, 4, 449–454.

Hardy, D. (2001) 'Creating through loss: an examination of how art therapists sustain their practice in palliative care.' *The International Journal of Art Therapy* 6, 23–31.

Hardy, D. (2005) 'Creating Through Loss: How Art Therapists Sustain Their Practice in Palliative Care.' In D. Waller and C. Sibbett (eds) *Art Therapy and Cancer Care (Facing Death)* (pp.23–31). London: Open University Press.

Hardy, D. (2013) 'Working with loss: an examination of how language can be used to address the issue of loss in art therapy.' *International Journal of Art Therapy 18*, 1, 29–37.

Harms, E. (1975) 'The Development of Modern Art Therapy.' *Leonardo 8*, 241–244.

Harper, D. (2002) 'Talking about pictures: a case for photo elicitation.' *Visual Studies 17*, 1, 13–26.

Hart, N. and Crawford-Wright, A. (1999) 'Research as therapy, therapy as research: Ethical dilemmas in new-paradigm research.' *British Journal of Guidance and Counselling 27*, 2, 205–214.

Hartley, N. and Payne, M. (2008) *The Creative Arts in Palliative Care*. London and Philadelphia: Jessica Kingsley Publishers.

Heidegger, M. (1962 [1927]) *Being and Time*. New York: Harper & Row.

Hellema, P. (2011) *'She Who Laughs Last…' The Meaning of Humour, as Described by Women in a Creative Arts Process*. MIECAT MA Thesis. Accessed on 11/03/2017 at https://goo.gl/060jOh.

Henley, D. (1997) 'Aesthetics in art therapy: theory into practice.' *The Arts in Psychotherapy 19*, 153–161.

Herman, J. (1992) *Trauma and Recovery: The Aftermath of Violence – from Domestic Abuse to Political Terror*. New York: Basic Books.

Higgs, G. (2008) 'Psychology: Knowing the Self through Arts.' In G. Knowles and A. Cole (eds) *Handbook of the Arts in Qualitative Research* (pp.545–556). Thousand Oaks: Sage.

Hiles, D. (2008) 'Transparency.' In L. M. Givens (ed.) (2008) *The Sage Encyclopaedia of Qualitative Research* (pp.890–892). Thousand Oaks: Sage.

Hill, A. (1945) *Art Versus Illness: A Story of Art Therapy*. London: George Allen and Unwin Ltd.

Hill, A. (1951) *Painting Out Illness*. London: William & Norgate Ltd.

Hilliker, L. (2006) 'Letting go while holding on: postmortem photography as an aid to the grieving process.' *Illness, Crisis, and Loss 14*, 3, 245–269.

Hocoy, D. (2007) 'Art Therapy as a Tool for Social Change: A Conceptual Model.' In F. Kaplan (ed.) *Art Therapy and Social Action* (pp.21–39). London and Philadelphia: Jessica Kingsley Publishers.

Hogan, S. (ed.) (1997) *Feminist Approaches to Art Therapy*. London and New York: Routledge.

Hogan, S. (2001) *Healing Arts: The History of Art Therapy*. London and Philadelphia: Jessica Kingsley Publishers.

Hogan, S. (ed.) (2003) *Gender Issues in Art Therapy*. London and Philadelphia: Jessica Kingsley Publishers.

Hogan, S. (2013) 'Your body is a battleground: art therapy with women.' *The Arts in Psychotherapy 40*, 415–419.

Hogan, S. and Martin, R. (2011) *Look at Me! Images of Women and Aging Project*. Accessed on 10/03/2017 at www.representing-ageing.com.

Hogan, S. and Warren, L. (2012) 'Dealing with complexity in research findings: how do older women negotiate and challenge images of ageing?' *Journal of Women and Ageing 24*, 4, 329–350.

Holmes, M. (2011) 'Gendered Identities.' In A. Elliott (ed.) *Routledge Handbook of Identity Studies* (pp.186–202). London and New York: Routledge.

# REFERENCES

Hubbard, G., Kidd, L. and Kearney, N. (2010) 'Disrupted lives and threats to identity: the experiences of people with colorectal cancer within the first year following diagnosis.' *Health 14*, 2, 131–146.

Husserl, E. (1970 [1954]) *The Crisis of European Sciences and Transcendental Phenomenology* [D. Carr trans.]. Evanston, IL: Northwestern University Press.

Husserl, E. (1977 [1929]) *Cartesian Meditations: An Introduction to Phenomenology* [D. Cairns trans.]. The Hague: Nijhoff.

Hutchison, I., Gilbert, M. and Farrand, P. (eds) (2000) *Saving Faces*. Nottingham: The University of Nottingham Press.

Inckle, K. (2010) 'Telling tales? Using ethnographic fictions to speak embodied "truth".' *Qualitative Research 10*, 1, 27–47.

Isserow, J. (2013) 'Between water and words: reflective self-awareness and symbol formation in art therapy.' *International Journal of Art Therapy 18*, 3, 122–131.

Jaremka, L., Fagundes, C., Glaser, R., Bennette, J. *et al.* (2012) 'Loneliness predicts pain, depression, and fatigue: understanding the role of immune dysregulation.' *Psychoneuroendocrinology 38*, 8, 1310–1317.

Jones, D. (1983) 'An art therapist's personal record.' *Art Therapy, Journal of the American Art Therapy Association 1*, 22–25.

Jones, D. (2006) 'Don Jones: Still Waters Run.' In M. Junge and H. Wadeson (eds) *Architects of Art Therapy: Memoirs and Life Stories* (pp.31–50). Springfield, IL: Charles C. Thomas Publisher Ltd.

Jones, J. (2010) 'The Deathbed Portrait's Unique Tribute.' *The Guardian*, 23 June, 2010. Accessed on 11/03/2017 at https://goo.gl/kB41U8.

Jones, M. (2003) 'From the Peninsula: The Geography of Gender Issues in Art Therapy.' In S. Hogan (ed.) *Gender Issues in Art Therapy* (pp.92–107). London and Philadelphia: Jessica Kingsley Publishers.

Jongeward, C. (2009) 'Visual Portraits: Integrating Artistic Process into Qualitative Research.' In P. Leavy (ed.) *Method Meets Art: Arts-Based Research Practice* (pp.253–265). London, New York: The Guilford Press.

Kierkegaard, S. [1844] (1944 trans. by Walter Lowrie) *The Concept of Dread*. Princeton: Princeton University Press.

Kinnvall, C. (2004) 'Globalization and religious nationalism: self, identity, and the search for ontological security.' *Political Psychology 25*, 5, 741–767.

Kinsella, E. (2006) 'Constructions of Self: Ethical Overtones in Surprising Locations.' In F. Rapport and P. Wainwright (eds) *The Self in Health and Illness* (pp.21–32). Abingdon: Radcliffe Publishing.

Kipling, R. (1892) 'Gunga Din.' In R. Kipling, *Barrack-Room Ballads and Other Verses* (pp.208–9). London: Methuen & Co.

Kirkengen, A. and Ulvestad, E. (2007) 'Heavy burdens and complex disease – an integrated perspective.' *Journal of the Norwegian Medical Association 127*, 3228–3231.

Klass, D., Silverman, P. and Nickman, P. (1996) *Continuing Bonds: New Understandings of Grief*. London: Routledge.

Klein, M. (1952) 'Some Theoretical Conclusions Regarding the Emotional Life of the Infant.' In M. Klein, P. Heimann, S. Isaacs and J. Riviere (eds) *Developments in Psycho-Analysis* (pp.61–93). London: Hogarth.

Kleinman, A. (1988) *The Illness Narratives: Suffering, Healing and the Human Condition*. New York: Basic Books.

Kleinman, A. (2012) 'Caregiving as moral experience.' *The Lancet 380*, 9853, 1550–1551.

Knill, P. (1995) 'The place of beauty in therapy and the arts.' *The Arts in Psychotherapy 22*, 1, 1–7.

Knill, P., Levine, E. and Levine, S. (2005) *Principles and Practice of Expressive Arts Therapy: Toward a Therapeutic Aesthetics.* London and Philadelphia: Jessica Kingsley Publishers.

Knowles, G. and Cole, A. (eds.) (2008) *Handbook of the Arts in Qualitative Research.* Thousand Oaks: Sage.

Koren, L. (1998) *Wabi-Sabi for Artists, Designers, Poets and Philosophers.* Berkeley, CA: Stonebridge Press.

Kramer, E. (1971) *Art as Therapy with Children.* London: Schocken Books Inc. Elek.

Kramer, E. (1986) 'The art therapist's third hand: reflections on art, art therapy and society at large.' *The American Journal of Art Therapy 24*, 71–86.

Kramer, E. (2000) 'The Art Therapist's Third Hand: Reflections on Art, Art Therapy and Society at Large'. In L. Gerity (ed.) *Art as Therapy Collected Papers: Edith Kramer* (pp.47–72). London and Philadelphia: Jessica Kingsley Publishers.

Kramer, E. (2004) *Art Tells the Truth.* (Film) Lenfim Studio. Accessed on 10/03/2017 at http://vimeo.com/33476299.

Kramer, E. (2006) 'Edith Kramer: Art as Therapy.' In M. Junge and H. Wadeson (eds) *Architects of Art Therapy: Memoirs and Life Stories* (pp.25–35). Springfield, IL: Charles C. Thomas Publisher Ltd.

Kubler-Ross, E. (1975) *Death: The Final Stage of Growth.* New Jersey: Prentis Hall.

Lachman-Chapin, M. (1983) 'The artist as clinician: an interactive technique in art therapy.' *American Journal of Art Therapy 23*, 13–25.

Lakoff, G. and Johnson, M. (1980) *Metaphors We Live By.* Chicago and London: University of Chicago Press.

Langer, S. (1953) *Feeling and Form.* London: Routledge & Kegan Paul.

Latimer, J. (2009) 'Unsettling Bodies: Frida Kahlo's Portraits and In/dividuality.' In J. Latimer and M. Schillmeier (eds) *Un/knowing Bodies.* Sociological Review Monograph Series (pp.46–62). Oxford: Wiley-Blackwell.

Lawler, S. (2008) *Identity: Sociological Perspectives.* Cambridge UK, Malden USA: Polity Press.

Lawton, J. (1998) 'Contemporary hospice care; the sequestration of the unbounded body and 'dirty dying'.' *Sociology of Health and Illness 20*, 2, 121–143.

Lazarus-Leff, B. (1998) 'Art therapy and the aesthetic environment as agents for change: a phenomenological investigation.' *Art Therapy: Journal of the American Art Therapy Association 15*, 2, 120–126.

Learmonth, M. (2002) 'Painting ourselves out of a corner.' *Newsbriefing, Newsletter of the British Association of Art Therapists*, June.

Leary, M. and Tangney, J. (eds) (2012) *Handbook of Self and Identity* (Second Edition). New York: The Guilford Press.

Leavy, P. (2009) *Method Meets Art: Arts-Based Research Practice.* New York: The Guilford Press.

Ledbury, P. (2009) Personal email to the author.

Lee, S. and Kristjanson, L. (2003) 'Human research ethics committees: issues in palliative care research.' *International Journal of Palliative Nursing 9*, 1, 13–18.

Lerner, E. (2005) 'The Healing Journey: A Ten-Week Group Focusing on Long-Term Healing Processes.' In D. Waller and C. Sibbett (eds) *Art Therapy and Cancer Care (Facing Death)* (pp.149–162). London: Open University Press.

Lett, W. (1998) 'Researching experiential self-knowing.' *The Arts in Psychotherapy 25*, 5, 331–342.

Little, M., Jordens, C.F., Paul, K., Montgomery, K. *et al.* (1998) 'Liminality: a major category of the experience of cancer illness.' *Social Science & Medicine 47*, 10, 1492–1493.

# REFERENCES

Luzzatto, P. (1998) 'From Psychiatry to Psycho-Oncology: Personal Reflections on the Use of Art Therapy with Cancer Patients.' In M. Pratt and M. Wood (eds) *Art Therapy in Palliative Care: The Creative Response* (pp.169–175). London, New York: Routledge.

Luzzatto, P. (2005) 'Musing with Death in Group Art Therapy with Cancer Patients.' In D. Waller and C. Sibbett (eds) *Facing Death: Art Therapy and Cancer Care* (pp.169–175). Maidenhead,: Open University Press.

Maclagan, D. (1989) 'The aesthetic dimension of art therapy: luxury or necessity?' *Inscape: Journal of the British Art Therapy Association*, Spring, 10–13.

Maclagan, D. (1998) 'Between the aesthetic and the psychological.' *International Journal of Art Therapy [Inscape]* 2, 40–51.

Maclagan, D. (2001) *Psychological Aesthetics*. London and Philadelphia: Jessica Kingsley Publishers.

Maclagan, D. (2005) 'Re-imagining art therapy.' *International Journal of Art Therapy* 10, 1, 23–30.

Maclagan, D. (2011) 'Between art and therapy: using pictures from the world of art as an imaginal focus.' *Art Therapy Online* 2, 2, 1–9.

Maiter, S., Simich, L., Jacobson, N. and Wise, J. (2008) 'Reciprocity: an ethic for community-based participatory action research.' *Action Research* 6, 305–325.

Malchiodi, C. (1999a) 'Artists and clinicians: can we be both?' *Art Therapy: Journal of the American Art Therapy Association* 16, 3, 110–111.

Malchiodi, C. (ed.) (1999b) *Medical Art Therapy with Adults*. London and Philadelphia: Jessica Kingsley Publishers.

Malchiodi, C. (2007) 'Invasive Art: Art as Empowerment for Women with Breast Cancer.' In S. Hogan (ed.) *Feminist Approaches to Art Therapy* (pp.49–64). London and New York: Routledge.

Mallinson, G. (1989) 'Life crises: when a baby dies.' *Nursing Times* 85, 9, 31–34.

Mandal, M. and Ambady, N. (2004) 'Laterality of facial expressions of emotion: universal and culture-specific influences.' *Behavioral Neurology* 15, 23–34.

Mander, R. and Marshall, R. (2003) 'An historical analysis of the role of paintings and photographs in comforting bereaved parents.' *Midwifery* 19, 3, 230–242.

Martin, R. (1986) 'Phototherapy.' In J. Spence (ed.) *Putting Myself in the Picture: A Political, Personal, and Photographic Autobiography* (pp.35–46). London: Camden Press.

Martin, R. (2009) 'Inhabiting the image: photography, therapy and re-enactment phototherapy.' *European Journal of Psychotherapy and Counselling* 11, 1, 35–49.

Martin, W., Grey, M., Webber, T., Robinson, L. *et al.* (2007) 'Balancing dual roles in end-of-life research.' *Canadian Oncology Nursing Journal* 17, 3, 141–147.

Mathieson, C. and Stam, H. (1995) 'Renegotiating identity: cancer narratives.' *Sociology of Health and Illness* 17, 3, 283–306.

Matho, E. (2005) 'A Woman with Breast Cancer in Art Therapy.' In D. Waller and C. Sibbett (eds) *Art Therapy and Cancer Care* (pp.102–118). London: Open University Press.

Matthews, E. (2006) *Merleau-Ponty: A Guide for the Perplexed*. London, New York: Continuum.

Mauthner, N.S. and Doucet, A. (1998) 'Reflections on a Voice-Centred Relational Method of Data Analysis: Analysing Maternal and Domestic Voices.' In J. Ribbens and R. Edwards (eds) *Feminist Dilemmas in Qualitative Research: Private Lives and Public Texts* (pp.119–146). London: Sage.

McCann, L. and Pearlman, L. (1990) 'Vicarious traumatization: a framework for understanding the psychological effects of working with victims.' *Journal of Traumatic Stress* 3, 1, 131–149.

McCreaddie, M. and Wiggins, S. (2007) 'The purpose and function of humour in health, health care and nursing: a narrative review.' *Journal of Advanced Nursing 61*, 6, 584–595.

McGraw, M. (1999) 'Studio-Based Art Therapy for Medically Ill and Physically Disabled Persons.' In C.A. Malchiodi (ed.) *Medical Art Therapy with Adults* (pp.243–363). London and Philadelphia: Jessica Kingsley Publishers.

McNiff, S. (1986) 'Freedom of research and artistic inquiry.' *The Arts in Psychotherapy 13*, 279–284.

McNiff, S. (1992) *Art as Medicine: Creating a Therapy of the Imagination.* Boston and London: Shambala.

McNiff, S. (2004) *Art Heals: How Creativity Cures the Soul.* Boston and London: Shambala.

McNiff, S. (2008) 'Art-based research.' In G. Knowles and A. Cole (eds) *Handbook of the Arts in Qualitative Research* (pp.29–40). Thousand Oaks: Sage Publishing.

McPherson, C., Wilson, K. and Murray, M. (2007) 'Feeling like a burden to others: a systematic review focusing on the end of life.' *Palliative Medicine 21*, 115–128.

Mercer, J. (2007) 'The challenge of insider research in educational institutions: wielding a double-edged sword and resolving difficult dilemmas.' *Oxford Review of Education 33*, 1, 1–17.

Merleau-Ponty, M. (2002 [1945]) *Phenomenology of Perception.* London: Routledge.

Meyer, J. and Land, R. (2003) 'Threshold concepts and troublesome knowledge: linkages to ways of thinking and practising within the disciplines.' *ETL project, Occasional Report 4*, pp.1–12. Accessed on 13/03/2017 at www.etl.tla.ed.ac.uk/docs/ETLreport4.pdf.

Miller, R. (2007) 'The role of response art in the case of an adolescent survivor of developmental trauma.' *Art Therapy: Journal of the American Art Therapy Association 24*, 4, 184–190.

Minar, V. (1999) 'Art Therapy and Cancer: Images of the Hurter and Healer.' In C. Malchiodi (ed.) *Medical Art Therapy with Adults* (pp.227–242). London and Philadelphia: Jessica Kingsley Publishers.

Moon, B. (1990) *Existential Art Therapy: The Canvas Mirror.* Springfield, IL: Charles C. Thomas Publisher.

Moon, C. (2002) *Studio Art Therapy: Cultivating the Artist Identity in the Art Therapist.* London and Philadelphia: Jessica Kingsley Publishers.

Moon, C. (2014) 'Theorizing from the margins.' *ATOL: Art Therapy OnLine 5*, 1, 1–12.

Moulder, C. (1998) *Understanding Pregnancy Loss.* London: Macmillan.

Moustakas, C. (1990) *Heuristic Research.* Newbury Park, CA: Sage.

Mullins, C. (2006) *Painting People: The State of the Art.* London: Thames & Hudson Ltd.

O'Brien, F. (2004) 'The making of mess in art therapy: attachment, trauma and the brain.' *International Journal of Art Therapy [Inscape] 9*, 1, 2–13.

O'Neill, M. (2008) 'Transnational refugees: the transformative role of art?' *Forum: Qualitative Social Research 9*, 2, 1–23.

Oyserman, D., Elmore, K. and Smith, G. (2012) 'Self, Self-Concept, and Identity.' In M. Leary and J. Price (eds) *Handbook of Self and Identity* (Second Edition) (pp.69–104). New York: The Guilford Press.

Padfield, D. (2003) *Perceptions of Pain.* Stockport, UK: Dewi Lewis Publishing.

Palmer, P. (2007 [1998]) *The Courage to Teach: Exploring the Inner Landscape of a Teacher's Life.* San Francisco: Jossey-Bass Publications.

Parry, G. (1997) 'Bambi fights back psychotherapy research and service improvement.' *International Journal of Art Therapy [Inscape] 2*, 1, 11–13.

Pearlman, L. and Saakvitne, K. W. (1995) *Trauma and the Therapist: Countertransference and Vicarious Traumatization in Psychotherapy with Incest Survivors.* New York: Norton.

# REFERENCES

Pereira, H. (2012) 'Rigor in phenomenological research: reflections of a novice nurse researcher.' *Nurse Researcher 19*, 3, 16–19.

Persons, R. (2009) 'Art therapy with serious juvenile offenders: a phenomenological analysis.' *International Journal of Offender Therapy and Comparative Criminology 53*, 433–453.

Pink, S. (2001) *Doing Visual Ethnography: Images, Media and Representation in Research.* London: Sage.

Pink, S. (2007) *Doing Visual Ethnography.* London, California, New Delhi and Singapore: Sage Publications.

Pink, S. (2009) *Doing Sensory Ethnography.* London, California, New Delhi and Singapore: Sage Publications.

Pink, S. (2012) *Advances in Visual Methodology.* London, California, New Delhi and Singapore: Sage Publications.

Pinker, S. (2002) *The Blank Slate: The Modern Denial of Human Nature.* London, New York, Victoria, Ontario, Auckland: Penguin Publications.

Pinkola Estes, C. (1992) *Women Who Run With the Wolves.* New York: Ballantine Books.

Pointon, M. (2013) *Portrayal and the Search for Identity.* Reaktion Books: London.

Pratt, M. and Thomas, G. (eds) (2002) *Guidelines for Arts Therapies and the Arts in Palliative Care Settings.* London: Help the Hospices.

Pratt, M. and Wood, M. (eds) (1998) *Art Therapy in Palliative Care: The Creative Response.* London: Harper Collins.

Puchalski, C., Ferrell, B., Virani, R., Otis-Green, S. *et al.* (2009) 'Improving the quality of spiritual care as a dimension of palliative care: the report of the Consensus Conference.' *Journal of Palliative Medicine 12*, 10, 885–904.

Quail, J. and Peavy, V. (1994) 'A phenomenologic research study of a client's experience of art therapy.' *The Arts in Psychotherapy 21*, 1, 45–57.

Rådestad, I., Nordin, C., Steineck, G. and Sjogren, B. (1996) 'Stillbirth is no longer managed as a nonevent: a nationwide study in Sweden.' *Birth 23*, 4, 209–217.

Radley, A. (2002) 'Portrayals of suffering: on looking away, looking at, and the comprehension of illness experience.' *Body and Society 8*, 3, 1–23.

Radley, A. (2009) *Works of Illness: Narrative, Picturing and the Social Response to Serious Disease.* Ashby-De-La-Zouche, UK: Inker Men Press.

Radley, A. and Bell, S. (2007) 'Artworks, collective experience and claims for social justice: the case of women living with breast cancer.' *Sociology of Health and Illness 29*, 3, 366–390.

Rando, T. (1991) 'Parental Adjustment to the Loss of a Child.' In D. Papadatou and C. Papadatos (eds) *Children and Death* (pp.233–254). London: Hemisphere Publishing Corporation.

Reason, P. (2006) 'Choice and quality in action research practice.' *Journal of Management Inquiry 15*, 2, 187–203. Reeve, J. (2010) *Interpretive Medicine: Supporting Generalism in a Changing Primary Care World.* Occasional Paper 88. London: The Royal College of General Practitioners Publications.

Reeve, J., Lloyd-Williams, M., Payne, S. and Dowrick, C. (2010) 'Revisiting biographical disruption: exploring individual embodied illness experience in people with terminal cancer.' *Health 14*, 178–195.

Rennie, D. L. (1994) 'Human science and counselling psychology: closing the gap between research and practice.' *Counselling Psychology Quarterly 7*, 3, 235–250.

Reynolds, F. and Lim, K. H. (2007) 'Contribution of visual art-making to the subjective well-being of women living with cancer: a qualitative study.' *The Arts in Psychotherapy 34*, 1–10.

Reynolds, F. (2003a) 'Conversations about creativity and chronic illness I: textile artists coping with long-term health problems reflect on the origins of their interest in art.' *Creativity Research Journal 15*, 4, 393–407.

Reynolds, F. (2003b) 'Reclaiming a positive identity in chronic illness through artistic occupation.' *OTJR: Occupation, Participation and Health 23*, 3, Summer, 118–127.

Reynolds, F. and Prior, S. (2003) '"A lifestyle coat-hanger": a phenomenological study of the meanings of artwork for women coping with chronic illness and disability.' *Disability and Rehabilitation 25*, 14, 785–794.

Rizzolatti, G., Fadiga, L., Gallese, V. and Fogassi, L. (1996) 'Premotor cortex and the recognition of motor actions.' *Cognitive Brain Research 3*, 131–141.

Robbins, A. (2000) *The Artist as Therapist*. London and Philadelphia: Jessica Kingsley Publishers.

Rodin, G., Craven, J. and Littlefield, C. (1991) *Depression in the Medically Ill: An Integrated Approach*. New York: Brunner/Mazel.

Rogers, C. (1951) *Client-Centred Therapy: Its Current Practices, Implications, and Theory*. New York: Houghton Miffin.

Rogers, C. (1957) 'The necessary and sufficient conditions of therapeutic personality change.' *Journal of Consulting Psychology 21*, 2, 95–103.

Rolls, A. (2013) Personal email to Susan Carr.

Rolls, A. (2014a) 'A Graceful Death: Part One.' *ehospice online*, 27 January. Accessed on 10/03/2017 at https://goo.gl/DahtnQ.

Rolls, A. (2014b) 'A Graceful Death: Part Two.' *ehospice online*, 28 January. Accessed on 11/03/2017 at https://goo.gl/6miHUS.

Rosenblum, B. (1991) 'I Have Begun the Process of Dying.' In J. Spence and P. Holland (eds) *Family Snaps: The Meaning of Domestic Photography* (pp.243–254). London: Virago.

Rosselli, H. (2009) *Face to Face: Looking at and Portraying Disfigurement*. Audio recording of the panel discussion, the Mall Galleries, Tuesday 19 May.

Rossetto, E. (2012) 'A hermeneutic phenomenological study of community mural making and social action art therapy.' *Art Therapy: Journal of the American Art Therapy Association 29*, 1, 19–26.

Rostron, J. (2010) 'On amodal perception and language in art therapy with autism.' *International Journal of Art Therapy 15*, 1, 36–49.

Sacks, O. (1984) *A Leg to Stand On*. New York: Touchstone.

Saunders, C. (1976) 'The Challenge of Terminal Care'. In T. Symington and R. Carter (eds) *Scientific Foundation of Oncology* (pp.673–679). London: Heinemann.

Saunders, C. (ed.) (1990) *Hospice and Palliative Care: An Interdisciplinary Approach*. Sevenoaks, UK: Edward Arnold Pubs.

Sawday, J. (1996 [1995]) *The Body Emblazoned: Dissection and the Human Body in Renaissance Culture*. London and New York: Routledge.

Seymour, W. (2002) 'Time and the body: re-embodying time in disability.' *Journal of Occupational Science 9*, 3, 135–142.

Schore, A. (2000) 'Attachment and the regulation of the right brain.' *Attachment and Human Development 2*, 1, 23–47.

Scruton, R. (2012) *Why Beauty Matters*. BBC Documentary, 8 December. Accessed on 21/07/2017 at www.youtube.com/watch?v=bHw4MMEnmpc.

Sibbett, C. (2004) 'Liminality: Living and Practising at the Threshold.' 3rd Global Conference: Making Sense of Health, Illness and Disease, July 2004, St Catherine's College, Oxford.

# REFERENCES

Sibbett, C. (2005a) 'Liminal Embodiment: Embodied and Sensory Experience in Cancer Care and Art Therapy.' In D. Waller and C. Sibbett (eds) *Facing Death: Art Therapy and Cancer Care* (pp.50–81). Maidenhead: Open University Press.

Sibbett, C. (2005b) 'Betwixt and Between: Crossing Thresholds.' In D. Waller and C. Sibbett (eds) *Facing Death: Art Therapy and Cancer Care* (pp.12–37). Maidenhead, UK: Open University Press.

Sibbett, C. (2005c) 'An Art Therapist's Experience of Having Cancer: Living and Dying with the Tiger.' In D. Waller and C. Sibbett (eds) *Facing Death: Art Therapy and Cancer Care* (pp.223–248). Maidenhead, UK: Open University Press.

Sibbett, C. and Thompson, W. (2008) 'Nettlesome knowledge, liminality and the taboo in cancer and art therapy experiences: implications for learning and teaching.' In R. Land, J. Meyer and J. Smith (eds) *Threshold Concepts within the Disciplines* (pp.227–242). Rotterdam: Sense Publishers.

Sinding, C., Gray, R. and Nisker, J. (2008) 'Ethical Issues and Issues of Ethics.' In G. Knowles and A. Coles (eds) *Handbook of the Arts in Qualitative Research* (pp.459–467). London, California, New Delhi, Singapore: Sage.

Skaife, S. (1993) 'Sickness, health and the therapeutic relationship.' *International Journal of Art Therapy [Inscape]*, Summer 1993, 24–29.

Skaife, S. (2001) 'Making visible: art therapy and intersubjectivity.' *International Journal of Art Therapy [Inscape]* 6, 2, 40–50.

Smith, C. (2008) 'Performing My Recovery: a play of chaos, restitution, and quest after traumatic brain injury.' *Forum: Qualitative Social Research* 9, 2, 30–35.

Smith, J. (2004) 'Reflecting on the development of interpretative phenomenological analysis and its contribution to qualitative research in psychology.' *Qualitative Research in Psychology* 1, 39–54.

Smith, J., Flowers, P. and Larkin, M. (2009) *Interpretative Phenomenological Analysis: Theory Method and Research*. London, California, New Delhi, Singapore: Sage.

Sontag, S. (1991) *Illness as Metaphor and Aids and Its Metaphors*. London: Penguin Books.

Sontag, S. (2003) *Regarding the Pain of Others*. New York: Picador.

Spaniol, S. (2005) 'Learned hopefulness: an arts-based approach to participatory action research.' *Art Therapy: Journal of the American Art Therapy Association* 22, 2, 86–91.

Spence, J. (1986) 'Phototherapy.' *Venue 14*, 48–49.

Spence, J. (2005) *Beyond the Perfect Image. Photography, Subjectivity, Antagonism. MACBA Exhibition catalogue*, Barcelona: 2005.

Spence, J. and Holland, P. (eds) (1991) *Family Snaps. The Meaning of Domestic Photography*. London: Virgo Press.

Spinelli, E. (1995) *The Interpreted World. An Introduction to Phenomenological Psychology*. London, California, New Delhi, Singapore: Sage.

Springham, N. (2008) 'Through the eyes of the law: what is it about art that can harm people?' *International Journal of Art Therapy* 13, 2, 65–73.

Springham, N. and Woods, A. (2014) 'Toolkit uses patient experiences to improve mental health services.' *Guardian Professional*, 7 January, 2014.

Stern, D. (1985) *The Interpersonal World of the Infant*. New York: Basic Books.

Stieglitz, A. (2000 [1922]) 'Is Photography a Failure?' [First published in *The Sun*, New York, 14 March 1922.] In A. Stieglitz, R. Whelan and S. Greenough (eds) *Stieglitz on Photography* (p.229). New York: Aperture.

Street, A. and Kissane, D. (2001) 'Discourses of the body in euthanasia: symptomatic, dependent, shameful and temporal.' *Nursing Inquiry* 8, 3, 162–172.

Strohm, K. (2012) 'When anthropology meets contemporary art: notes for a politics of collaboration.' *Collaborative Anthropologies* 5, 98–124.

Stuckley, H. and Nobel, J. (2010) 'The connection between art, healing, and public health: a review of current literature.' *American Journal of Public Health 100*, 2, 254–263.

Sullivan, G. (2010) *Art Practice as Research: Inquiry in Visual Arts* (Second Edition). London, New York, Singapore, New Delhi: Sage Publishing.

Svenaeus, F. (2000) 'Das Unheimliche – towards a phenomenology of illness.' *Medicine, Health Care and Philosophy 3*, 3–16.

Svenaeus, F. (2001) *The Hermeneutics of Medicine and the Phenomenology of Health*. Linköping: Springer.

Svenaeus, F. (2011) 'Illness as unhomelike being-in-the-world: Heidegger and the phenomenology of medicine.' *Medicine Health Care and Philosophy 14*, 333–343.

Svenaeus, F. (2012) 'Organ transplantation and personal identity: how does loss and change of organs affect the self?' *Journal of Medicine and Philosophy 37*, 139–158.

Taylor, C. (1989) *Sources of the Self: The Making of Modern Identity*. Cambridge: Cambridge University Press.

Taylor, C. (1991) *The Ethics of Authenticity*. Cambridge, MA, and London, UK: Harvard University Press.

Tembeck, T. (2008) 'Exposed wounds: the photographic autopathographies of Hannah Wilke and Jo Spence.' *RACAR XXXIII*, Numbers 1–2, 87–100. Accessed on 10/03/2017 at https://goo.gl/5nn6R6.

Thorne, D. (2011) 'Raising questions about art therapy: reflections on the recent ATPRN symposium and the BBC2 "Art for Heroes" Programme.' *British Association of Art Therapy Newsbriefing*, Autumn, pp.26–29.

Tjasink, M. (2010) 'Art psychotherapy in medical oncology: a search for meaning.' *International Journal of Art Therapy 15*, 2, 75–83.

Toombs, S. (1988) 'Illness and the paradigm of lived body.' *Theoretical Medicine 11*, 227–241.

Toombs, S. (1990) 'The temporality of illness: four levels of experience.' *Theoretical Medicine 11*, 3, 227–241.

Toombs, S. (1992) *The Meaning of Illness: A Phenomenological Account of the Different Perspectives of Physician and Patient*. Dordrecht: Kluwer Academic Publishers.

Toombs, S. (ed.) (2001) *Handbook of Phenomenology and Medicine*. Dordrecht: Kluwer Academic Publishers, Springer.

Trotsky, L. (2005 [1924]) *Literature and Revolution* (W. Keach (ed.) trans. R. Strunsky), Chicago, IL: Haymarket Books.

Turner, V. (1969 [1995]) *The Ritual Process: Structure and Anti-Structure*. New York: Aldine de Gruyter.

Turner, V. (1982) *From Ritual to Theatre: The Human Seriousness of Play*. New York: Performing Arts Journal Publications.

Ulman, E. (1980) 'Symposium: Integration of Divergent Points of View in Art Therapy.' In E. Ulman and C. Levy (eds) *Art Therapy Viewpoints* (pp.6–17). New York: Schoken.

van Alphen, E. (1997) 'The Portrait's Dispersal: Concepts of Representation and Subjectivity in Contemporary Portraiture.' In W. Joanna (ed.) *Portraiture: Facing the Subject* (pp.240–241). Manchester: Manchester University Press/St. Martin's.

van der Kolk, B. (1987) *Psychological Trauma*. Washington, DC: American Psychiatric Press.

van der Kolk, B. (1988) 'The trauma spectrum: the interaction of biological and social events in the genesis of the trauma response.' *Journal of Traumatic Stress 1*, 273–290.

van der Kolk, B. (2003) 'Frontiers in Trauma Treatment.' Presented at the R. Cassidy Seminars, St. Louis, MO, 2004.

van Gennep, A. (1960) *The Rites of Passage*. Chicago, IL: The University of Chicago Press.

# REFERENCES

van Lith, T. (2008) 'A phenomenological investigation of art therapy to assist transition to a psychosocial residential setting.' *Art Therapy, Journal of the American Art Therapy Association 25*, 1, 24–31.

van Manen, M. (1990) *Researching Lived Experience*. Ontario, Canada: The State University of New York Press.

Vaughan, K. (2005) 'Pieced together: collage as an artist's method for interdisciplinary research.' *International Journal of Qualitative Methods 4*, 1, Article 3, 1–15.

Vecchi, B. (2004) Interview. In Z. Bauman (ed.) *Identity: Conversations with Benedetto Vecchi*. Cambridge and Malden: Polity Press.

Vick, R. (2000) 'Creative dialog: a shared will to create.' *Art Therapy: Journal of the American Art Therapy Association 17*, 3, 216–219.

Volkan, V. (1997) *Bloodlines: From Ethnic Pride to Ethnic Terrorism*. Boulder, CO: Westview.

Wahrendorf, M., Ribet, C., Zins, M., Goldberg, M. *et al*. (2010) 'Perceived reciprocity in social exchange and health functioning in early old age: prospective findings from the GAZEL study.' *Aging & Mental Health 14*, 4, 425–432.

Waller, D. (ed.) (2002) *Arts Therapies and Progressive Illness: Nameless Dread*. Hove and New York: Brunner-Routledge.

Waller, D and Sibbett, C. (eds) (2005) *Art Therapy and Cancer Care*. Maidenhead: Open University Press.

Watts, J. (2009) 'Meanings of spirituality at the cancer drop-in.' *International Journal of Qualitative Studies on Health and Well-Being 4*, 2, 86–93.

Weisfeld, G. (1993) 'The adaptive value of humor and laughter.' *Ethology and Sociobiology 14*, 2, 141–169.

Werner-Seidler, A. and Moulds, M. (2011) 'Autobiographical memory characteristics in depression vulnerability: formerly depressed individuals recall less vivid positive memories.' *Cognition & Emotion 25*, 6, 1087–1103.

Wertz, F. (2005) 'Phenomenological research methods for counselling psychology.' *Journal of Counselling Psychology 52*, 2, 167–177.

West, S. (2004) *Portraiture*. Oxford: Oxford University Press.

Whicher, S., Spiller, R. and Williams, W. (eds) (1964) *The Early Lectures of Ralph Waldo Emerson*. Cambridge, MA: Harvard University Press.

Wilkinson, R. and Chilton, G. (2013) 'Positive art therapy: linking positive psychology to art therapy theory, practice, and research.' *Art Therapy: Journal of the American Art Therapy Association 30*, 1, 4–11.

Williams, B. (2002) 'Using collage art work as a common medium for communication in interprofessional care.' *Journal of Interprofessional Care 16*, 1, 53–58.

Winnicott, D. (1971) 'Mirror-role of the Mother and Family in Child Development.' In D. Winnicott (1971) *Playing and Reality* (pp.111–118). London: Tavistock.

Wix, L. (2000) 'Looking for what's lost: the artistic roots of art therapy: Mary Huntoon.' *Art Therapy: Journal of the American Art Therapy Association 17*, 3, 168–176.

Wood, M. (1990) 'Art therapy in one session, working with people with AIDS.' *International Journal of Art Therapy [Inscape]*, Winter 1990, 27–33.

Wood, M. (1998) 'The Body as Art: Individual Session with a Man with AIDS.' In M. Pratt and M. Wood (eds) *Art Therapy in Palliative Care: The Creative Response* (pp.140–152). London, New York: Routledge.

Wood, M. (2005) 'Shoreline: The Realities of Working in Cancer and Palliative Care.' In D. Waller and C. Sibbett (eds) *Art Therapy and Cancer Care* (pp.82–101). London: Open University Press.

Wood, M., Molassiotis, A. and Payne, S. (2011) 'What research evidence is there for the use of art therapy in the management of symptoms in adults with cancer? A systematic review.' *Psycho-Oncology 20*, 135–145.

Wood, M., Low, J., Molassiotis, A. and Tookman, A. (2013) 'Art therapy's contribution to the psychological care of adults with cancer: a survey of therapists and service users in the UK.' *International Journal of Art Therapy 18*, 2, 42–53.

Wright, K. (2005) 'The shaping of experience.' *British Journal of Psychotherapy 21*, 4.

Wright, K. (2009) *Mirroring and Attunement: Self-Realisation in Psychoanalysis and Art.* London, New York: Routledge.

Yin, R. (2009) *Case Study Research: Design and Methods* (Fourth Edition). Thousand Oaks CA, London, New Delhi, Singapore: Sage Publications.

Yin, R. (2012) *Applications of Case Study Research.* Thousand Oaks CA, London, New Delhi, Singapore: Sage Publications.

Young, M. (1988) 'Understanding identity disruption and intimacy: one aspect of post-traumatic stress.' *Contemporary Family Therapy 10*, 1, 30–43.

# Websites

Dying Matters Coalition. Accessed on 10/03/2017 at http://dyingmatters.org/overview/about-us.

Farrand, P. (2000) *Portraiture as Therapy.* Saving Faces website. Accessed on 10/03/2017 at www.savingfaces.co.uk/news-media/art-project/35-news-media/art/133-dr-paul-farrand-medical-psychologist.

Gilbert, M. (2000) 'Portraiture as Therapy.' Saving Faces Website. Accessed on 10/03/2017 at www.savingfaces.co.uk/news-media/art-project/35-news-media/art/133-dr-paul-farrand-medical-psychologist.

'How Cancer Saved my Life' by John D. Edwards. Accessed on 24/03/3017 at www.howcancersavedmylife.co.uk.

Hutchison, I., Farrand, P. and Gilbert, M. (2000) *Portraiture as Therapy.* Saving Faces website. Accessed on 10/03/2017 at www.savingfaces.co.uk/news-media/art-project/35-news-media/art/133-dr-paul-farrand-medical-psychologist.

# AUTHOR BIOGRAPHY

**Susan Carr** was born in Winchester, but she moved with her family to Gibraltar when she was seven years old. Growing up in the beautiful surroundings of Gibraltar gave Susan an appreciation for different cultures and an eye for detail. Susan began painting portraits when she was at school; however, her journey as an artist has taken her to many rich and varied areas, including sculpture, illustration, community art, printmaking and mixed media. Susan has recently developed a love for painting *en plein air*, enjoying the challenge and spontaneity of painting from life, outdoors.

Susan's professional journey began with a BA (Hons) degree in Design/Illustration from Cranfield University, followed by two years as artist in residence at a secondary school in Swindon. Through working with some of the pupils in the 'exclusion unit' Susan began to see how art could be used as therapy, and enrolled at the University of Hertfordshire to study for an MA in Art Therapy. Susan has 12 years' experience of working as an art therapist in palliative care, during which time she also completed her PhD at Loughborough University, developing Portrait Therapy as an intervention for people who experience illness as a disruption to their sense of self-identity. Susan has published articles in *The International Journal of Art Therapy* and presented papers at many national and international conferences, as well as facilitating workshops and teaching events. Susan has now begun her own art therapy and portrait therapy private practice, as well as continuing with her artistic and writing careers.

Susan is planning a touring exhibition of the portraits depicted within this book, beginning with an exhibition at Swindon Museum and Art Gallery during the summer of 2017.

# SUBJECT INDEX

abandonment
  in childhood 112, 164
  and loss of self-identity 112
  and lack of a secure
    attachment 164
  and transformation of 172
acceptance 117, 119, 158,
    197
  adaptive 205
  of 'being-towards-death'
    (Heidegger) 190
'Active Documentâtion
  Sketchbook' (ADS) (De
  Freitas) 209, 214–215
  and reflexivity and self-
    reflective processes 234
  and creating a statement of
    intention 218
adaption
  and change 117
  through increased flexibility
    and agency 117
  and changes in perception
    of control 117
  and closure 112
  and creating emotional
    distance and connection
    102
  and creativity 19
  and identity transition 196,
    230
  and liminality 19
  and mourning losses 105
  through self-care and
    agency 238
  through transforming
    meaning & changing
    perspectives 91
  and visible mending 126

'aesthetic resonance' (Carr)
    160
  adding meaning, complexity
    and coherence to
    portraits 127
  and art therapy training 246
  attaching to portraits 160,
    161–166
  and beauty 127, 160
  and coherence 162
  and collage and prose poems
    217
  empathically attuned 244
  excluded in self-portraits
    242
  and holding dualities within
    the portraits 244
  and 'mirroring and
    attunement' (Wright)
    240
  and mitigation 156
  as a powerful healing force
    244
  and 'third hand' (Kramer)
    interventions 246
'aesthetic response' (Knill)
    51, 244
  within arts therapy 51
aesthetics 50
  beauty and healing 49
  challenge of, in art therapy
    49–52
  power 49, 51
agency
  and adaption through
    increased flexibility and
    control 117–126
  and collaborative
    relationship 112
  and death 39

and helplessness 147
increased 91, 126, 239
lived experience of 120
and portraits 27
renewed sense of 133, 140,
    194, 240
self-care and 238, 239
self-worth and 137
and subjects within portraits
    37
as theme in art therapy and
  palliative care literature
    59
agoraphobic fears 140
alchemy
  of art 27, 35
  of portraiture 204
ambivalence 133, 148
amelioration of suffering 33,
    72, 245, 248
analysis
  and 'Active Documentation
    Sketchbook' (ADS) (De
    Freitas) 214
  Arts-based Life/world
    Phenomenological
    Analysis (ALPHA)
    226–230
  cross-case 225–226
  and essence statements
    119, 138, 185, 196,
    229–230
  and emergent themes 122,
    194, 225
  evaluating portrait therapy
    223–235
  a phenomenological
    approach to 52,
    226–228
  and participants 86, 87, 222

## SUBJECT INDEX

of portraits 62, 63, 64, 197
and unexpected themes 93
visual analysis matrix 229
visual methods 161, 185, 226
voice centred interpersonal analysis 231–233
'voice centred relational analysis' (Brown & Gilligan) 231
of voice recordings 196, 231–233
anger, as catharsis 157
antidepressants 22, 245, 248
anxiety 35, 44
  attacks 84
  and depression 44, 244
  and emotional affect 89
  existential 168, 177
  and fear of death 24
  and raising painful issues with patients in palliative care 88
  reducing 89, 210, 215
  and suicidal ideation 83
  in the therapist 36
  and 'third hand' (Kramer) interventions 197
  transforming unbearable 24
appropriation 217–218, 219, 234
art
  the alchemy of 27, 35, and portraiture 204
  creation of 16, 31
  portraits 27, 62, 115
  and healing 51, 98, 128, 178, 241, 242
  how life imitates, and renewed personal agency 132
  and 'making special' (Dissanayake) 35, 40, 167–177, 239
  see also 'made special' (Dissanayake) 34, 104, 170
  transformational power of 27, 30, 73
  and transforming meanings 16, 31,91–98
art therapist/s,
  and 'aesthetic response' (Knill) 51
  and aesthetics and art therapy (Maclagan) 50

and artist identities merged 16
British Association of Art Therapists (BAAT) 86
clinical supervision 53, 249
clinical theory development 224
collaborative relationships 17, 33, 53
collaboration with artists 66
containment 24
creative art practice 16
embodied countertransference and vicarious traumatization 77, 89–90
empathic understanding 87, 128
equalizing therapeutic relationships 17, 53
expressions of pain and trauma 50
facing death 36
as 'good enough (m)other' (Winnicott/Wright)
holding experiences or affect 24, 58
humour 98–99
'liminality' (Caryl) 34–36
painting portraits of patients 58–61, 220–221
  analysis of 223–235
  co-designing of 198
  as collaborative intervention 77
  demonstrating 'care' 59, 249
  and depicting subjectivity 36–43
  exhibitions of 191, 243
  and 'mirroring and attunement' (Wright) 220, 241, 248
  and self-identity 59, 70
  statement of intention for 218
  and time and attention 198, 205, 239
  a therapist's manual 209–222
  and the therapeutic relationship 58, 249
  and training 248
  and vulnerability 242
  and witnessing 58, 59, 89, 247, 249

and placements 15, 36
and reflexivity 53
and relational meaning 85
and research in palliative care 58–61, 87
and resonance 214
and response art, 160, 215
and self-identities
  multiple 88, 250
  construction of 85
  student 15, 36, 246
and 'studio art therapy' (Moon)
and subjective responses 53
and training 50, 88, 249
and the 'third hand' (Kramer) 30–33, 241, 242, 248
and the third space 85
using a phenomenological approach 52–54
verbal and facial responses of 25
art therapy
  accessible 30, 33
  limitations and problems 31
  and an 'aesthetic response' (Knill) 41, 244
  and aesthetics 49–52
  and AIDS 55
  and the art world
  and 'beauty' (McNiff) 50–52
  benefits in life-threatening and chronic illnesses (literature) 59–61
  and calls for research in life threatening & chronic illnesses 33
  in cancer care 59–60
  case study research 225
  clinification of 25
  collaboration with users of 85, 89
  confidentiality 86, 209
  dys-engagement with aesthetics, rejection of art world 52
  equalizing power structures within 85
  externalizing problems and the art therapist's 'third hand' (Kramer) 202
  focus on art 16
  and gender 43–45

— 277 —

art therapyy *cont.*
  and health and wellbeing 16
  and imagination 91
  and the medical model 50
  and a phenomenological approach to illness 52–54
  person centred 65
  and portraiture and palliative care 58–61
  psychodynamic & psychoanalytic 25
  and self-identity 61
  and spirituality 168
  and 'studio art therapy' (Moon) 16
  and Surrealism 51
  and theory building 224, 241
  and time 65
  and training 246, 248
arts-based Life/World Phenomenological Analysis (ALPHA) 223, 226–230
  and 'phenomenological hermeneutic interpretation' (Heidegger) 226
  and 'phenomenological reduction' (Husserl) 226
  and primary pre-reflective knowing 226
  and secondary reflective learning 226
  the six steps of 227–228
attunement' (Stern) 24
authenticity 22, 178, 180
  therapists 216
autonomy 146
  disruption to 84, 141
  increase in 91, 136, 238
  perceptions of control and 117, 126

balance 150, 151, 152, 162, 170
  in the portraits and collages 134, 135, 153, 159
beautiful, recapturing a sense of self as 29, 127, 160, 163, 165, 166, 181
beauty 28, 29, 50, 144
  adding to portraits 160, 217, 240
  and aesthetics 49–52

to assuage pain and suffering 50
a challenging kind 39
and illness 67
as a metaphor for recovery and self-reclamation 162
and positive art therapy 244
and redemption 51
and revisioning self-identity 160
and its capacity of to move and heal 49, 50
as truth and goodness 51
universal need of human beings for 51
*see also* aesthetic resonance 160, 217, 240, 244
'becoming' (Kinnvall) 247
  as autonomy 190, 196
  *see also* agency
  and self-identity formation 194
  as turning points within the portraits 236
being-held-in-mind
  by the art therapist 198
  and the art therapist's 'third hand' (Kramer) 242
  and portraiture 112, 198, 205, 239
being known at end of life 246–249
  and humour 102, 238
  and portraits 127, 137, 140, 177, 202
  and spirituality 176
  to themselves 131, 247, 248
  *see also* self-knowledge
'being-towards-death' (Heidegger) 48
  and acceptance of 190
  and adaption 105
  recognition of 157
  within the portraits 187
  *see also* death
belonging
  and connection 190, 239
  increasing a sense of 167
  and remembering within portraits 177–190
  a search for 47
  stories of 180
bereavement 81, 106
  and accepting loss 112
  and childbirth 114

and closure 117, 238
and Dying Matters Coalition 49
and feelings of guilt 112, 249
and helplessness 117
and illness 117
and loss 106
of baby and childhood abandonment 112–117
memento mori 116
and mourning 69
and portraits 114, 115, 244
and relational self-identity 117
and stories of 114
*see also* grief
betrayal of the body
  as container for disease and revealing disease 20, 131
body language 27
  reading 127
body-centred counter-transference and vicarious traumatization 89–90
  *see also* embodied counter-transference 77, 221
body-image
  and illness 59
  problematized 43
  and self-identity 22
  and stigma 43
body
  and beauty 49
  and cancer treatments 44
  central role of, in 'perception' (Merleau-Ponty) 20, 43
  and death 39
  a diseased 168
  and gender 43
  and healing 128
  idealized 44
  and illness 20, 33, 38, 40, 43, 44, 56, 70, 106, 131, 197
  language 27, 127
  and loneliness 247
  medicalisation of 71–72
  and neuroscience 191, 201
  as object reclaimed 199
  objectification of 20
  paying attention to 60
  photographing 102
  and politics 43

# SUBJECT INDEX

and portraiture 246
as portrait 55
problematized 43, 44
self-hatred 44
and soul 167
and 'stigma' (Goffman) 43
and the sick role 44
trapped within 157
the 'unbounded' (Lawton) 157, 158
boundaries,
pushing the 32, 219, 241
and client confidentiality 61
maintaining 78, 209
secure 249
and humour 99
and self-concept 131
Bourgeois, Louise 188, 261
bracketing out 54, 234, 241
and phenomenology 54
within the 'six steps' for ALPHA 227
British Association of Art Therapists (BAAT)
Code of Ethics and Principles of Practice 86
brittle asthma 97, 83
burden on patients 86, 88–89, 115
button elicitation task 117, 129, 210, 211
button sculpt 211
and emotional distancing 213, 214
and stories of self-identity 236
and art therapy training 246

cancer
art therapy with patients living with 157, 250
and liminality 34
and death 83
living with a diagnosis of 18, 33, 41
terminal 27, 37
mastectomy 66–67
patient 42, 79, 81, 82
research in art therapy and 59–60
treatments 44
case-studies
portrait therapy patients 75–171
and bracketing out 54
and generalisation

multiple case-study design 224–226
cathartic 65
and the aesthetic 244
content of portraits 158
for the therapist 221
celebrity
and fame and popular culture 70, 202
and patient 99, 185
chemotherapy 38, 44, 79, 81, 82
childhood
difficulties in 82, 104, 119, 149, 161, 163
redefining and reclaiming 166, 240
and distress 152
and over-protection and under-protection 118, 120, 149, 150, 159
positive 154, 194
transitional moments in 28, 29
Chronic Obstructive Pulmonary Disorder (COPD) 79, 81, 84
clinical theory development 244
and portrait therapy 224, 237, 241–242
clinification of art therapy 16, 25
closure
and the therapist 250
and bereavement 112, 116, 117, 173, 174, 238
clothes
as external props 43, 60
in portraits 137, 147, 187–189
signifying temporality 188
co-designing 17
and agency 112
with patients 29, 118, 119, 151, 187, 195, 217–220
as intersubjective process 85, 170
and lived experience of 'control' 117
portraits patients needed to see 102
portraits patients needed others to see 102, 142
and strengthening self-identity 32

and time and attention 198
Cognitive Behavioural Therapy (CBT) 223
'cognitive dissonance' (Festinger)
confusion and disorientation 47
dissipating within portraits holding dualities 139, 241
coherence
and aesthetic resonance 160, 162
adding within portraits 127, 163, 166, 240, 248
and inner and outer landscapes portrayed within portraits 158
and sense of self-identity 131, 159
collaborative
case-studies 75–171
co-designing process 32, 220
intersubjective relationship 17, 53, 87, 88–89, 112, 210, 248, 250
intervention 33
process 116, 156,
research process 85, 249
collage and prose poems 217
and art therapy training 246
as cathartic process in therapist 221
as containers of duality 146–159
exploring difficult feelings 112, 113, 169, 199–200
and gender 45
and healing 242
intersubjective validation of self-identity 127, 240
and love 192, 205
and metaphor 118, 189
and narrative 129
as 'response art' (Fish) 56, 215–217, 234
and stories of self-identity 111
companioning 247
*see also* witnessing
conceptual
art 51
artists 52
confidentiality 86–87, 209
and anonymity 243

confidentiality *cont.*
  and boundaries 61
  counterproductive 243
  and limits to 86, 209, 249
  as universal requirement within art therapy 224, 242, 243
confrontation 72, 73, 141
'containment' (Bion) 24
  bodily 157
  self 157
  a sense of 95
  *see also* holding
'continuing bonds' (Klass, Silverman & Nickman) 105
contrapuntal voices
  listening for 96, 124, 196, 231, 232
control
  and autonomy 91, 126, 238
  and illness 60, 123
  of information around illness 44, 148
  lack of 60
  over images 89, 102
  perceptions of 117, 122
  regaining a sense of 72
  and self-identity 56
  and social stigma 44
creative capacity to adapt to illness 91
  and empowerment 238
  negative impact of illness on 18
  increasing 95, 97, 125, 238
counter-transference
  body-centred and vicarious traumatization 89–90
  *see also* embodied countertransference 77, 221

de-personalisation and healthcare 44
death
  and absence of subjectivity 39
  being-towards 48, 105, 157, 169, 187, 190
  in birth 114, 115
  and change and uncertainty 35
  cheating 26, 167, 205, 239
  and closure 122, 166, 117, 173, 174, 238, 250

denial of, 48, 106, 111, 205, 245
  facing 106
  and rituals 172, 174, 250
  fear of 24, 48
  as 'final stage of growth' (Kubler-Ross) 49
  'a graceful death' (Rolls) 67
  a good death 22
  as homecoming 187
  impending 72, 158, 247
  as last taboo
  and legacy 204
  life and 139, 197
  and liminal entities 35
  metaphor and symbolism of 60, 147
  and mourning 189
  and portraiture 38–40, 70
  reunited in 112
  and self-identity 168
  unboundedness and 36
  and unfinished business 29, 250
  *see also* annihilation
denial
  and death 48, 106, 111, 205, 245
  and inability to 'hold' 145
  and illness 180, 197
dependent
  and illness 19, 84, 131
depression 104, 158
  and anxiety 83, 84, 244
  and the body 44
  and portrait therapy 204, 237, 244
  postnatal 114
  and social isolation 18
  and suicidal ideation 83
despair
  feelings of 145, 174
  hope and 45, 139, 146, 147, 149, 159, 162, 163, 187, 241
  and illness 160
disability
  illness and 47, 144
  physical 244
disease
  and betrayal of the body and revealing 20
  biomedical model of 46
  and the body 20, 70, 168, 199

life-threatening 69, 79
  multi-layered nature of 41
  pain of 66
  and stigma 43
discursive language 56, 127
  and communication issues 127
discursive selves 16
disempowerment
  and illness 21
  and self-identity disruption 17
disrupted self-identities 17–19
  and antidepressants 22, 248
  and illness 18, 20, 21, 32, 55, 78, 245, 246
  and ontological security 46
  and stigma of 194
  and trauma 244, 246
  *see also* self-identity disruption
dual-role conflict 86
  and 'insider' research 88
dualities
  adaptive 102–104
  contradictory 170
  holding of within portraits 131, 139, 147, 149, 241
  belonging and separation 187
  beauty and suffering 244
  breathing and suffocation 139
  denial and acceptance 197
  fear and courage 154, 158
  good and evil 159
  helplessness and agency 147
  hope and despair 45, 139, 146, 147, 149, 159, 162, 163, 187, 241
  hope and hopelessness 197
  idealisation and vilification 154
  imprisonment and freedom 159
  inner and outer realities 156, 159, 241
  life and death 187, 197
  past and future 187
  power and helplessness 154

## SUBJECT INDEX

truth and deception 153
under and over protected 159
within collages and prose poems 150
Dying Matters Coalition 49

eating disorder 44
elicitation tasks 129
  button 210–211
  LEGO ® 211–212
  photo 212–214
embodied empathy 197
  and renewed sense of self-love 190
embodiment
  of experience in cancer 60
  of illness 30, 55
  of lost-self 136
  of pain and suffering in portraits 237
  and self-identity disruption 17, 122, 131
emotional connection and distancing 102–104
empathic 30, 32
  attuning other 17, 24
  engagement 191, 197
  focused attention 242, 246
  listening 241
  therapeutic relationship 58, 248
  understanding 87
  therapist 89, 128
empathy
  embodied 190, 197
  and imagery 191
  and portraits 64
  and self-love 205
End of Project Interviews (EPIs) 222, 237, 255–256
essence(s)
  or 'air', of a person 26, 27, 56, 64, 109, 130
  reducing to 146, 226, 227–230
  of human experience 52
  of self-identity 196
  statements 77, 111, 109, 138, 148, 156, 161, 174, 185, 195
ethic of care 50, 88
ethical
  approval 86
  considerations and portrait therapy 86–90

confidentiality 86–87
exploitation 87–88
dual-role conflict or 'insider' research 88
burden on patients 88–89
body-centred counter-transference
  and vicarious traumatization 89–90
National Research and Ethics Service (NRES) 86
Evidence Based Practice (EBP) 232
exclusion criteria for portrait therapy 79
exhibitions 67, 202, 243
existential
  anxiety 177
  and fear of annihilation 168
  reduction in 168
  search for meaning 59
  questions 96, 215
  need to do more for patients 221
externalising objects 238

faces
  examining 26
  familiar, preference for 127
  as markers of identity 56
  and mirrors and self-recognition 17, 128
  and portraits 26
  saving 64, 65, 129, 240
facial expressions 27, 127, fear
  agoraphobic 140, 240
  of annihilation 221
  containment of within portraits 103
  of death 24, 48
  of hospice 36
  and illness 29, 141
  memories of 215
  portrayal of 150, 157, 158
  stories of 178
  of the unknown 168, 198
focus group 32, 84, 85
forgiveness 188
'frames of identity' (Taylor) 21, 177
further research into portrait therapy 64, 214
  implications for 244–246

gender
  and a cohesive self-identity 22
  and cultural influences 60
  and problematized bodies 43–45
generalisations
  and case studies 255
  and research outcomes 237
'good enough (m)other' (Winnicott/Wright) 33, 128, 188, 241, 250
good enough artist 33, 128
grief
  and illness 18
  containment of 173
  and ritual 174
  see also bereavement
guardian angel 170

healing
  and the creative imagination 98
  and a focus on aesthetics 51
  and holding in mind 216
  and memories, ritual and meaning making 115
  and the power of the arts 51, 128, 174, 241
  through portrait therapy 116, 117, 170
'health within illness' (Carel) 33, 46, 125, 241
helplessness
  and agency 147
  power and 154, 159, 241
  feelings of 38, 60,
  reducing feelings of 50, 112, 117, 126
  terror of 168
holding
  in art 58
  baby 110, 115, 172
  back 96
  burdensome secrets and power 155
  and containing hidden pain and suffering 104
  containing, and transforming unbearable anxiety 24
  dualities within the portraits 131, 139, 147, 149, 241
  belonging and separation 187

— 281 —

holding *cont.*
  beauty and suffering 244
  breathing and suffocation, denial and acceptance 197
  fear and courage 154, 158
  good and evil 159
  helplessness and agency 147
  hope and despair 45, 139, 146, 147, 149, 159, 162, 163, 187, 241
  hope and hopelessness 197
  idealisation and vilification 154
  imprisonment and freedom 159
  inner and outer realities 156, 159, 241
  life and death 187, 197
  past and future 187
  power and helplessness 154
  truth and deception 153
  under and over protected 159
  dualities within collages and prose poems 150
  hands 48, 137, 139, 179,
  hidden pain and suffering 238
  hope 159, 197, 241
  in life or death 169
  soft toy/teddy 40, 41, 42
  and validating self-identity 241
holding in mind 216, 274
  *see also* being-held-in-mind
holistic
  care and the empowerment of the individual 245
  impact on health of therapist 89
  paradigm 16
home visits 209
'homelike-being-in-the-world' (Svenaeus)
  and illness 19, 238
  and liminality 135
  and ontological security 167–205
  and portraits 48, 169, 175, 177, 185, 190, 205, 239
  *see also* 'unhomelike-being-in-the-world' (Svenaeus)

hope 133, 168
  and aesthetic resonance 160
  and fear 153
  in the face of adversity 47
  and grace 155
  holding 156, 197, 241
  loss of 89
  of recovery 197
  within portraits 148, 157, 158, 159, 241
  hope and despair, dualities of 45, 139, 146, 147, 149, 159, 162, 163, 187, 241
hopeless 84
hopelessness 59, 197, 90, 197
humour
  as an adaptive and imaginative way of being-in-the-world 98–102, 238
  and being known 102, 238
  benefits of 102
  and boundaries 99
  black 98
  and emotional distance 98
  and laughter as humanising dimension 99
  as a 'ludic' defence mechanism (Turner) 98
  as an 'imaginative way of being' (Hellema) 98
  and the intersubjective relationship 99
  and liminality 98
  and male patients 99, 101, 179, 201
  misinterpretation of 98
  in palliative care 98
  patient led 99
  and ritual 102
  and trust 99
  within portrait therapy sessions 99, 101, 179, 201

'I-thou' relationship (Buber) 45, 159
idealisation and vilification 154, 156
identities
  to authenticate 57
  disrupted 33, 245
  past and present 22
  and future 199

  merging of in the therapist 16, 88
  *see also* self-identities
illness
  and bereavement 117
  the body compromised by 20, 47, 81, 82, 141, 197, 245
  and changes in self-perception 20, 144
  and control over 121, 148
  to conceal 43, 131
  and death 43, 158
  'deep' (Frank) 18, 106
  denial of 180
  disruption caused by 20, 199
  and embodiment 30, 43, 55, 131
  effects of 59, 60, 79
  experiences of 20, 21, 29, 32, 55, 60, 85, 104, 126
  fears and anxieties 29
  finding 'health within' (Carel) 33, 46, 241
  and humour 98–99
  and increasing the patients' creative capacity
  to adapt to 18, 33, 91–130, 98, 123, 238
  and information control 44
  invisible 40, 41, 100, 144, 156, 157
  lived experience of 54 (literature), 246
  and meaning 21, 34
  and medicalisation 23
  narrative 42
  the nature of 34
  and phenomenology 52–54
  and photography 70–73
  and portraiture 38, 46, 56, 63–70, 89, 111, 140, 145, 146, 166, 175, 200
  psychological 204
  as punishment 44
  representations of 243
  romanticised 163
  and self-identity 17, 55, 61, 87, 117, 128, 129, 142, 145, 146, 198, 210, 211, 212, 220
  and spirituality 168, 169
  stigma in 131, 194, 245

## SUBJECT INDEX

terminal 88, 185
and treatment 46
as 'unhomelike being-in-the-world' 19–22
'world and works of' (Radley) 6, 92, 101, 202
and liminality' (Sibbett) 34–36, 96, 249
*see also* life threatening and chronic illness
images
and ambiguity 58
dangers of 42
drawing towards 218
and interpretation 56, 58, 224
relationships, with each other 57
vivid and positive 195, 198
imagination
and adaption 91–98
and art therapy (Maclagan) 91–92
creative 32, 98
and empathy 190
lack of 95, 96, 97
increase in 169
and neuroscience 92
and the past 187
and reality 123
and 'safety' 161
and 'third hand' interventions (Kramer) 30
imaginative 237
engagement 213
humour as 98–102
ideas and the PRA 219
portraits 57, 71, 97, 111
'potential' (Higgs) 91, 95, 97, 98
thinking 238
immortality 55, 202
immortalizing the 'sitter' or subject within a portrait 26, 197
inclusive, portrait therapy as 33
independence 84, 132
maintaining 125
individuality 44, 46, 61, 225
'indwelling' (Moustakas) 192, 227, 232
informed consent 78, 87

inner and outer landscapes 156, 158
inner and outer realities combined in portrait 123, 131, 156, 157, 159, 241
validated 131
insider research 88
'instrumental reason' (Levinas) 45
intentionality 25, 141, 146
made visible 194
intersubjective 43, 46
collaborative way of working 85, 87, 170, 217
embodied 190
knowing 159
and humour 98
and meaning 247
'mirroring and attunement' and (Wright) 240–241
portraits patients needed others to see 140–159, 240
relationship 17, 24–25, 38, 45, 53, 65, 71, 88, 98, 99, 102, 178, 229
symbolic capacity 159
and symbolic ways of knowing, being and relating 131–166
and validation of self-identity 140–146
*see also* intrasubjective
interpretation
and meanings 222, 228
collaboratively created 25, 226
'hermeneutic' (Heidegger) 226
by therapist/researcher 226
intrasubjective
and mourning 105
and self-identity 105, 127
portraits patients needed to see 128
and validation of self-identity 131–140, 240
intuition
within ALPHA 227
of the therapist 134, 224
intuitive resonant response 216

invisible
illness 40, 41, 100, 144, 156, 157
made visible 40, 157
invisibility
and portraiture 141
and illness 55, 122,
isolation
and illness 18, 40, 157
negative impact upon body and immune system 247
social 18, 40, 47, 84
and collage 132
and vulnerability 186

Kahlo, Frida
appropriation of self-portraits by 100, 137, 138, 156, 218
and embodiment 101
and suffering 100, 137, 158
and the 'world of illness' (Radley) 101

legacy
and portraiture 30, 167, 197–205
and alchemy 204
and future self-identity 239
and mortality 203
LEGO® elicitation task 129, 211–212, 213, 214, 215, 234
emotional distancing 213
and stories of self-identity 236
and art therapy training 246
life threatening and chronic illness
and antidepressants 22, 245, 248
and artists 36
painting portraits of people living with 62–70
using portrait photography with people living with 70–73
and art therapy 16 (literature), 33, 59, 61
'being known' through the portraits

life threatening and chronic illness *cont.*
   and the body/embodiment 60, 131, 245
   and containment 95
   and ethical considerations 86–90
   and empathic relationship 248
   and exclusion 33
   and existential anxiety 168
   and gender 44, 45, 60
   and impact on life/world 52
   and social isolation 18
   and stigmatization 245
   and 'liminality' (Sibbett) 19
   love and acceptance, need for within 158, 194
   and meaning 168
   and mourning losses 117
   and ontological insecurity 46, 47
   and 'ontological security' (Giddens) 46–47
   and portrait therapy 48
      and empowerment, adaption and growth 238
      introducing the patient-researchers 80–84
      mitigating against sense of despair 160
      selecting the patient-researchers for the study 77–78
      home visits 210
   and the psychological needs of patients 21
   and rituals 35
   self-identity 234
      disruption 17, 21, 33, 248
         and lack of self-recognition 105
         and perceptions of time and the future 197
      as 'unhomelike being-in-the-world' (Svenaeus) 19–22,
   and vulnerability 18, 36, 41, 67, 158, 186

'liminality' (Van Gennep) 19
   the challenge of and the 'world of illness' (Radley) 34–36
   and humour 98, 238
   and illness (Little) 35, 36
   and life threatening and chronic illnesses 19
   and people 36
   and place 19, 34
      and hospice 36
   and play 175
   in portraiture 101
   'world of' (Sibbett) 35
liminars 36
listening for 'Contrapuntal Identity Voices' (Gilligan) 96, 124, 196, 231, 232
lived experience 42, 46, 64, 158, 182
   of agency 120
   and the body 199
   and case studies 225, 235
   of control 117
   and elicitation tasks 234
   embodied 45
   give voice to 34
   held 24
   'homelike-being-in-the-world' (Svenaeus) 238
   and 'ontological security' (Giddens) 238, 239
   of illness 246
   and phenomenology 52, 53, 54, 223, 226, 232
   of portrait therapy 222
   and portraiture 52, 101
   subjective 41
loneliness 247
   and antidepressants 245
loss(es) 47, 163
   to accept 112
   bereavement 106, 117, 189, 238
   burden on patients 88
   and closure 238
   and death 48, 49, 113, 114, 172, 174
   and grief 18
   and guilt 112
   identity-affirming opportunities 45
   and illness 33, 60, 117, 160
   of innocence 155
   of meaning 18, 89
   mourning 95, 105–117, 172, 238
   and portraits 145, 178, 189, 238, 244
   and self-acceptance 191
   to self-identity 24, 94, 105, 106, 117, 250
   of subjectivity 43
   uncontrollable 126
love(d) 40, 107, 162, 193, 240
   and acceptance 158
   and agency 136, 140
   and portraits 29, 30, 94, 110, 115, 153, 154, 155, 157, 174, 191, 194, 197
   for the self 155, 190–197, 205, 239
      and narcissism 197
      and self-identity 23
   within the therapeutic relationship 192, 197

'making special' (Dissanayake) 35
making meaning 167–177, 169, 173, 174
   spiritual 239
   as alchemy 35
   in portraits 40
   as unique function of art 35
memories 93, 117
   difficult childhood 163
   and death 115, 116
   elicitation of 212, 213
   fearful 215
   and imagination 92
   and portraits 69, 129, 205, 239
   positive 166, 204, 205, 239
   vivid 198
   traumatic 154
Mental Capacity Act 243
mentalisation
   positive 121, 195
Mercury, Freddie 146, 191
   and a sense of belonging and connection to 190
   *Bohemian Rhapsody* 141
   identification with 183, 184, 185, 239
'metaphor and symbolism' (Lakoff & Johnson) 57
   and aesthetic resonance 217
   appropriation 218
   and death 169
   ways of knowing, being and relating, 130
   and meanings, hidden 169
   and mirroring 160

# SUBJECT INDEX

within portraits 130, 146, 160, 163, 165
and self-identity 220
and statement of intention 218
and tacit knowledge 58
mimesis
and attunement 24
in portraiture 26, 201
'mirror neurons' (Rizzolatti et al.) 191, 197
'mirroring and attunement' (Wright)
and aesthetic resonance 160, 240
and art therapy training 246
and agency 240
and the art therapist's 'third hand' (Kramer) 240
and the formation of self-identity 23–25
and portraits 127–128, 104, 152, 154, 220, 240, 241, 245
and psychodynamic and psychoanalytic art therapy 25
and 'response art' (Fish) 215
and revisioning self-identities 128–131
and self-portraits 242
theory of 23–24
mortality
and illness 145
and imagery 72
and legacy 203
and portraits 241
and temporality 197
see also death and 'being-towards-death' (Heidegger)
Motor Neuron Disease (MND) 30, 79, 80, 147, 197
mourning
and adaption 105–117, 238
and accepting change 105
and the death of loved ones 106, 114, 174, 189
and empathy 174
and illness 105
and photographs 116
and portraits 24, 69, 95, 105, 114, 147, 189
and rituals 115
and self-identity 24
father of 106

mother of 106
multiple case-study design 224–226
and cross-case analysis 225, 226, 232
and triangulation 225

narcissism 197
National Portrait Gallery 26
Native American Indian 115
Black Foot Tribe/Clan 137, 164, 175
and identity 137, 165, 175
and metaphor and symbolism 163
and portraits 115, spirituality 84, 169, 174
and smudging ceremony 177, 238
neuroscience and imagination 92
non-pathologising 33, 89
non-stigmatising 89

'object relations theory' (Klein) 24, 25
objective 22, 37
objectivity 37
'ontological security' (Giddens) 47–48
and continuity of self 190
and 'homelike-being-in-the-world' (Svenaeus) 167–205, 238–239
and portrait therapy 48, 171, 238–239
religion 169
'open studio model' of art therapy (Allen) 16
'otherness' (Svenaeus) and illness 20, 21

pain 39
and aesthetics 244
and art therapy 50, 51, 244
and beauty 50
and counter-transference 89
expression of 50, 156
hidden 73, 102, 104, 238
inner 100, 241
and illness 38, 81, 111
in portraits 101, 120, 129, 145, 151, 157, 158, 159, 178, 237
witnessing 72

painting 221
and ethical considerations 86–90
from life 220, 234
using photographic reference 26
portraits for patients/clients 32, 58, 250
making preparatory sketches 97, 101, 218, 220
palliative care 15, 22, 31, 78, 86, 88, 190
and art therapy 59–60, 88, 242
the Creative Response 85
placements 36, 246
and portraiture and 58–61
and 'third hand' 242
and training 246
and witnessing 89
anxiety and emotional affect 89
and death 48, 250
ethos of 16, 54
and fear of annihilation 221
and humour 98
and need to do more for patients 221
and research 87, 223, 241
and self-identity 198
and spirituality 168
and witnessing 89
patient selection
for the study 77–79
criteria 78, 79
patient-researchers, introducing 80–84
patient-expert divide 224
patients' voices 232
being heard 77
identifying in the analysis 232, 235
patriarchy 45
and domination in early life 150, 154
'performance' (Goffman) 40, 70, 141
personalised care, lack of 23
see also de-personalised care 45
phenomenology 52–53
approach to aesthetics 50
art therapy and illness 52–54

— 285 —

phenomenology *cont.*
  and depicting subjectivity 34
  and portrait therapy 54
  analysis and research 223
  '4 'R's' of good (Finlay) 234
  and Merleau-Ponty 20, 52, 127
  and Heidegger 48–49, 52, 169, 226, 228
  and hermeneutic interpretation, 234
  and Husserlian 227
    bracketing out 54, 214, 227, 234
    reduction to essences 226–228
    transcendental 52, 227, 234
  methodological congruence 233
  reliability and validity 225, 233–235
  and trustworthiness 233
  and 'approach to illness' (Carel) 54
photo elicitation task 151, 169, 212–214
photographs 37
  as reference material for portraits 27, 28, 38, 101, 109, 162, 184, 187, 210, 212–213, 221
  and depictions of illness 40–42, 70–73
  requested by patients of their portraits 142, 146, 170, 171, 177, 238
'Phototherapy' (Spence & Martin) 60
  and autopathographic self-portraiture 71–73
Picasso, Pablo 122, 123, 141, 147, 148, 197, 153
portrait effect 129, 248
portraits 25–27
  the 'as if' nature of 201, 204, 205, 226
  co-designing process 17
  and agency 112
  with patients 29, 118, 119, 151, 187, 195, 217–220
  as intersubjective process 85, 170

and lived experience of 'control' 117
portraits patients needed to see 102
portraits patients needed others to see 102, 142
and strengthening self-identity 32
and time and attention 198
historical 37, 38, 70, 72, 105, 185, 188, 202, 212, 219
holding and containing duality 131, 139, 147, 149, 241
belonging and separation 187
beauty and suffering 244
breathing and suffocation 139
denial and acceptance 197
fear and courage 154, 158
good and evil 159
helplessness and agency 147
hope and despair 45, 139, 146, 147, 149, 159, 162, 163, 187, 241
hope and hopelessness 197
idealisation and vilification 154
imprisonment and freedom 159
inner and outer realities 156, 159, 241
life and death 187, 197
past and future 187
power and helplessness 154
truth and deception 153
under and over protected 159
immortalizing the sitter/cheating death 26, 197
and intentionality 25, 141, 146, 194
and 'mirroring and attunement' (Wright) 127–128, 104, 152, 154, 220, 240, 241, 245
as representations of patient's past, present and future self-identities 25, 171–190

strengthening self-identity
knowing the self through being known 248
increasing a sense of worthwhileness 112, 106, 171, 187, 197, 239, 240
increasing creative capacity to adapt to illness 95, 97, 125, 238
increasing 'ontological security' (Giddens) 48, 171, 238–239
and making meaning 167–177, 169, 173, 174
and improving/increasing quality of life 16, 54, 59, 91, 245, 248
as subject-object 199, 240
as surrogate adaptive mother 24, 241
postmodernism 56
positive art therapy 244
positive focused attention 198, 205, 239, 241
positive memories 166, 198, 205, 239
postmodern society 47
power
  and aesthetics 244
  of art 31, 51, 131, 132, 236, 242
  discrepancy between patient and therapist 61, 85, 102, 226
  of health professionals 46, 245
  and portraits 55, 59, 70, 103, 131, 144, 154, 159, 170, 188, 199, 202, 241, 248
  and self-identity 56
  *see also* empowerment
prose poems 56, 215–217
psychoanalytic 25
psychodynamic 25

quality of life
  and impact of illness 18
  improvement to 16, 54, 59, 91, 245, 248

Raphael 66
Randomised Controlled Trials (RCTs) 223

## SUBJECT INDEX

reflexive 53
and the 'active documentation sketchbook' (ADS) De Freitas 214, 215
approach 53, 88
and case-studies 225
and decision making process 226
and phenomenological research 234
resonance 54, 227, 234
and self-identity 23
reliability in research 225, 233
religion 51
belief in 21, 202
eclectic beliefs 168
Rembrandt 66, 219, 252
reparation and forgiveness (Louise Bourgeois) 188
representation
human 57
and illness 243
self 31
and gender 44
and subjectivity 38, 53
visual 35, 137, 219, 236
of aging 60, 61
research 77, 79, 191, 212
arts based 215, 224
and art therapy 16, 33, 34, 58, 59, 60, 61
and bereavement 106
and life-threatening and chronic illnesses 19, 35, 59, 64, 70
and portraiture 36, 45, 56, 58, 62, 70, 85, 86, 87, 89, 167
dual-role conflict or 'insider' 88
phenomenological 53–54, 78, 223, 226–235
further, into portrait therapy 214, 244–246
and semi-structured end of project interviews (EPIs) 222
qualitative 224, 225
resonance 128
aesthetic 127, 156, 242
and portraiture 160–166, 217, 244, 246

and 'mirroring and attunement' (Wright) 240
reflexive 54, 214, 227, 234
and ritual 170
'response art' (Fish) 215
and art therapy 160, 216
collage and prose poems as 56, 178, 215–217
and 'mirroring and attunement' (Wright)
and 'third hand' (Kramer) 194
'revisioning' self-identities (Carr) 24, 85, 102, 117, 139, 160, 199, 217, 236
and 'mirroring and attunement' (Wright) 128–131
rites of passage 19, 35
ritual 35, 40, 57, 102, 115, 117, 160, 169, 170, 172, 174, 175, 177, 239
adaptive 238
and formulating experience 169
and the therapist 250
romanticised 155, 181
Rossetti, Dante Gabriel [1828–1882] 154, 155, 254
Rubens 66

science 66, 224
and lack of meaning in illness 45, 168
and self-identity 22
and suffering 21, 45
Second World War 178
self-acceptance 141
self-care 84, 135, 136, 239
self-esteem
and autonomy 136
increase to 205
*see also* self-worth
self-identities/self-identity 22–23
and analysis of research 223, 228, 229, 232–233
and art therapy 53, 59, 61
and childhood abandonment 112
and coherence 25, 47, 131, 153, 159, 239, 248
and death 168

disruption of 17–19, 22–23, 32, 55, 94, 142
and antidepressants 248
and life-threatening and chronic illnesses 13, 19, 21, 59, 89, 129, 194, 234, 238, 246
and portraiture 17, 55, 68, 69, 70, 97, 102, 104, 115
and time 197
and trauma 244, 246
and embodiment 20, 33, 194, 245
and faces 128
formation of 23–25, 46, 57, 85, 126
*see also* 'mirroring and attunement' (Wright)
and gender 43, 44
and narrative 111, 127, 128, 129, 130, 213, 215, 216, 217, 248
and meaning 21, 91
and mourning 105, 106, 109, 112, 117, 146
multiple 88, 161, 196, 231, 236, 240, 248
re-imagining of 91–98
revisioning of 24, 66, 85, 102, 117, 128–131, 139, 160, 199, 217, 236
past, present, future 25, 112, 145, 166, 167, 171, 177–190, 199, 202, 239
and portraiture 56, 59, 111, 117, 129, 134, 137–140, 145, 146, 166, 192, 241, 244
exhibitions of 202
patients as experts on 220
stronger sense of 237
and subjectivity 37, 39
validation of 18, 23, 42, 46, 128, 241, 243, 245
intersubjective 140–146
intrasubjective 131–140, 240
virtual 200
voices of 124, 225, 231, 232–233
and witnessing 178, 243
*see also* identity
self-love 191, 194, 204

see also self-esteem
self-perception and illness 20
self-portraiture 56, 57
  and illness 70, 71, 72, 100, 101, 156
  and patients 32, 55, 242
  as personal therapy 71
self-referential images 32
self-worth 198
  enhanced 135, 177, 187, 199
  affirmed 187
  and 'ontological security' (Giddens) 47
  see also self-esteem
shame
  and fear 152
  and dependence 36
  and the sick role 19
smudging ceremony 172, 173, 174, 177, 238
social isolation 47, 84, 132, 186
  and reduced immune function 18, 247
  and depression 18
  and shortened life expectancy 18
spiritual/spirituality 51, 84,
  and holistic paradigm 16, 46
  being 'held' 171
  Buddhist 169
  loss of 51
  meaning-making 168, 239
  Native American Indian 84, 168, 174, 175
  and portraiture 172, 176, 177
  presence 195, 230
  and religion 169
  support 116
statement of emergent knowing, creation of 228–229
statement of emergent learning, creation of 228–229
statement of intention 217–218
Statement of Reflexive Resonance, creation of 227
stigma and illness 19, 43, 44, 131, 194, 245, 248
stillbirths and miscarriages 83, 115

stories
  of bereavement 114
  episodic and fragmented 236
  and illness 21
  listening to 46
  performing 60
  reflecting back 178, 215, 216, 234
  of self-identity 104, 109, 111, 128, 129, 130, 180, 213, 215
  and subjectivity 38
  of survival 165
  witnessing 178
  untold, waited a lifetime to tell 131, 240, 248
  see also narrative
stories of self-identity 109, 129, 213
  and elicitation tasks 215
  empathically engage with 128
  the 'portrait effect' (Carr) 129, 130, 131, 248
  reflecting back, as response art
  collages and prose poems 215–217
'studio art therapy' (Moon) 16
subjectivity 37, 53
  challenge of depicting 36–43
  and absence of 39, 220
  and hiding 41
  portraiture 26, 119, 240, 250
  portrayal of 52, 250
  validation of a person's 42
  see also intersubjectivity
'sublimation' (Kramer) 30
suffering 81, 157, 178
Surrealism 51
symbolic capability within patients 146, 159, 240
symbolism and metaphor 58, 165, 169
  see also metaphor and symbolism

tacit knowledge 58, 210
temporality 22, 188, 218
  and legacy 197–205
  within portraits 202
  see also time
testimony 170
  making 247

  of presence 25
  of time and attention 198
therapeutic relationship 48, 58, 249
  and aesthetic 51
  and collaboration 28
  and humour 98
  intersubjective 65
  and self-identity 210
  and time and attention 198
  psycho- 51
'third hand' (Kramer) 30–33, 84, 192, 214, 234, 241
  benefits of as therapeutic tool 84, 194, 197, 241, 242, 245, 246
  and emotional distance and connection 102
  and 'mirroring and attunement' (Wright) 240
  and research 245, 249
  and 'sublimation' (Kramer) 30
  and time 65
  and art therapy training 246, 248
time 193
  and creative tasks 213
  to freeze 202
  and death 48, 72
  and illness 40, 146, 197–198
  and palliative care 22, 61, 68, 88, 132
  and portraiture 26, 27, 39, 42, 39, 62, 65, 68, 69, 71, 78, 79, 112, 134, 138, 139, 145
  captured through 205, 239
  and self-identity 197
  and the therapeutic process 221, 249
  and the art therapist's 'third hand' (Kramer) 65
  see also 'being-held-in-mind'
training
  art therapy and the aesthetic 50
art therapists, implications for 246
  and ethical considerations 88
health-care professionals 245
  and vulnerable people 66

## SUBJECT INDEX

transitional moments 28, 29
trapped, feeling of being 84,
    117, 119, 157, 199, 200
trauma 21
traumatic experiences 22,
    46, 149
  expressions of 50
  and diagnosis 34
  and humour 98
  and portrait therapy 244,
    246
  and transformation 22
'triangulation' (Yin) 223
truth
  and deception 153
  fact and fiction within
    58, 91
  and goodness and beauty 51
  and photography 72
  and portraiture 68
  and 'truth effect' 73

'Unbounded' body (Lawton)
    157
  and death 36
  and escape 157
  and the inner self 157, 158
  and portraits 157, 158
  and vulnerability 36
'unconditional positive regard'
    (Rogers/Petruska)
'unhomelike being-in-the-
    world' (Svenaeus) 19–22
  and humour 102
  and liminality 238
  metaphor for 164

unprotected 149
unwelcome contradictions
    114, 172

validation
  of self-identity 23, 24, 46
  intersubjective 127,
    140–146, 240
  intrasubjective 127,
    131–140, 240
  and portraits 24, 42
valuable, patients' recapturing
    a sense of themselves as
    127, 160, 166, 197, 239,
    240
vicarious traumatization
  and body-centered counter-
    transference 89–90
  *see also* embodied counter-
    transference
visibility
  and invisibility 55, 141
  and tension between 122
visible mending
  bereavement 106
  in portraits 117, 123, 126,
    180
visual analysis matrix
    229–230
visual
  anthropology 57
  communication 127
'vivid positive memories'
    (Werner-Seidler &
    Moulds) 198

Voice-centred Interpersonal
    Analysis 231–233
  listening for contrapuntal
    voices 96, 124, 196
void, between past, present
    and future self-identities
    198
vulnerability
  and illness 18
  and isolation 186
  within portraits 41, 67, 158
  and unboundedness 36

war experiences
  aestheticized or
    romanticized 181
  and heroism 178, 181
  within portraits 181–182
  preoccupation with 180
  and self-identity 180
  witnessing 178, 178
wise woman/elder 175
witness 35
  and illness 55, 72
  and portraits 58, 59, 89,
    119, 145, 146, 240,
    247, 249
  to anonymise 243
  and photographic 60
  and therapy 248, 249
  stories of self-identity 178,
    192
'world of illness' (Radley) and
  liminality 34–36, 67, 96,
    101, 238, 249

# AUTHOR INDEX

Achterberg, J. 128
Achterberg, J., Dossey, B. and Kolkmeier, L. 169
Adams, A. 6, 27
Adamson, E. 16
Addington-Hall, J. 88
Aita, V., Lydiatt, W. and Gilbert, M. 62–65, 194, 239–241, 244, 245, 248
Akhtar, S. and Samuel, S. 22
Alea, N. and Bluck, S. 129
Allen, P. 16, 25
Anzieu, D. 157, 180
Arnheim, R. 59
Awan, F. 213

Balan, N. 231, 234
Barnett, M. 88
Barrett, E. and Bolt, B. 224
Barthes, R. 26, 37, 109
Balboni, T., Vanderwerker, L., Block, S., Paulk, E. 168
Bauman, Z. 22, 47, 167, 168
Becker, E. 48
Bell, J. 219
Bell, S. 16, 24, 53, 54, 71, 72, 168
Benner, P. 45
Benner, P. and Wrubel, J. 45
Betensky, M. 53
Bion, W. 24
Blows, E., Bird, L., Seymour, J. and Cox, K. 35
Bolen, J. 17
Bolton, G. 66
Booth, A., Trimble, T. and Egan, J. 89, 221
Brilliant, R. 69
Brockelman, T. 215
Brough, J. 131
Brown, C. 16, 58

Brown, J. 39, 40
Brown, L., Argyris, D., Attanucci, J., Bardige, B. 231
Brown, L. and Gilligan, C. 231
Broyard, A.Bruce, V. and Young, A. 160
Buber, M. 45, 159
Buckner, R. and Carroll, D. 92
Burt, H. 92
Butler, J. 44, 105, 106, 117
Butler-Kisber, L. 215

Cahn, E. 16
Canals, R. 57
Cancienne, M. and Snowber, C. 43
Carel, H. 18, 19, 20, 33, 46, 49, 54, 56, 131, 199, 241, 245, 247
Carr, S. 24, 25, 26, 30, 32, 92, 129
Carr & Hancock 85, 127
Cauvel, J. 27
Chambers, E. 42, 71
Charmaz, K. 17, 91
Charmaz, K. and Rosenfeld, D. 43, 122, 131, 141
Clark, A. 86
Clayton, J., Hancock, K., Parker, S., Butow, P. 146
Clayton, J., Butow, P., Arnold, R. and Tattersall, M. 146
Cohen, M. 169
Cole, A. and Knowles, G. 224
Collier, J. Jnr. 212, 213
Connell, C. 16, 59, 60
Cooper, A. 22
Costello-Du Bois, J. 58
Corbin, J. and Strauss, A. 17

Corbin, J. 60
Craig, G. 53
Crewe, N. 18
Crossley, M. 197

Darwent, C. 188
Davis, D. 215
Dean, R., Kinsman, A. and Gregory, D. 98, 99
De Freitas, N. 214
Denzin, N. 224
Dissanayake, E. 16, 34, 35, 160, 169, 170, 239
Douglass, M. 169
Duesbury, T. 190

Edwards, D. 221
Edwards, D. 223, 225
Edwards, J, D. 18, 19
Eisner, E. 46, 92, 132
Elkins, J. 42, 127, 128, 190
Elliott, A. 22
Etherington, K. 22, 53, 88
Evans, K. 22, 23, 36, 43, 44, 167, 168, 199
Exley, C. and Letherby, G. 145

Falk, B. 90, 168
Farelly-Hansen, M. 168
Farrand, P. 65, 66, 129, 248
Faulkner, S. 216
Falvo, D. 18
Fenton, J. 59
Festinger, L. 139, 241
Field, N. 89
Fine, M. and Glendinning, C. 36
Finlay, L. 190, 225, 226, 232, 234

# AUTHOR INDEX

Finley, S. and Knowles, G. 88
Fish, B. 90, 194, 215
Frank, A. 18, 72
Franklin, M. 58
Fraser, G. and Gordon, L. 19
Freeland, C. 25–27, 33, 37, 56, 57, 58, 109, 128, 140, 203, 220
Fuller, P. 24
Furman, R., Langer, C., Davis, C., Gallardo, H. 215

Gablik, S. 248
Gadamer, H. 226
Gallese, V. and Lakoff, G. 191
Gauntlett, D. 22, 211
Gauntlett, D. and Holzwarth, P. 22
Gemmell, G. 217, 218
Giddens, A. 21, 22, 23, 24, 47, 167, 190
Gilbert, M. 62–66, 129, 201
Gilligan, C. 231
Gilligan, C., Spencer, R., Weinberg, M.K. and Bertsch, T. 232, 234
Gilroy, A. 85, 224, 249
Giorgi, A. 233
Goffman, E. 43, 70
Gormley, A. 137
Grau, C. 22, 248
Grey, C. and Malins, J. 215, 263
Grice, E. 66, 263

Hansen, D., Rosholm, J., Gichangi, A. and Vach, W. 168, 245. 262
Hardy, D. 59
Harper, D. 212, 213
Harms, E. 49
Hart, N. and Crawford-Wright, A. 85, 86
Hartley, N. and Payne, M. 66
Heidegger, M. 48, 49, 52, 169, 226, 228
Hellema, P. 98
Henley, D. 50
Herman, J. 17
Higgs, G. 91
Hiles, D. 53
Hill, A. 16, 49, 59, 182
Hilliker, L. 105
Hocoy, D. 21, 245

Hogan, S. 35, 44, 51, 54, 59, 218, 225
Hogan, S. and Martin, R. 61
Hogan, S. and Warren, L. 60, 61, 180
Holmes, M. 44
Hubbard, G., Kidd, L. and Kearney, N. 33
Husserl, E. 52, 226, 227
Hutchison, I., Gilbert, M. and Farrand, P. 64, 65, 240

Inckle, K. 58
Isserow, J. 60

Jaremka, L., Fagundes, C., Glaser, R., Bennette, J. 18, 247
Jones, D. 58
Jones, J. 39, 40
Jones, M. 58
Jongeward, C. 58, 224

Kierkegaard, S. 168
Kinnvall, C. 47, 177, 187, 247
Kinsella, E. 46
Kipling, R. 179
Kirkengen, A. and Ulvestad, E. 54
Klass, D., Silverman, P. and Nickman, P. 105
Klein, M. 24
Kleinman, A. 21, 46
Knill, P. 51, 244
Knowles, G. and Cole, A. 224
Kramer, E. 16, 30, 32, 33, 49, 58, 59, 194, 241, 248, 249
Koren, L. 50
Kubler-Ross, E. 49, 169

Lachman-Chapin, M. 160
Lakoff, G. and Johnson, M. 58
Langer, S. 25
Latimer, J. 101, 137
Lawler, S. 22
Lawton, J. 36, 157, 158
Lazarus-Leff, B. 53
Learmonth, M. 66
Leary, M. and Tangney, J. 22
Leavy, P. 216, 224
Ledbury, P. 69, 70
Lee, S. and Kristjanson, L. 78
Lerner, E. 59, 60

Lett, W. 154, 227, 228, 234
Little, M., Jordens, C.F., Paul, K., Montgomery, K. 35, 36
Luzzatto, P. 16, 31, 59, 157

Maclagan, D. 31, 50, 91, 242
Maiter, S., Simich, L., Jacobson, N. and Wise, J. 88
Malchiodi, C. 16, 59
Mallinson, G. 116
Mandal, M. and Ambady, N. 127
Mander, R. and Marshall, R. 115
Martin, R. 60, 71, 72
Martin, W., Grey, M., Webber, T., Robinson, L. 86, 88
Mathieson, C. and Stam, H. 18
Matho, E. 59, 60, 61
Matthews, E. 20
Mauthner, N.S. and Doucet, A. 226, 231, 234
McCann, L. and Pearlman, L. 89
McCreaddie, M. and Wiggins, S. 99
McGraw, M. 59
McNiff, S. 16, 50, 51, 98, 223, 224, 249
McPherson, C., Wilson, K. and Murray, M. 89
Merleau-Ponty, M. 20, 43, 52, 127
Mercer, J. 88
Meyer, J. and Land, R. 35
Miller, R. 215
Minar, V. 59
Moon, B. 58
Moon, C. 16, 50, 56, 58, 87, 91, 224, 245, 249
Moulder, C. 116
Moustakas, C. 227, 232
Mullins, C. 26, 58

O'Brien, F. 16
O'Neill, M. 35, 128, 154
Oyserman, D., Elmore, K. and Smith, G. 22

Padfield, D. 156
Palmer, P. 22, 23
Parry, G. 232, 234

Pearlman, L. and Saakvitne, K. W. 89
Pereira, H. 234
Persons, R. 53
Pink, S. 53, 87, 89, 212, 224
Pinker, S. 47
Pinkola Estes, C. 251
Pointon, M. 27, 45, 55, 56, 57, 70, 71, 72, 188
Pratt, M. and Thomas, G. 60
Pratt, M. and Wood, M. 16, 59
Puchalski, C., Ferrell, B., Virani, R., Otis-Green, S. 168

Quail, J. and Peavy, V. 53, 233

Rådestad, I., Nordin, C., Steineck, G. and Sjogren, B. 115, 116
Radley, A. 66, 72, 101, 202, 238, 243, 247
Radley, A. and Bell, S. 22
Rando, T. 106, 223
Reason, P. 16
Reeve, J., Lloyd-Williams, M., Payne, S. and Dowrick, C. 18, 33, 46, 88
Rennie, D. L. 85
Reynolds, F. and Lim, K. H. 207
Reynolds, F. and Prior, S. 53
Reynolds, F. 59
Rizzolatti, G., Fadiga, L., Gallese, V. and Fogassi, L.
Robbins, A. 16
Rodin, G., Craven, J. and Littlefield, C. 18
Rolls, A. 67–69
Rosenblum, B. 37–38
Rosselli, H. 66–67
Rossetto, E. 53
Rostron, J. 53

Sacks, O. 168, 198
Saunders, C. 16
Sawday, J. 157
Seymour, W. 162, 197, 198
Schore, A. 127
Scruton, R. 51, 160
Sibbett, C. 19, 34, 35, 36, 37, 60, 98, 101, 102, 169, 185, 238
Sibbett, C. and Thompson, W. 35
Sinding, C., Gray, R. and Nisker, J. 86
Skaife, S. 24, 53, 60, 88
Smith, C. 18, 19, 20
Smith, J. 225
Smith, J., Flowers, P. and Larkin, M. 78, 225
Sontag, S. 34, 38, 39, 42
Spaniol, S. 87
Spence, J. 41, 42, 71, 72,
Spence, J. and Holland, P. 36
Spinelli, E. 227
Springham, N. 86
Springham, N. and Woods, A. 85, 87
Stern, D. 24
Stieglitz, A. 73
Street, A. and Kissane, D. 36
Strohm, K. 86
Stuckley, H. and Nobel, J. 16
Sullivan, G. 224
Svenaeus, F. 20, 21, 48, 54, 164, 190, 198, 199, 238

Taylor, C. 21, 22, 45, 130, 177, 185, 202
Tembeck, T. 71, 72
Thorne, D. 158
Tjasink, M. 53
Toombs, S 18, 54, 156
Trotsky, L. 236
Turner, V. 19, 35, 36, 98, 101, 175, 185, 238

Ulman, E. 158
van Alphen, E. 36
van Gennep, A. 35
van der Kolk, B. 21, 257
van Lith, T. 53
van Manen, M. 52, 53
Vaughan, K. 215
Vecchi, B. 22
Vick, R. 87
Volkan, V. 105

Wahrendorf, M., Ribet, C., Zins, M., Goldberg, M. 88
Waller, D. 59
Waller, D and Sibbett, C. 16, 21, 33, 60, 168
Watts, J. 46, 47
Weisfeld, G. 98
Werner-Seidler, A. and Moulds, M. 117, 195, 198
Wertz, F. 190
West, S. 26, 202
Whicher, S., Spiller, R. and Williams, W. 27
Wilkinson, R. and Chilton, G. 244
Williams, B. 215
Winnicott, D. 24, 35, 250
Wix, L. 16
Wood, M. 31, 55, 59, 61, 66, 249, 250
Wood, M., Molassiotis, A. and Payne, S. 33, 59, 61, 223
Wood, M., Low, J., Molassiotis, A. and Tookman, A. 59
Wright, K. 23, 24, 25, 33, 56, 127, 128, 129, 146, 215, 241

Yin, R. 223, 224, 225
Young, M. 17, 19